Precision Medicine in Stroke

Ana Catarina Fonseca • José M. Ferro
Editors

Precision Medicine in Stroke

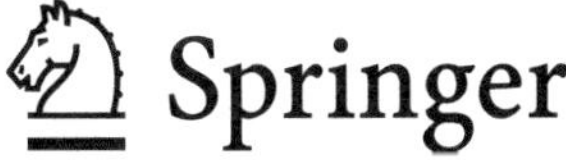 Springer

Editors
Ana Catarina Fonseca
Neurology
University of Lisbon
Lisbon
Portugal

José M. Ferro
Department of Neurosciences
University of Lisbon
Lisbon
Portugal

ISBN 978-3-030-70763-7   ISBN 978-3-030-70761-3   (eBook)
https://doi.org/10.1007/978-3-030-70761-3

This Springer imprint is published by the registered company Springer Nature Switzerland AG
The registered company address is: Gewerbestrasse 11, 6330 Cham, Switzerland

Preface

In this book, we intend to provide the reader with a comprehensive coverage of the state of the art of Precision Medicine in stroke. The first chapters are dedicated to the basic and current concepts regarding precision medicine and the rationale for its application in stroke medicine. The second part of the book addresses current use of precision medicine in ischemic and hemorrhagic stroke. Monogenic stroke disease, pharmacogenomics, and acute stroke treatment are the areas that have been most influenced by the application of precision medicine to stroke. Advanced brain imaging methods have started to help us to know more about individual thresholds to brain ischemia and to personalize therapeutic time windows for endovascular treatments. The third part of the book explores future applications of precision medicine in stroke. A review of the ongoing studies and of the different biomarkers that are being studied is provided. The expectation is that the use of different types of biomarkers will in the future enhance early stroke diagnosis and estimation of prognosis that will allow an adapted treatment for each patient. The fourth part of the book provides an in-depth exposition of how different interdisciplinary areas like artificial intelligence, molecular biology, and genetics are contributing to this area. Also, a description of the different tools used in the interdisciplinary areas and that can be applied to further enhance the study of precision medicine in stroke is given. Concepts regarding registry-based stroke research and how it can be used to contribute to precision medicine research are also provided.

Finally, Dr. Louis Caplan provides a very needed reflection regarding the differences and similarities between personalized and precision medicine and reminds us that our main objective is to know and help the individual that presents in front of us.

With this book, we intend to provide the reader with a comprehensive coverage of where we currently stand regarding precision medicine in stroke and to show how future stroke care may be influenced by it. If after reading this book or some of its chapters some of the readers become motivated or interested to contribute even more to the development and application of stroke medicine to stroke, we will have managed to achieve the ultimate objective that led us to edit and write this book. Advancement and application of precision medicine to stroke medicine will hopefully lead to a better and individualized care of stroke patients, which will contribute to reduce the burden of stroke.

We would like to thank our colleagues that contributed with their time and expertise to this book.

Lisbon, Portugal   Ana Catarina Fonseca
Lisbon, Portugal   José M. Ferro

Contents

Part I

Precision Medicine

Introduction

1

José M. Ferro

José was a 77-year Caucasian old male, retired, active and fully independent, with hypertension and diabetes, on aspirin, statin, amlodipine, valsartan and carvedilol. One night, after having dinner, he experienced the sudden onset of left hemiparesis, facial asymmetry and speech disturbance. His wife called the national emergency number 112. The paramedics transported him to the reference hospital offering hyperacute stroke treatment, where he arrived 1:32 after symptom's onset. He scored 15 in the NIHSS. CT showed no early infarct signs (ASPECTS 10). CT angiography showed a M1 left MCA occlusion. The patient had no contraindications for rtPA. So, while preparing the endovascular procedure, rtPA bolus was started with no improvement. Mechanical thrombectomy successfully opened the artery in single catheter pass. The patient immediately improved to a NIHSS of 4, with no aphasia, mild right upper limb paresis and minimal lower limb weakness. He is admitted to the stroke unit. On the second hospital, he developed fever. He had clinical and radiological signs of pulmonary infection. He received paracetamol and antibiotics for 7 days and low-molecular-weight heparin, in prophylactic dosage, for prevention of deep venous thrombosis of the lower limbs. The search for the cause of stroke included carotid and vertebral ultrasound, which showed bilateral <50% heterogeneous, partly calcified carotid stenosis. The echocardiogram disclosed a dilated left atrium and left ventricular hypertrophy. 24-Hour Holter monitoring identified paroxysmal atrial fibrillation for 4:43 h. At this stage, the patient continued statin and antihypertensive and was prescribed a direct anticoagulant. Rehabilitation was started. The patient was discharged on day 7 after admission,

J. M. Ferro (✉)
Serviço de Neurologia, Department of Neurosciences and Mental Health,
Hospital de Santa Maria—CHULN, Lisbon, Portugal

Instituto de Medicina Molecular, Faculdade de Medicina, Universidade de Lisboa,
Lisbon, Portugal
e-mail: jmferro@medicina.ulisboa.pt

A. C. Fonseca, J. M. Ferro (eds.), *Precision Medicine in Stroke*,
https://doi.org/10.1007/978-3-030-70761-3_1

with the diagnosis of ischemic stroke, of cardioembolic cause, scoring 3 points on the NIHSS and achieving grade 2 on the modified Rankin scale.

This apparently simple clinical vignette is a typical example of a patient with ischemic stroke successfully treated by thrombectomy. However, if we look closely, it is much more than that. The vignette describes the demographic, biological and health features which are components of the unique individual of José: he is a male, 77 years old, retired, active, independent, hypertensive and diabetic. We know the medications he was on. He could, if needed, include hundreds of other variables from his health and other records and databases to describe him in much more detail. The clinical and imagiological features of the disease are reported and scores quantify the severity of the stroke. He has no contraindications to rtPA and presents a large vessel occlusion, making him a candidate for thrombectomy. Results of vascular and cardiac ancillary procedures unveil several "abnormal" results. The chain and process of care are detailed: recognition of symptoms, reaction, transportation, hospital admission, confirmation of the diagnosis, hyperacute care, treatment of complications, secondary prevention, rehabilitation and discharge. At almost each step of the chain, his condition changes from the previous one, adding more information on the description of his uniqueness. Would he be a different person, with a different type and severity of stroke, and the choices at each step of the process would also probably be different.

Along the process of care, the management of the patient depends on key dichotomous decisions, in order to apply or not several logistic (e.g. transport and admission), diagnostic and therapeutic interventions, which can result in benefit or harm to the patient. Each intervention and step of care contributes to the main desired outcome (complete cure, full return to previous health and functional status) and a multitude of secondary outcomes. Before deciding for each intervention, can we predict with robustness and confidence if the intervention will result in benefit or harm to the patient and if the desired outcomes will be reached?

At the current stage of knowledge, many of the clinical decisions related to therapeutic interventions are supported by scientific evidence, whose quality varies from high to very low. Such evidence was generated by experimental studies, often randomised controlled trials and meta-analysis of randomised controlled trials. The results of these studies are presented for the whole group of participants, without considering its individual variability. Large randomised controlled trials and meta-analysis with thousands of participants can have enough statistical power to analyse a priori identified subgroups, described by the presence and absence of one or two variables. However, they almost never have the statistical power to analyse subgroups defined by combinations of variables, such as those which describe José. Furthermore, subjects are enrolled in clinical trials following the trial protocol inclusion and exclusion criteria. These criteria are chosen to maximise the possibility of finding a significant result on the efficacy outcomes and avoiding severe adverse events, thus protecting patient safety. Inevitably, many patients with the disease and the intervention being tested are left out of the trial. Therefore, the results of a trial cannot be applied to individuals not meeting the inclusion and exclusion criteria of a trial. In the case of José, that would imply at least that he complies with the inclusion-exclusion criteria of randomised controlled trials evaluating the benefit of rtPA, thrombectomy, admission to a stroke unit and heparin to prevent deep venous thrombosis in acute stroke and of direct anticoagulants for secondary prevention of stroke in patients with atrial fibrillation.

For several other clinical decisions we do not have evidence from randomised clinical trials (e.g. should the patient be transported in a seated position or lying down?). In this situation, it is often claimed "we need a randomised clinical trial". Some of these trials are really needed, are feasible and must be done. But for several other clinical questions, especially in less common disease (e.g. rare types or causes of stroke), such trials are not feasible, because of the huge number of required participants and centres involved, the corresponding high cost of launching such a trial and the difficulty of finding a sponsor or agency to fund the study. Other trials will be considered unethical, because the component of care to be tested is already implemented in current practice, and there is no equipoise regarding its efficacy and safety.

When we do not have evidence from clinical trials, how can we help José? We can rely on results from observational studies, which however have a high risk of bias to evaluate interventions. In fact, in daily clinical practice, interventions are not prescribed randomly, and in general, more severe patients tend to receive more intervention and more aggressive ones. Even if we adjust for all baseline imbalance between groups, we will not be able to control for the implicit information due to clinical experience and the emotional factors that lead to prescription of an intervention to an individual patient.

If observational information is not available, we had to decide based on clinical experience and opinions. Clinical experience accumulates in individual doctors, in those more talented, with a peculiar expertise or with higher leadership, such as heads of clinical units and opinion leaders but also in clinical organisations, such as clinical units, medical societies and expert consensus. Clinical experience and opinion have several biases, including cognitive and emotional factors, that lead to the registration and evocation of some cases and events but not of others and are also influenced by intellectual conflicts of interest with previous opinions and convictions. Nevertheless, clinical experience is a very valuable and useful natural human intelligence creation, which from the accumulation of information from numerous clinical cases produces recognition patterns for almost instantaneous diagnosis and binary questions for rapid management decisions.

For diagnostic decisions on diagnostic procedures, i.e. which tests or sequence of tests should be performed in an individual patient, there is an additional methodological problem. Almost all studies evaluating diagnostic tests looked at outcomes such as sensitivity, specificity and accuracy or compared a new diagnostic method with the currently used "gold standard". Very few studies investigated if performing or not a diagnostic test changes the outcome of the patient or causes harm, including anxiety while waiting for performing the test or for or from the test results.

In summary, to be able to help José and other patients, by advising and prescribing diagnostic and therapeutic interventions which benefit them and do not produce arm, we have now at our disposal accumulated knowledge from clinical trials, meta-analysis of clinical trials, observational studies and clinical experience, and we must integrate all this information and use it judiciously.

Currently we can make a detailed description of individuals using thousands of variables. We also have robust information to make assumption for groups of patients regarding several important clinical questions. Unfortunately we are yet quite weak to identify which individuals will benefit most from an intervention or even more to detect those who will be harmed or experience significant adverse events.

Precision medicine is the next step in the scientific approach to the practice of clinical medicine. Precision medicine's final aim is to identify for each disease a tailored diagnosis and therapy for each individual. Such an aim can be achieved through a collection of a multitude of clinical, biological and imaging data points and by the synthesis of individualised data into clinical usable end points. Refinement of statistical approaches, namely using artificial intelligence techniques, will allow the individualised prediction of recurrence risk, medication effects and recovery [1, 2]. A leap forward will be the integration of precision medicine with public health and population health management [3].

Precision medicine is already a reality in clinical practice in oncology, haematology and rheumatology, and in other specialities managing inflammatory conditions and monogenic diseases. Slower, but already significant, progresses have been achieved in other chronic non-communicable diseases, including stroke [1, 2, 4].

This book's main purpose is to cover the current and future applications of precision medicine in stroke. The book is introduced by a definition of precision medicine and its need to improve stroke care. Specific chapters will describe the state of the art of precision medicine in monogenic causes of stroke, pharmacogenetics of drugs commonly used to treat or prevent ischemic stroke and acute stroke imaging. Two other chapters will detail how precision medicine is already used in the management of haemorrhagic stroke, including subarachnoid haemorrhage. The future applications of precision medicine in stroke are focused in two chapters dealing, respectively, with early stroke diagnosis and prognosis determination.

The implementation of precision medicine needs an interdisciplinary approach. Advances in genetic and molecular biology will be pivotal to identify new diagnostic markers and therapeutic targets. The construction of big data banks and the analysis of big data will be done mostly using artificial intelligence technique and other advanced statistical methods. The book includes three chapters detailing these issues. The final chapter by Prof. Louis Caplan offers a broad perspective of the care of the individual person, and discusses the differences and overlaps between the concepts of personalised and precision medicine [5, 6].

References

1. Hinman JD, Rost NS, Leung TW, Montaner J, Muir KW, Brown S, Arenillas JF, Feldmann E, Liebeskind DS. Principles of precision medicine in stroke. J Neurol Neurosurg Psychiatry. 2017;88(1):54–61. https://doi.org/10.1136/jnnp-2016-314587.
2. Acosta JN, Brown SC, Falcone GJ. Genetic underpinnings of recovery after stroke: an opportunity for gene discovery, risk stratification, and precision medicine. Genome Med. 2019;11(1):58. https://doi.org/10.1186/s13073-019-0671-5.

3. Grossman DC, Larson EB, Sox HC. Integrating personalized medicine with population health management: the path forward. JAMA. 2020; https://doi.org/10.1001/jama.2020.1406.
4. Simpkins AN, Janowski M, Oz HS, Roberts J, Bix G, Doré S, Stowe AM. Biomarker application for precision medicine in stroke. Transl Stroke Res. 2020;11(4):615–27. Published online 2019 Dec 18. https://doi.org/10.1007/s12975-019-00762-3.
5. Sandercock PA. Does personalized medicine exist and can you test it in a clinical trial? Int J Stroke. 2015;10(7):994–9. https://doi.org/10.1111/ijs.1259.
6. Bello NA, Miller EC, Cleary KL, Wapner R. Cases in precision medicine: a personalized approach to stroke and cardiovascular risk assessment in women. Ann Intern Med. 2019;171(11):837–42. https://doi.org/10.7326/M19-1601.

Precision Medicine: Enabling Healthcare Progress in the Twenty-First Century

2

Maria Carmo-Fonseca

2.1 Introduction

The genomic revolution marked the beginning of the twenty-first century in biology and medicine. Completion of the Human Genome Project in 2003 brought a flood of discoveries that transformed biology. The Human Genome Project also fostered technological innovations that enabled decoding the entire genetic information in health and disease, leading to the concept of personalized genomic medicine and the foundation of the precision medicine movement [1]. By 2012, the new label "precision medicine" gained momentum [2] and since then it has been increasingly used by key opinion leaders in scientific headlines and journal articles [3].

A decisive seal of approval to the movement was given when the President of the United States launched the "Precision Medicine Initiative" in 2015 with the intent to merge genomic, biological, behavioral, environmental, and other data on individuals to identify drivers of health that might support personalized healthcare decision-making [4]. Given the enormous potential and promise for new medical breakthroughs based on this "emerging approach for disease treatment and prevention that takes into account individual variability in genes, environment, and lifestyle for each person," several other countries have developed dedicated precision medicine programs on a national scale. For example, the United Kingdom initiated the sequence of 100,000 genomes from National Health Service patients, and China announced the "China Precision Medicine Initiative" in 2017. In Europe, Nordic region countries and Switzerland have proposed road maps for similar initiatives [5, 6].

M. Carmo-Fonseca (✉)
Instituto de Medicina Molecular João Lobo Antunes, Faculdade de Medicina, Universidade de Lisboa, Lisbon, Portugal
e-mail: carmo.fonseca@medicina.ulisboa.pt

© Springer Nature Switzerland AG 2021
A. C. Fonseca, J. M. Ferro (eds.), *Precision Medicine in Stroke*,
https://doi.org/10.1007/978-3-030-70761-3_2

In the twentieth century, the growing impact of the scientific method on clinical practice led to the concept of evidence-based medicine, wherein clinical decision-making is based on evidence obtained from randomized controlled trials [7]. The first randomized controlled clinical trial was conducted in 1946 and demonstrated the efficacy of streptomycin for treating tuberculosis [7]. This was followed by a period of rapid methodological progress in the design and analysis of clinical trials as well as observational studies. Randomized clinical trials have provided strong scientific evidence on useful interventions, thanks to double-blind treatment application and tests for treatment associations with clinical outcomes. Contrasting with evidence-based medicine's empirical associations, precision medicine in the twenty-first century strives for developing a new taxonomy of human disease that results from the convergence of scientific data obtained through multi-"omics" approaches, advanced imaging, and information technology. Although precision medicine was conceptualized based on the power of genomics, its overarching aim is to enable a new era of medicine that integrates molecular, physiological, behavioral, and environmental data on individuals. According to this non-reductionist perspective, treatment selections should be based on molecular biomarkers as well as on demographic and physiological measurements, comorbid conditions, individual patient preferences, and lifestyle.

This chapter illustrates current state-of-the-art applications of the precision medicine concept, from new trends in genetic diagnostics and the advent of RNA therapeutics, gene therapy, and genome editing to breakthroughs in cancer treatment and the microbiome as a new research frontier.

2.2 New Trends in Genetic Diagnosis

At present, the catalog of Mendelian or rare genetic disorders is still far from complete. Clinical application of high-throughput DNA sequencing technologies (whole-exome and whole-genome sequencing) to cases undiagnosed by conventional approaches currently enables the identification of new disease/genetic associations at a rate of approximately 260 per year [8]. However, DNA sequence alone is not sufficient for diagnosis of all patients due to two main limitations. First, the clinical relevance of many gene variants remains unknown and, second, the clinical impact of variation in noncoding regions of the genome is still poorly understood. By combining DNA sequencing with additional technologies such as metabolomics and transcriptomics, the discovery rate of new genetic based diagnosis is predicted to increase to approximately 500 per year in the near future. For example, detection of abnormal levels of particular metabolites in serum using recently developed mass spectroscopy techniques (which expanded by at least 100-fold the ability to detect small molecules in circulation) complements the interpretation of sequence variants found in genes that encode enzymes involved in a particular metabolic pathway [9]. Application of RNA sequencing can also help to shed light on the possible pathogenicity of variants of unknown significance identified through DNA sequencing by revealing transcriptional alterations [10].

Speed of precision diagnosis is critical particularly in childhood disorders, since corrective therapies have their greatest efficacy when used early. In this regard, the recently developed ability to sequence fetal genomic DNA in the mother's circulation, which is used to screen for chromosomal aneuploidy as well as to diagnose specific defects in fetal genes [11], underscores the potential for in utero precision medicine. In a recently reported case, diagnosis of adrenal hyperplasia led to in utero fetal hormonal replacement therapy, anticipating in utero screening for genetic diseases for which there are treatment options [9].

2.3 The Advent of RNA Therapeutics, Gene Therapy, and Genome Editing

In 2000, Francis Collins, the then director of the genome agency at the National Institutes of Health, suggested, "Over the longer term, perhaps in another 15 or 20 years, you will see a complete transformation in therapeutic medicine" [12]. Indeed, by 2020, breakthroughs in RNA therapeutics, gene therapy, and genome editing have reinforced the vision and aspiration for the precision medicine movement.

Spinal muscular atrophy (SMA) used to be one of the most common genetic causes of infant mortality and a major cause of childhood morbidity due to muscle weakness, until innovative drugs changed the disease outcome for the first time [13]. SMA is caused by deletions or loss-of-function mutations in the *SMN1* gene. However, the human genome has a highly homologous gene called *SMN2*, which differs from *SMN1* by 11 nucleotides but has an identical coding sequence. One of the altered nucleotides weakens a splice site, resulting in skipping of exon 7 in the messenger RNA (mRNA). Approximately 80–90% of the transcripts derived from the *SMN2* gene skip exon 7, leading to a protein product that is rapidly degraded. Thus, forcing the inclusion of exon 7 in *SMN2* mRNA should suffice to produce a fully functional SMN protein that compensates for loss of the *SMN1* gene [14]. Nusinersen (Spinraza®), the first drug that received approval for treatment of SMA, is an antisense oligonucleotide that is administered intrathecally and increases SMN protein concentration by modifying the splicing of the *SMN2* mRNA. Another approved splicing modifier is Evrysdi™ (risdiplam), a small molecule that is administered orally and is the first medicine for SMA that can be taken at home. An alternative recently approved treatment strategy for SMA is gene replacement therapy. Onasemnogene abeparvovec (Zolgensma®) is an adeno-associated viral vector-based gene therapy designed to deliver a functional copy of the *SMN1* gene to the motor neurons through a single intravenous infusion [13].

In addition to children with SMA, several other patients affected by incurable diseases are benefiting from specific gene and RNA therapies. Namely, Luxturna® is a gene therapy for an inherited retinal disease that leads to progressive visual loss and ultimately total blindness. The disease is caused by biallelic loss-of-function mutations in the *RPE65* gene that destroy the ability of retinal pigment epithelium cells to react to light. The drug is applied intraocularly by a subretinal injection and consists of an adeno-associated viral vector that carries a functional copy of the *RPE65* gene [15].

Excitement over potentially curative gene therapy options for nonmalignant hematological disorders is also growing. For the X-linked bleeding disorders hemophilia A (factor VIII deficiency) and hemophilia B (factor IX deficiency), near-to-complete correction has been achieved in patients injected with engineered recombinant adeno-associated virus vectors that deliver the functional sequence of the defective coagulation factor gene to the liver [16]. More recently, a gene therapy for transfusion-dependent beta-thalassemia received regulatory approval [17]. In this case, hematopoietic stem cells are collected from the peripheral blood, maintained in culture in the laboratory (i.e., ex vivo), and modified by transduction with an engineered lentiviral vector carrying the therapeutic DNA sequence; next, the corrected stem cells are infused intravenously into the patient, who was previously treated with myeloablative chemotherapy [18]. The success seen in beta-thalassemia motivated efforts to extend the therapy to sickle cell patients [17].

Altogether, gene replacement therapies currently approved and in development use engineered viruses to deliver an extra DNA sequence that replaces the defective gene. Thus, this treatment strategy is restricted to autosomal recessive disorders, which are caused by biallelic loss-of-function mutations. Treating autosomal dominant diseases often requires silencing the expression of the mutated gene, which encodes a toxic protein. A very promising gene-silencing approach is RNA interference (RNAi), which involves the delivery into cells of short synthetic double-stranded RNAs (called small interfering RNAs or siRNAs) that activate a cellular enzymatic machine to degrade the mutant mRNA. Because siRNAs can in principle downregulate any human mRNA, they should be ideal to eradicate the expression of disease-causing genes. A breakthrough was achieved in 2018 with the first-ever siRNA product (patisiran) approved as a therapy [19]. Onpattro® (patisiran) is being used to treat adult patients with familial polyneuropathy caused by transthyretin-mediated amyloidosis [20]. This autosomal dominant, progressive, multisystemic, and life-threatening disease is caused by mutations in the gene encoding transthyretin (TTR). The mutant TTR protein accumulates as amyloid in peripheral nerves, heart, kidney, and gastrointestinal tract giving rise to polyneuropathy and cardiomyopathy. The drug is a double-stranded small interfering RNA encapsulated in a lipid nanoparticle for delivery to hepatocytes. By specifically binding to a conserved sequence region common to mutant and wild-type TTR mRNA, patisiran causes its degradation via RNA interference and subsequently a reduction in serum TTR protein levels and tissue TTR protein deposits [19, 20].

As an alternative to gene replacement and RNA-targeted therapies, the CRISPR gene-editing tool holds great promise in treating a wide range of genetic disorders. In 2020, Emmanuelle Charpentier and Jennifer Doudna were awarded the Nobel Prize in Chemistry for developing the prokaryotic CRISPR (Clustered Regularly Interspaced Short Palindromic Repeats) immune system into a simple easy-to-use programmable gene-editing tool with a guide RNA molecule that directs the bacterial Cas9 endonuclease to cleave sequence-specific regions of DNA. Just 8 years after their groundbreaking paper [21], CRISPR has transformed molecular biology research and is pushing medicine to enter a new age. The hype surrounding CRISPR is certainly high, but the first results from ongoing clinical trials suggest that real cures are already taking shape. For example, patients with either beta-thalassemia or sickle cell disease were successfully treated with an "ex vivo" therapy that uses CRISPR to modify hematopoietic stem cells. When reintroduced to the patient, the edited stem cells establish a permanent supply of red blood cells containing fetal hemoglobin. Despite the difference in oxygen affinity when compared to adult hemoglobin, fetal hemoglobin is still functional in adults and can rescue the defect caused by the mutations [22].

More recently, CRISPR gene editing was performed directly in the human body. The CRISPR therapy EDIT-101 was injected in the eye to treat congenital blindness caused by a mutation in the CEP290 gene [23]. EDIT-101 uses a construct containing an adeno-associated viral vector with two guide RNAs to identify the location of the mutation, combined with DNA encoding the Cas9 enzyme under a promoter specific to photoreceptor cells [24]. Another CRISPR treatment, NTLA-2001, was injected intravenously to treat patients with familial polyneuropathy caused by transthyretin-mediated amyloidosis [25]. NTLA-2001 consists of lipid nanoparticles designed to deliver to the liver a guide RNA specific to the disease-causing gene and messenger RNA that encodes the Cas9 protein. Preclinical data showed robust and long-lasting transthyretin reduction following knockout of the *TTR* gene in vivo [25].

In conclusion, therapeutic genome editing has reached the clinic, with several applications under development at rapid pace. This represents a profound opportunity to change healthcare for many patients, but there are still many challenges ahead. Further developments in regulatory action are also critical to ensure that the new technology is used safely and responsibly [26].

2.4 Precision Oncology

Genomics has revolutionized cancer research and transformed our understanding of how cancer arises. Thus, oncology was expected to benefit the most in the near term from the precision medicine approach [4]. Indeed, in recent years cancers have been reclassified based on the mutations that drive the disease, a multitude of new drugs were developed that target specific molecular features of the tumor, and constant technological advances have expanded the ability to characterize cancer patients beyond sequencing the tumor DNA.

Successful innovative treatment strategies have emerged, such as chimeric antigen receptor T-cell (CAR-T) therapy. This technique involves an ex vivo genetic modification of the patient's T cells to recognize the B-cell protein CD19. Once the modified T cells are returned to the patient, they bind to and destroy B cells expressing CD19. The first CAR-T product approved in 2017 (tisagenlecleucel; Kymriah®) resulted in a remission rate of 81% in pediatric and adolescent patients with refractory or relapsed B-cell acute lymphoblastic leukemia [27]. A second CAR-T product (axicabtagene ciloleucel; Yescarta®) was also approved in 2017 for use in relapsed or treatment-resistant large B-cell lymphoma [28].

Another innovative treatment approach that is attracting much attention is the use of mRNA to develop cancer vaccines [29]. Comprehensive catalogs of all acquired somatic mutations in individual tumors are being explored to determine which mutations may be particularly potent vaccination targets as they can create neoantigens that are not subject to central immune tolerance. Using machine learning approaches to reliably predict highly immunogenic epitopes expressed in each cancer in order to design and manufacture a vaccine unique for each patient, two studies reported exciting immunologic and clinical results after treatment of melanoma patients [30, 31]. Although one study administered the neoantigens in the form of peptides [30] and the other administered mRNAs [31], in both cases vaccination expanded preexisting neoantigen-specific T-cell populations and induced a broader repertoire of new T-cell specificities in cancer patients.

Despite the availability of several drugs targeting specific molecular features of tumors, only a minority of cancer patients currently benefit from targeted therapies. Three recent studies assessed how comprehensive molecular profiles of the tumor improve the outcome of patients with incurable recurrent and/or metastatic cancer [32–34]. The first study included analysis of circulating tumor DNA (ctDNA) to guide therapy [32], the second study included drug combinations [33], and the third study included RNA sequencing in addition to DNA analysis [34]. The authors of the first study found a high concordance rate between mutations identified in ctDNA and in the tumor tissue. An actionable molecular alteration was identified in 41 patients (41%), among whom 11 patients (11%) were treated with a matched therapy. Four patients experienced an objective response, which represents 36% of the treated patients and 4% of the whole included population. The second study focused on several actionable molecular alterations to propose drug combinations (including immunotherapy) under the premise that simultaneous targeting of more than one molecular alteration in the tumor may delay relapse. The study enrolled 149 patients, of which 73 were treated with matched therapy. Seventeen patients experienced an objective response, which represented 23% of the patients treated with matched therapy and 11% of the whole cohort. The third study identified 158 patients (52%) with an actionable molecular alteration, and 69 patients received matched therapy determined on the basis of DNA alterations. An additional 38 patients received therapy selected on the basis of changes in RNA expression. Twelve patients experienced an objective response, which represented 11% of the patients treated with matched therapy and 4% of the whole cohort. The clinical benefit of precision medicine approaches for pediatric patients with refractory/relapsed/progressive malignant disease was also recently assessed [35]. For a cohort of 525 children, 28% were candidates to receive targeted therapies. Although overall survival was the same for all participants, the 20 children with targets ranked highest in priority had a median progression-free survival of 204 days, compared with 114 days for all other 505 patients [35].

In striking contrast to the small number of patients that benefited from targeted therapies in the above studies, an inhibitor of the neurotrophic tropomyosin receptor kinase (NTRK), larotrectinib, was associated with durable objective responses across a wide range of cancers (75%) independent of their location [36]. Both larotrectinib and another inhibitor of the same target, entrectinib, are currently used in the clinic for any advanced solid tumor with a NTRK gene fusion, in adults and children. Why larotrectinib and entrectinib induce such high response rates, regardless of which NTRK gene fusion is being targeted, is still unknown. NTRK gene fusions are unusual, occurring in less than 1% of common cancers, but they are found much more frequently in rare cancers, such as secretory breast cancers and infantile fibrosarcoma. Although these drugs will only help a small number of people, they demonstrate the value of continued drug development targeting oncogenic molecules.

How can precision oncology therapies help more people with cancer? Possibly, we are still too limited in the ability to identify dominant oncogenic drivers and in the targeted drug armamentarium. In this regard, the paradigm in precision oncology is to take into account the molecular and cellular features of a tumor as well as those of its microenvironment and additional traits of the individual, such as genetics and lifestyle, to create a tailor-made treatment [37]. In addition to new technology to detect more molecular biomarkers, real-world data in the rapidly expanding electronic health records may further assist in identifying new options for targeted treatments. Cloud-based machine learning systems are already helping clinicians to devise more effective treatment plans for cancer patients [38].

Finally, it is important to emphasize that even the most common forms of standard cancer treatment, i.e., surgery, chemotherapy, and radiotherapy, are improving all the time and becoming increasingly precise. For example, the new generation of linear accelerators have a built-in magnetic resonance imaging scanner that allows to closely monitor the patient anatomy and adapt the treatment plan to reduce the risk of radiation side effects [39]. Moreover, radiation oncologists are studying how to adapt treatments to the molecular profile of each individual. An association was recently found in breast cancer patients between radiation side effects and variants of two genes linked with circadian rhythm [40]. Whether radiation doses can be optimized based on molecular signatures of radiation sensitivity is currently under investigation [39].

2.5   A New Frontier in Precision Medicine: The Microbiome

In recent years, advances in genome sequencing technologies and metagenomic analysis resulted in an explosion of studies on the human microbiome. Most importantly, microbiome research is changing our perception of human biology in health and disease [41]. It is estimated that over 10,000 species of microorganisms, including bacteria, fungi, protozoa, and viruses, are present in the human body. Tremendous variation in a person's microbiome occurs depending on diet, medication, age, stress levels, or disease. The microbiome is also implicated in the direct biotransformation of drugs. In particular, bacterial drug metabolism is a general mechanism through which the microbiome in the gastrointestinal and reproductive tracts, and perhaps even within diseased tissue, alters drug response [41]. Namely, variation in the efficacy of cancer immunotherapeutic drugs was linked with differences in the gut microbiome [42–44].

Therapeutic manipulation of the microbiome is a rapidly advancing field [41]. One approach to microbiome modification is to selectively deplete strains with undesirable activities, such as those that act on drugs to form toxic metabolites. Another is to introduce engineered strains into the host as live bacterial therapeutics. Two recent studies described engineering *Escherichia coli* to express genes that could complement absent host functions in human metabolic diseases caused by genetic mutations [45, 46]. Other efforts aim to genetically edit bacteria that are actively colonizing the human body. Progress toward precision modification of the human microbiome holds great potential as a novel approach for managing certain human diseases.

2.6 Conclusions and Outlook

Precision medicine explicitly prioritizes the individualization of patient care through mechanistic reasoning and integration of distinct methodologies. How to advance knowledge for precision medicine is fundamentally different from evidence-based medicine, which focuses on population-based studies. Population-based data will certainly remain important for understanding health and disease, but should no longer be considered as sufficient. A major challenge for precision medicine will be to integrate molecular data with aspects of lifestyle and environment, as promised in its definition. Success will depend on constant development of new technology, and approaches for rapid incorporation of the evolving medical knowledge into clinical practice. The ability to measure, store, share, and analyze health-related data is rapidly expanding. Electronic health records will provide a dynamic overview of health outcomes at various stages of life. Increased availability of personal devices such as smartphones, activity monitors, and wearable GPS units, as well as electronic data capture tools to monitor behavior and exposure to environmental cues, offers unprecedented opportunities for behavioral interventions and real-time assessment of individual health. Progress in artificial intelligence will be transformative. Improved machines will acquire better medical images. Advanced "multi-omics" technologies will provide comprehensive molecular profiles of individuals. Engineered tissues and organs will enable mechanistic dissection of biological pathways driving disease and innovative drug design. In conclusion, the current precision medicine movement is just starting to reveal how medical knowledge and healthcare will develop in the future.

References

1. Collins FS. Shattuck lecture—medical and societal consequences of the human genome project. N Engl J Med. 1999;341:28–37. https://doi.org/10.1056/NEJM199907013410106.
2. Mirnezami R, Nicholson J, Darzi A. Preparing for precision medicine. N Engl J Med. 2012;366:489–90. https://doi.org/10.1056/NEJMp1114866.
3. Katsnelson A. Momentum grows to make 'personalized' medicine more 'precise'. Nat Med. 2013;19:249. https://doi.org/10.1038/nm0313-249.

  4. Collins FS, Varmus H. A new initiative on precision medicine. N Engl J Med. 2015;372:793–5. https://doi.org/10.1056/NEJMp1500523.
  5. Njolstad PR, Andreassen OA, Brunak S, Borglum AD, Dillner J, Esko T, et al. Roadmap for a precision-medicine initiative in the Nordic region. Nat Genet. 2019;51:924–30. https://doi.org/10.1038/s41588-019-0391-1.
  6. Meier-Abt PJ, Lawrence AK, Selter L, Vayena E, Schwede T. The Swiss approach to precision medicine. Swiss Med Wkly. 2018; https://doi.org/10.3929/ethz-b-000274911.
  7. Kosorok MR, Laber EB. Precision medicine. Annu Rev Stat Appl. 2019;6:263–86. https://doi.org/10.1146/annurev-statistics-030718-105251.
  8. Boycott KM, Rath A, Chong JX, Hartley T, Alkuraya FS, Baynam G, et al. International cooperation to enable the diagnosis of all rare genetic diseases. Am J Hum Genet. 2017;100:695–705. https://doi.org/10.1016/j.ajhg.2017.04.003.
  9. Caskey T. Precision medicine: functional advancements. Annu Rev Med. 2018;69:1–18. https://doi.org/10.1146/annurev-med-041316-090905.
 10. Marco-Puche G, Lois S, Benítez J, Trivino JC. RNA-Seq perspectives to improve clinical diagnosis. Front Genet. 2019;10:1152. https://doi.org/10.3389/fgene.2019.01152.
 11. Hui L, Bianchi DW. Noninvasive prenatal DNA testing: the vanguard of genomic medicine. Annu Rev Med. 2017;68:459–72. https://doi.org/10.1146/annurev-med-072115-033220.
 12. Wade N. A decade later, genetic map yields few new cures. The New York Times. 12 Jun 2010. https://www.nytimes.com/2010/06/13/health/research/13genome.html. Accessed 15 Jan 2021.
 13. Kirschner J, Butoianu N, Goemans N, Haberlova J, Kostera-Pruszczyk A, Mercuri E, et al. European ad-hoc consensus statement on gene replacement therapy for spinal muscular atrophy. Eur J Paediatr Neurol. 2020;28:38–43. https://doi.org/10.1016/j.ejpn.2020.07.001.
 14. Rigo F, Hua Y, Krainer AR, Bennett CF. Antisense-based therapy for the treatment of spinal muscular atrophy. J Cell Biol. 2012;199:21–5. https://doi.org/10.1083/jcb.201207087.
 15. Ciulla TA, Hussain RM, Berrocal AM, Nagiel A. Voretigene neparvovec-rzyl for treatment of RPE65-mediated inherited retinal diseases: a model for ocular gene therapy development. Expert Opin Biol Ther. 2020;20:565–78. https://doi.org/10.1080/14712598.2020.1740676.
 16. Perrin GQ, Herzog RW, Markusic DM. Update on clinical gene therapy for hemophilia. Blood. 2019;133:407–14. https://doi.org/10.1182/blood-2018-07-820720.
 17. Kunz JB, Kulozik AE. Gene therapy of the hemoglobinopathies. Hema. 2020;4:e479. https://doi.org/10.1097/HS9.0000000000000479.
 18. Thompson AA, Walters MC, Kwiatkowski J, Rasko JEJ, Ribeil J-A, Hongeng S, et al. Gene therapy in patients with transfusion-dependent β-thalassemia. N Engl J Med. 2018;378:1479–93. https://doi.org/10.1056/NEJMoa1705342.
 19. Adams D, Gonzalez-Duarte A, O'riordan WD, Yang C-C, Ueda M, Kristen AV, et al. Patisiran, an RNAi therapeutic, for hereditary transthyretin amyloidosis. N Engl J Med. 2018;379:11–21. https://doi.org/10.1056/NEJMoa1716153.
 20. Wood H. FDA approves patisiran to treat hereditary transthyretin amyloidosis. Nat Rev Neurol. 2018;14:570. https://doi.org/10.1038/s41582-018-0065-0.
 21. Jinek M, Chylinski K, Fonfara I, Hauer M, Doudna JA, Charpentier E. A programmable dual-RNA-guided DNA endonuclease in adaptive bacterial immunity. Science. 2012;337:816–21. https://doi.org/10.1126/science.1225829.
 22. Frangoul H, Altshuler D, Cappellini MD, Chen Y-S, Domm J, Eustace BK, et al. CRISPR-Cas9 gene editing for sickle cell disease and β-thalassemia. N Engl J Med. 2020; https://doi.org/10.1056/NEJMoa2031054.
 23. First CRISPR therapy dosed. Nat Biotechnol. 2020;38:382. https://doi.org/10.1038/s41587-020-0493-4.
 24. Maeder ML, Stefanidakis M, Wilson CJ, Baral R, Barrera LA, Bounoutas GS, et al. Development of a gene-editing approach to restore vision loss in Leber congenital amaurosis type 10. Nat Med. 2019;25:229–33. https://doi.org/10.1038/s41591-018-0327-9.
 25. First systemic CRISPR agent in humans. Nat Biotechnol. 2020;38:1364. https://doi.org/10.1038/s41587-020-00773-8.

26. Doudna JA. The promise and challenge of therapeutic genome editing. Nature. 2020;578:229–36. https://doi.org/10.1038/s41586-020-1978-5.
27. Ucks G, Rheingold SR. The journey to CAR T cell therapy: the pediatric and young adult experience with relapsed or refractory B-ALL. Blood Cancer J. 2019;9:10. https://doi.org/10.1038/s41408-018-0164-6.
28. Mohty M, Dulery R, Gauthier J, Malard F, Brissot E, Aljurf M, et al. CAR T-cell therapy for the management of refractory/relapsed high-grade B-cell lymphoma: a practical overview. Bone Marrow Transplant. 2020;55:1525–32. https://doi.org/10.1038/s41409-020-0892-7.
29. Pardi N, Hogan MJ, Porter FW, Weissman D. mRNA vaccines—a new era in vaccinology. Nat Rev Drug Discov. 2018;17:261–79. https://doi.org/10.1038/nrd.2017.243.
30. Ott PA, Hu Z, Keskin DB, Shukla SA, Sun J, Bozym DJ, et al. An immunogenic personal neoantigen vaccine for patients with melanoma. Nature. 2017;547:217–21. https://doi.org/10.1038/nature22991.
31. Sahin U, Derhovanessian E, Miller M, Kloke B-P, Simon P, Löwer M, et al. Personalized RNA mutanome vaccines mobilize poly-specific therapeutic immunity against cancer. Nature. 2017;547:222–6. https://doi.org/10.1038/nature23003.
32. Rothwell DG, Ayub M, Cook N, Thistlethwaite F, Carter L, Dean E, et al. Utility of ctDNA to support patient selection for early phase clinical trials: the TARGET study. Nat Med. 2019;25:738–43. https://doi.org/10.1038/s41591-019-0380-z.
33. Sicklick JK, Kato S, Okamura R, Schwaederle M, Hahn ME, Williams CB, et al. Molecular profiling of cancer patients enables personalized combination therapy: the I-PREDICT study. Nat Med. 2019;25:744–50. https://doi.org/10.1038/s41591-019-0407-5.
34. Rodon J, Soria J-C, Berger R, Miller WH, Rubin E, Kugel A, et al. Genomic and transcriptomic profiling expands precision cancer medicine: the WINTHER trial. Nat Med. 2019;25:751–8. https://doi.org/10.1038/s41591-019-0424-4.
35. van Tilburg CM, Pfaff E, Pajtler KW, Langenberg KPS, Fiesel P, Jones BC, et al. The pediatric precision oncology study INFORM: clinical outcome and benefit for molecular subgroups. J Clin Oncol. 2020;38(18_Suppl):LBA10503.
36. Drilon A, Laetsch TW, Kummar S, DuBois SG, Lassen UN, Demetri GD, et al. Efficacy of larotrectinib in TRK fusion–positive cancers in adults and children. N Engl J Med. 2018;378:731–9. https://doi.org/10.1056/NEJMoa1714448.
37. Yates LR, Seoane J, Le Tourneau C, Siu LL, Marais R, Michiels S, et al. The European Society for Medical Oncology (ESMO) precision medicine glossary. Ann Oncol. 2018;29:30–5. https://doi.org/10.1093/annonc/mdx707.
38. Pishvaian MJ, Blais EM, Bender RJ, Rao S, Boca SM, Chung V, et al. A virtual molecular tumor board to improve efficiency and scalability of delivering precision oncology to physicians and their patients. JAMIA Open. 2019;2:505–15. https://doi.org/10.1093/jamiaopen/ooz045.
39. Keener AB. Making radiation oncology more personal. Nature. 2020. https://www.nature.com/articles/d41586-020-02677-8.
40. Johnson K, Chang-Claude J, Critchley A-M, Kyriacou C, Lavers S, Rattay T, et al. Genetic variants predict optimal timing of radiotherapy to reduce side-effects in breast cancer patients. Clin Oncol. 2019;31:9–16. https://doi.org/10.1016/j.clon.2018.10.001.
41. Lam KN, Alexander M, Turnbaugh PJ. Precision medicine goes microscopic: engineering the microbiome to improve drug outcomes. Cell Host Microbe. 2019;26:22–34. https://doi.org/10.1016/j.chom.2019.06.011.
42. Gopalakrishnan V, Spencer CN, Nezi L, Reuben A, Andrews MC, Karpinets TV, et al. Gut microbiome modulates response to anti-PD-1 immunotherapy in melanoma patients. Science. 2018;359:97–103. https://doi.org/10.1126/science.aan4236.
43. Matson V, Fessler J, Bao R, Chongsuwat T, Zha Y, Alegre M-L, et al. The commensal microbiome is associated with anti-PD-1 efficacy in metastatic melanoma patients. Science. 2018;359:104–8. https://doi.org/10.1126/science.aao3290.
44. Routy B, Le Chatelier E, Derosa L, Duong CPM, Alou MT, Daillère R, et al. Gut microbiome influences efficacy of PD-1-based immunotherapy against epithelial tumors. Science. 2018;359:91–7. https://doi.org/10.1126/science.aan3706.

45. Isabella VM, Ha BN, Castillo MJ, Lubkowicz DJ, Rowe SE, Millet YA, et al. Development of a synthetic live bacterial therapeutic for the human metabolic disease phenylketonuria. Nat Biotechnol. 2018;36:857–64. https://doi.org/10.1038/nbt.4222.
46. Kurtz CB, Millet YA, Puurunen MK, Perreault M, Charbonneau MR, Isabella VM, et al. An engineered *E. coli* Nissle improves hyperammonemia and survival in mice and shows dose-dependent exposure in healthy humans. Sci Transl Med. 2019;11:eaau7975. https://doi.org/10.1126/scitranslmed.aau7975.

Do We Need Precision Medicine in Stroke?

3

Ana Catarina Fonseca

Precision medicine is broadly defined as tailored diagnosis and therapy for each individual patient [1]. From an initial standpoint where treatment for a disease was needed and therefore a "one-size-fits-all" approach was used, we are now changing to a tailored approach with treatment suited for the particular characteristics of each individual.

This change in paradigm has been possible due to changes that occurred during the last decade. Widely available genetic and functional assays have revolutionized diagnostic and therapeutic options across various disciplines [2] and this sweeping change is also starting to impact stroke diagnosis and treatment and will further continue in years to come.

The term stroke encompasses a syndrome with a range of different manifestations that can affect distinctive parts of the brain and may be caused by diverse mechanisms. Rather than being a single disease, stroke is actually the common endpoint of several diseases. It is important to identify the underlying mechanism accurately in individual patients in order to choose the best treatment approach and reduce the risk of recurrence [3].

Currently, small attention is paid to different phenotypes and similar subtypes of stroke tend to be treated in a similar way in randomized clinical trials. Clinical trials take into account a normal distribution of the population and do not consider specificities of each individual. Therefore, we know that there is a part of the population that will not respond to treatment indicated by the current treatment guidelines. Results from clinical trials give the same prescription to patients with the same diagnosis. Among the patient group that receive this treatment four main groups can be defined: patients in which the drug will be toxic and not beneficial, patients in which the drug is toxic but beneficial, patients in which the drug is not toxic and not

A. C. Fonseca (✉)
Department of Neurosciences and Mental Health (Neurology), Hospital Santa Maria—CHLN, Faculdade de Medicina, Universidade de Lisboa, Lisbon, Portugal

© Springer Nature Switzerland AG 2021
A. C. Fonseca, J. M. Ferro (eds.), *Precision Medicine in Stroke*,
https://doi.org/10.1007/978-3-030-70761-3_3

21

beneficial, and patients in which the drug is not toxic but is beneficial. Knowing exactly in which group each patient fits would greatly improve stroke care. Some patients may suffer harm and therefore we need better ways to identify those who might benefit the most.

3.1　Acute Ischemic Stroke Treatment

Currently acute ischemic stroke treatment is similar in all patients. Intravenous thrombolysis (IV rtPA) with 0.9 mg/kg alteplase is given to all patients that present within 4.5 h of ischemic stroke independently of stroke etiology if all inclusion and exclusion criteria are fulfilled [4]. Established blood pressure and glucose limits that should be maintained as well as alteplase dosages are similar in all individuals independently of their personal history, extension of white matter disease, or presence of microbleeds. The major risk of using intravenous thrombolysis is intracranial hemorrhage that may be fatal in some patients. Knowing which patients are at a higher risk of this complication and if different dosages of alteplase adapted to each individual could potentially contribute to further enhancement of the benefit while reducing risk would be valuable.

The randomized clinical trials that aimed to expand the current therapeutic time window of 4.5 h in patients with IV rtPA that had a stroke at wake-up or unknown time of onset, using advanced imaging methods, like the EXTEND [5] and WAKE-UP [6] trials, have further helped to personalize acute ischemic stroke treatment. They take into account that tissue resistance to ischemia may vary from individual to individual. Another possible treatment strategy in acute ischemic stroke to enhance individualized treatment could be to optimize the brain tissue protection responses to ischemia. There are two main mechanisms of protection: collateral circulation and hypoxia-inducible factor (HIF) response [7]. These responses to cerebral ischemia vary from individual to individual and may be dependent on genetic and environmental factors. A better understanding of these mechanisms may move us further towards the goals of precision medicine, enabling physicians to customize treatments using personalized time windows for each patient and to use specific treatments that could enhance the endogenous responses to ischemia [8]. Individualization of treatment will ultimately contribute to increasing the number of patients that will be able to receive treatment and to maximizing the benefit/risk balance.

3.2　Diagnostic Strategies

Recently, similar considerations have been done regarding diagnosis evaluation of covert brain infarction (CBI) [9]. Different phenotypes may warrant different diagnostic approaches. For example, a patient with a lacune and severe white matter hyperintensities might primarily benefit from blood pressure control because the pathophysiology is probably hypertensive small vessel disease. Patients with multiple cortical CBIs without signs of white matter disease might benefit from long-term rhythm monitoring to detect subclinical atrial fibrillation which could be treated with oral anticoagulation. However for patients with multiple CBIs in one vascular territory noninvasive angiography of the supra-aortic vessels and revascularization or best medical treatment of large-artery stenotic disease might be the best option [10].

3.3 Stroke Prevention

Individual response to antithrombotics, statins, and even drugs commonly used to treat blood pressure and diabetes mellitus is often tested through a trial-and-error approach. Statins are among the most effective and widely used drugs for the primary and secondary prevention of cardiovascular disease and its complications. However, studies show that there is considerable individual variation in the low-density lipoprotein cholesterol (LDL) reduction at all doses of simvastatin, atorvastatin, and rosuvastatin [10]. Variability in drug response exists regardless of the measured phenotype, and genetic variability may be a contributing factor [11]. Novel approaches to pharmacogenetics have extended statin pharmacogenetic observations to new phenotypes and candidate genes [11]. In the future, genotyping could be used to routinely guide statin treatment. This could help to improve the benefit while reducing the risk of adverse events.

Currently ischemic stroke secondary prevention is broadly divided into two main groups: cardioembolic and noncardioembolic etiology. Cardioembolic strokes are treated with anticoagulants. For anticoagulation resumption after stroke from cardioembolic stroke, there is a balance of benefit/risk that needs to be taken into account: although the risk of early recurrent ischemic stroke is high, early oral anticoagulation is suspected to increase the risk of potentially harmful intracranial hemorrhage, including hemorrhagic transformation of the infarct [12]. Clinical trials are currently being conducted to try to determine what is the best time to start anticoagulation after ischemic stroke [12]. Most of these trials take into account the size of the infarct or the severity of the neurological deficit to randomize patients. However, it is comprehensible that patients may present with individual peculiarities that may further influence their risk of early stroke recurrence or hemorrhagic transformation of the infarct and influence this benefit/risk balance. Also, we know that the higher the CHADS2-VASC score a patient with atrial fibrillation presents, the higher the probability of having a stroke. However, currently all patients are equally treated with anticoagulants. More data is needed to know if this different stroke risk can be addressed with different treatment strategies.

Another field in which we are progressively seeing a change in the "one-size-fits-all" approach regards secondary stroke prevention of noncardioembolic strokes. According to the European Stroke Organization guidelines, clopidogrel is a first-line antiplatelet for secondary stroke prevention [13, 14]. However, it is known that there is significant heterogeneity across individuals regarding clopidogrel metabolism. Clopidogrel is an inactive prodrug that needs hepatic bioactivation by several enzymes, including CYP2C19 [15]. The prodrug is converted via a two-step process involving several cytochrome P450 (CYP) enzymes to an active metabolite. This resulting active metabolite irreversibly inhibits the platelet ADP receptor, P2Y12 [15]. Genetic variants that diminish the activity of the enzyme will cause shunting of the prodrug to the esterase-mediated degradation pathway to form inactive metabolites. This will lead to decreased levels of the active metabolite and less inhibition of platelets, leading to a greater risk of cardiovascular events. While the *1 allele of CYP2C19 has full enzymatic activity, the *2 (rs4244385) variant is the most common of the reduced-function variants and produces a complete loss of enzymatic activity resulting in a lower amount of active metabolite and attenuated clopidogrel-induced platelet inhibition [15]. With the *2 allele, a gene-dose effect is seen, where an increasing number of reduced-function alleles results in a decreasing amount of platelet inhibition. Apart from *2, other loss-of-function variants exist. These variants are rare but produce similar enzymatic defects as the *2 allele [15].

The Food and Drug Administration (FDA) agency requires a black-box warning for reduced effectiveness in persons who are poor metabolizers of clopidogrel. However, testing for CYP2C19 genotype to aid clinical management is not currently routinely done. For carriers of *2, one potential treatment strategy could be to consider higher doses of clopidogrel than usually used. Genetic variants affecting clopidogrel metabolism may identify nonresponders and reduce side effects, but these approaches have not yet been widely adopted in clinical practice.

Studies like the CHANCE [16] and POINT [17] clinical trials showed that patients with high-risk TIA (ABCD2 >3) or NIHSS <4 benefit from short-term dual-antiplatelet therapy with clopidogrel and aspirin. However, in the POINT study compared to the CHANCE trial, major hemorrhage occurred significantly more frequently in patients treated with clopidogrel + aspirin than in the placebo + aspirin arm. Also, one of the reasons why the POINT study was prematurely stopped was because the prespecified safety threshold for major hemorrhage had been crossed in the clopidogrel + aspirin arm in the interim analysis. One possible explanation was that CHANCE only included Chinese patients and these are known to have nonfunction allelic variants of CYP2C19 that may decrease the risk of bleeding.

Another important question is whether all stroke subtypes presenting with TIA or minor stroke should receive dual-antiplatelet therapy, or whether it is more effective in some stroke subtypes [3]. A subgroup analysis in the CHANCE trial showed an apparently greater effectiveness of dual-antiplatelet therapy in people with intracranial stenosis than in those without stenosis [18]. In the SOCRATES trial, ticagrelor was comparably effective to aspirin in early secondary prevention, but was more effective than aspirin in a subgroup analysis in patients with large artery stroke [3, 19]. This suggests that more intensive antiplatelet regimens are particularly effective in patients with TIA and stroke due to large artery stenosis. However, there is some uncertainty regarding the use of dual-antiplatelet therapy with aspirin and clopidogrel in patients with lacunar stroke. These patients were included in the CHANCE and POINT trials. However, the SPS3 study showed that in long-term prevention after lacunar stroke, dual-antiplatelet therapy was associated with no additional reduction in ischemic events, but with a significantly increased risk of bleeding [3, 20]. More data is needed to know which specific patients benefit the most from certain interventions.

3.4 Conclusions

The examples that were given only scratch the surface of possible applications of precision medicine in stroke. Application of precision medicine to stroke will improve the benefit of current treatments while minimizing their risk. It will also allow the development of treatments aimed at specific targets.

In order to further proceed, one of the challenges will be the collection of standardized clinical, biological (genomic, serological, and novel), and imaging data [21]. This will need cerebrovascular expertise on big data approaches to clinically relevant paradigms. Stroke precision medicine will also need experienced and rational valuation of these multiple data points and appropriate statistical methodology to obtain individualized decision-making [21].

References

1. Hamburg MA, Collins FS. The path to personalized medicine. N Engl J Med. 2010;363:301–4.
2. Joyner MJ, Paneth N. Promises, promises, and precision medicine. J Clin Investig. 2019;129:946–8.
3. Markus H. Personalising secondary prevention: different treatments for different strokes. Pract Neurol. 2020;20(1):34–8.
4. Powers WJ, Rabinstein AA, Ackerson T, Adeoye OM, Bambakidis NC, Becker K, Biller J, Brown M, Demaerschalk BM, Hoh B, Jauch EC, Kidwell CS, Leslie-Mazwi TM, Ovbiagele B, Scott PA, Sheth KN, Southerland AM, Summers DV, Tirschwell DL. Guidelines for the early management of patients with acute ischemic stroke: 2019 update to the 2018 guidelines for the early management of acute ischemic stroke: a guideline for healthcare professionals from the American Heart Association/American Stroke Association. Stroke. 2019;50:e344–418.
5. Ma H, BCV C, Parsons MW, Churilov L, Levi CR, Hsu C, Kleinig TJ, Wijeratne T, Curtze S, Dewey HM, Miteff F, Tsai CH, Lee JT, Phan TG, Mahant N, Sun MC, Krause M, Sturm J, Grimley R, Chen CH, Hu CJ, Wong AA, Field D, Sun Y, Barber PA, Sabet A, Jannes J, Jeng JS, Clissold B, Markus R, Lin CH, Lien LM, Bladin CF, Christensen S, Yassi N, Sharma G, Bivard A, Desmond PM, Yan B, Mitchell PJ, Thijs V, Carey L, Meretoja A, Davis SM, Donnan GA, EXTEND Investigators. Thrombolysis guided by perfusion imaging up to 9 hours after onset of stroke. N Engl J Med. 2019;380:1795–803.
6. Thomalla G, Simonsen CZ, Boutitie F, Andersen G, Berthezene Y, Cheng B, Cheripelli B, Cho TH, Fazekas F, Fiehler J, Ford I, Galinovic I, Gellissen S, Golsari A, Gregori J, Günther M, Guibernau J, Häusler KG, Hennerici M, Kemmling A, Marstrand J, Modrau B, Neeb L, Perez de la Ossa N, Puig J, Ringleb P, Roy P, Scheel E, Schonewille W, Serena J, Sunaert S, Villringer K, Wouters A, Thijs V, Ebinger M, Endres M, Fiebach JB, Lemmens R, Muir KW, Nighoghossian N, Pedraza S, Gerloff C, WAKE-UP Investigators. MRI-guided thrombolysis for stroke with unknown time of onset. N Engl J Med. 2018;379:611–22.
7. Shi H. Hypoxia inducible factor 1 as a therapeutic target in ischemic stroke. Curr Med Chem. 2009;16:4593–600.

8. Bang OY, Goyal M, Liebeskind DS. Collateral circulation in ischemic stroke: assessment tools and therapeutic strategies. Stroke. 2015;46:3302–9.

9. Meinel TR, Kaesmacher J, Roten L, Fischer U. Covert brain infarction: towards precision medicine in research, diagnosis, and therapy for a silent pandemic. Stroke. 2020;51(8):2597–606.

10. Karlson BW, Wiklund O, Palmer MK, Nicholls SJ, Lundman P, Barter PJ. Variability of low-density lipoprotein cholesterol response with different doses of atorvastatin, rosuvastatin, and simvastatin: results from VOYAGER. Eur Heart J Cardiovasc Pharmacother. 2016;2(4):212–7.

11. Zineh I. Pharmacogenetics of response to statins. Curr Atheroscler Rep. 2007;9(3):187–94.

12. Seiffge DJ, Werring DJ, Paciaroni M, Dawson J, Warach S, Milling TJ, Engelter ST, Fischer U, Norrving B. Timing of anticoagulation after recent ischaemic stroke in patients with atrial fibrillation. Lancet Neurol. 2019;18:117–26.

13. European Stroke Organisation (ESO) Executive Committee, ESO Writing Committee. Guidelines for management of ischaemic stroke and transient ischaemic attack 2008. Cerebrovasc Dis. 2008;25:457–507.

14. CAPRIE Steering Committee. A randomised, blinded, trial of clopidogrel versus aspirin in patients at risk of ischaemic events (CAPRIE). CAPRIE Steering Committee. Lancet. 1996;348:1329–39.

15. Anderson CD, Biffi A, Greenberg SM, Rosand J. Personalized approaches to clopidogrel therapy: are we there yet? Stroke. 2010;41:2997–3002.

16. Wang Y, Wang Y, Zhao X, Liu L, Wang D, Wang C, Wang C, Li H, Meng X, Cui L, Jia J, Dong Q, Xu A, Zeng J, Li Y, Wang Z, Xia H, Johnston SC, CHANCE Investigators. Clopidogrel with aspirin in acute minor stroke or transient ischemic attack. N Engl J Med. 2013;369(1):11–9.

17. Johnston SC, Easton JD, Farrant M, Barsan W, Conwit RA, Elm JJ, Kim AS, Lindblad AS, Palesch YY, Clinical Research Collaboration, Neurological Emergencies Treatment Trials Network, POINT Investigators. Clopidogrel and aspirin in acute ischemic stroke and high-risk TIA. N Engl J Med. 2018;379(3):215–25.

18. Liu L, Wong KSL, Leng X, et al. Dual antiplatelet therapy in stroke and ICAS: subgroup analysis of chance. Neurology. 2015;85:1154–62.

19. Amarenco P, Albers GW, Denison H, et al. Efficacy and safety of ticagrelor versus aspirin in acute stroke or transient ischaemic attack of atherosclerotic origin: a subgroup analysis of SOCRATES, a randomised, double-blind, controlled trial. Lancet Neurol. 2017;16:301–10.

20. Benavente OR, Hart RG, McClure LA, et al. Effects of clopidogrel added to aspirin in patients with recent lacunar stroke. N Engl J Med. 2012;367:817–25.

21. Hinman JD, Rost NS, Leung TW, Montaner J, Muir KW, Brown S, Arenillas JF, Feldmann E, Liebeskind DS. Principles of precision medicine in stroke. J Neurol Neurosurg Psychiatry. 2017;88(1):54–61.

Monogenic Stroke Diseases

4

Elisabeth Tournier-Lasserve

4.1 Introduction

Stroke is in most cases multifactorial with hypertension as a major risk factor, particularly in elderly patients. However, several rare monogenic diseases, affecting either the cerebral arteries, veins, or capillaries, lead to stroke. This group is highly heterogeneous on both a clinical and a genetic point of view. Monogenic diseases affecting mainly cerebral vessel's wall include small and large vessel diseases, cerebrovascular malformations, and dysplasia. In addition, stroke can be one of the manifestations of several monogenic diseases leading to cardioemboli, prothrombotic states, or various metabolic disorders.

Several genes whose mutations lead to monogenic CSVD, inherited cerebral cavernous angiomas, or arteriovenous malformations have been identified. Tremendous progress has also been done in the understanding of the mechanisms of some of these diseases and several excellent reviews have been published recently on these topics [1–6].

In this chapter we focus on eight monogenic CSVD for which causative genes and mutations have been identified in the last 20 years, helping to decipher this highly heterogeneous group of diseases.

4.2 Monogenic CSVD Diagnosis Challenges

Most CSVD are sporadic and their main risk factor is hypertension. However, several monogenic CSVD leading to stroke as their main manifestations have now been molecularly characterized with important implications for diagnosis, genetic

E. Tournier-Lasserve (✉)
AP-HP, Department of Genetics, Saint-Louis Hospital, INSERM U1141, Paris University, Paris, France
e-mail: elisabeth.tournier@aphp.fr

© Springer Nature Switzerland AG 2021
A. C. Fonseca, J. M. Ferro (eds.), *Precision Medicine in Stroke*,
https://doi.org/10.1007/978-3-030-70761-3_4

counseling, and clinical care. Gene identification also allowed the development of mouse models for several of these diseases such as CADASIL or COL4A1/A2-related diseases, paving the way to a better understanding of their mechanisms and the development of preclinical trials [4]. It also allowed a better understanding of sporadic CSVD which share many features with monogenic CSVD.

As regards to CSVD diagnosis in routine practice the clinician faces three main questions: (1) When and how to suspect that stroke is the consequence of a monogenic CSVD in my patient? (2) Which gene is involved? (3) What are the clinical implications of these findings for my patient and his/her relatives?

Detailed clinical phenotyping of the proband and careful collection of familial information are key to suspect a genetic cause. Indeed, an unusually young age at onset, an absence of vascular risk factors, a familial aggregation, a consanguinity, and/or the presence of suggestive extraneurological manifestations should lead to suspect a genetic cause. However, true genetic cases can sometimes present as sporadic cases; this may be the case for autosomal recessive disorders, dominant disorders with incomplete penetrance, and de novo mutations. A monogenic disease can also occur in the presence of vascular risk factors.

Once a monogenic CSVD has been suspected, which molecular screening should be performed? The advent of high-throughput sequencing, also called next-generation sequencing (NGS), now allows an easy and cost-effective screening of many genes at once. Screening of all known CSVD genes using genomic DNA extracted from blood is highly preferable when suspecting a monogenic CSVD since mutations in distinct genes can lead to similar phenotypes. This screening allows to detect point mutations whatever their nature but sometimes needs to be completed by additional techniques, either to analyze the functional consequence of a genomic variant of unknown significance or to search for mutations undetectable by exonic sequencing.

4.3　CADASIL and NOTCH3 Gene Mutations

Cerebral autosomal dominant arteriopathy with subcortical infarcts and leukoencephalopathy (CADASIL) is the most frequent monogenic CSVD. It is caused by highly stereotyped mutations of NOTCH3, a gene encoding a transmembrane receptor including 34 epidermal growth factor receptor (EGFR) motifs, each of them containing 6 cysteine residues [7]. CADASIL-type mutations lead to an odd number of cysteine residues in any one of these EGF receptor motifs leading to an aggregation of the NOTCH3 extracellular domain and the sequestration of multiple proteins from the extracellular matrix of cerebral small vessels [8].

Clinical, MRI, pathological, and genetic features of this adult-onset CSVD as well as pathophysiological data obtained in transgenic mouse models have been recapitulated in excellent reviews [8, 9]. Therefore, we will emphasize herein only the main features of this CSVD and a few points that emerged recently as regards the prevalence of CADASIL and its expressivity since these data will be of great importance for patients' care and genetic counseling.

In our routine diagnostic experience, 10–15% of patients referred for a familial vascular leukoencephalopathy with lacunar infarcts have a NOTCH3 pathogenic mutation. Age at onset is around 45–50 years in most patients. However, late onset (>70 years) is observed in some patients. The earliest, but inconstant, clinical manifestations are attacks of migraine with aura. Lacunar infarcts occur in at least two-thirds of patients. Additional manifestations include severe episodes of mood disturbances, apathy, cognitive impairment, and dementia [9]. Magnetic resonance imaging's (MRI) main features associate symmetrical white matter hypersignals (WMH), lacunes, microbleeds, and enlarged Virchow-Robin spaces (Fig. 4.1,

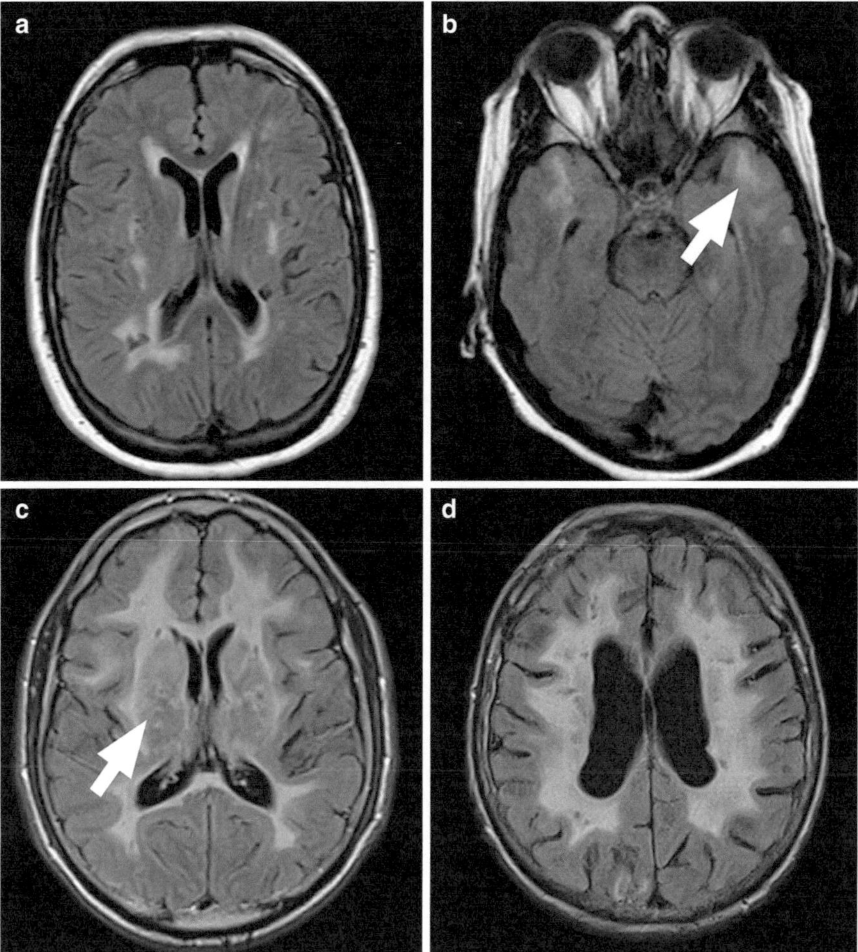

Fig. 4.1 CADASIL, CARASIL, and HTRA1 autosomal dominant CSVD. (**a, b**) Axial FLAIR images of a 59-year-old CADASIL patient. (**c, d**) Axial FLAIR images of a 59-year-old CARASIL patient. (**e, f**) T2-weighted and axial FLAIR images of a 69-year-old patient with a pathogenic heterozygous mutation within HTRA1

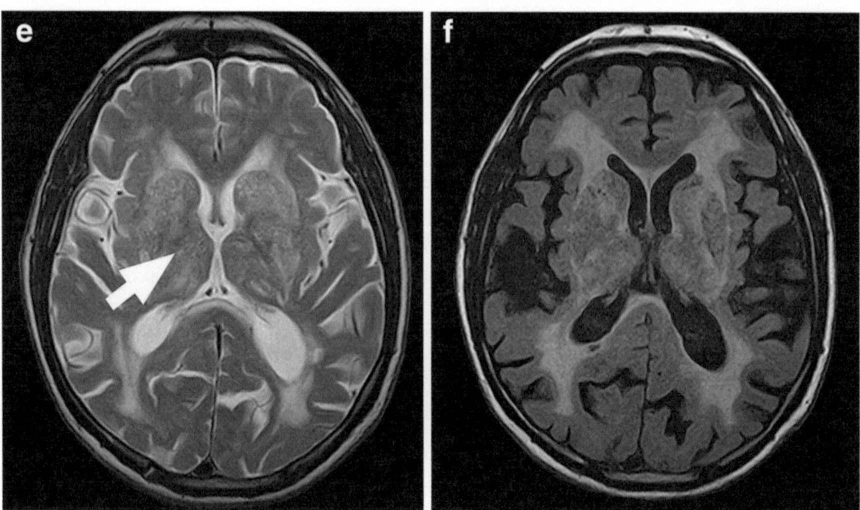

Fig. 4.1 (continued)

panels a, b). WMH of the anterior temporal lobes are frequently encountered but can be lacking and can also be observed in distinct CSVD. Once suspected, NGS sequencing of all NOTCH3 exons establishes the diagnosis when it detects a heterozygous mutation leading to an odd number of cysteine residues within one of the 34 EGFR motifs. There has been a long debate as regards to the causality of missense mutations that do not affect the number of cysteine residues. In most cases these mutations are not associated with another specific biomarker of CADASIL, namely the presence of granular osmiophilic deposits (GOM) in the vascular smooth muscle cells of skin vessels; they should therefore not be considered as CADASIL mutations. We cannot however totally exclude the role of a few very rare "noncysteine" missense mutations that would be associated with GOM. NGS sometimes detects heterozygous nonsense (stop codon) variants. These loss-of-function variants are not associated with GOM and are not CADASIL-type mutations. Several case report studies of CSVD patients showing heterozygous NOTCH3 nonsense mutations have been published with discordant conclusions as regards the causality of these mutations; additional work on larger series of patients and familial segregation analysis of these mutations with the affected phenotype are needed to conclude. Interestingly, several patients with a childhood onset of stroke and homozygous nonsense NOTCH3 mutations have been reported [10].

CADASIL population prevalence was previously estimated in the UK, based on epidemiological data, as being close to 2 per 100,000 [11]. However, Rutten et al. showed recently that the prevalence of NOTCH3 typical CADASIL mutations reached 1 per 300 in the 60,706 individuals from the Exome Aggregation Consortium (ExAC) control database [12]. A follow-up study by the same authors strongly suggested that CADASIL-type mutations located within the 7–34 EGR receptor motifs might lead to a milder phenotype [13]. It would be very important for clinical care and genetic counseling to characterize the individual penetrance and expressivity of the various mutations located in these 7–34 EGFR mutations. Indeed, R1231C and R544C represent 75% of the mutations identified in the ExAC control database and R1231C is also the most frequent CADASIL-type mutation identified in the UK biobank [14]. These data strongly suggest that a few typical CADASIL mutations, such as R1231C, might have a very low penetrance or are associated with a much later age of onset. These data would be of importance for medicine precision, genetic counseling, and inclusion criteria in future clinical trials.

4.4 CARASIL- and HTRA1-Associated CSVD

4.4.1 CARASIL

Cerebral autosomal recessive arteriopathy with subcortical infarcts and leukoencephalopathy is a very rare and severe autosomal recessive cerebral vasculopathy initially described in Japan [15]. Neurological, clinical, and MRI manifestations are quite similar to the ones observed in CADASIL (Fig. 4.1, panels c, d). However, several features should lead to suspecting of this disorder, namely the earlier age at the onset of neurological manifestations (30–40 years), the specific association with an early-onset alopecia, a spondylosis deformans and consanguinity, when present [16]. Initially, parents of affected individuals were reported to be asymptomatic and, in some families. CARASIL gene identification in 2009 by Hara et al. provided a biological marker of this disease, allowing its identification not only in Japan but also in China and various European countries [17]. The gene encodes for the high temperature requirement A (HTRA1) serine peptidase 1. Both alleles are mutated in CARASIL patients, either in a homozygous or in a compound heterozygous state. CARASIL mutations lead to a complete or almost complete loss of function of this homo-trimeric enzyme and it has been suggested that they cause a TGF-beta pathway deregulation but the precise pathophysiological mechanisms of this disease are largely unknown [17]. Although this disease is very rare in Caucasians, it might be underdiagnosed if a systematic search for extraneurological manifestations is not performed. A NGS targeted sequencing of all known CSVD genes when suspecting a monogenic cause will avoid missing these rare cases.

4.4.2 Autosomal Dominant CSVD Associated with HTRA1 Heterozygous Mutations

In addition to biallelic loss-of-function variants causing CARASIL, heterozygous missense HTRA1 variants have been reported to cause an autosomal CSVD [18]. This CSVD is milder than CARASIL, with a much later age of onset (around 60 years). In most cases it is not associated with extraneurological manifestations and has a dominant pattern of inheritance. Its clinical phenotype is quite similar to sporadic CSVD with the exception of the familial nature of this CSVD [18, 19]. Its

MRI phenotype is similar to CADASIL or CARASIL (Fig. 4.1, panels e, f). The prevalence of this dominant disease is much higher than CARASIL. Indeed, 2–5% of patients screened for a familial cerebral vascular leukoencephalopathy harbor a rare variant predicted to be pathogenic by in silico pathogenicity prediction tools [18, 19].

However, not all rare HTRA1 variants predicted to be pathogenic are causative and the analysis of the functional consequences of any new rare variant is requested before stating that this variant is causative. In addition to loss of protease activity, Nozaki et al. have shown that pathogenic variants exert a dominant negative effect on the HTRA1 trimer [19]. Some of them are not able to form trimers and others, although they form trimers, affect trimer-associated HTRA1 activation. Altogether, these data and molecular data from CARASIL patients' analysis strongly suggest that the severity and pattern of inheritance of HTRA1-associated diseases depend upon the level of HTRA1 residual activity (null in CARASIL patients, lower than normal but not null in heterozygous patients). A recent review of the literature summarizes functional data obtained for various heterozygous missense HTRA1 variants [20]. Collaborative additional work is needed to pursue the functional characterization of all candidate rare HTRA1 variants identified all over the world to establish their causality or absence of causality. These data are requested to avoid false-positive diagnosis.

4.5 COL41/COL4A2-Associated CSVD

4.5.1 CSVD Associated with Glycine and Stop Codon Mutations

COL4A1 and COL4A2 encode the alpha 1 and alpha 2 chains of type IV collagen, the major basement component in all tissues, including blood vessels. Type IV collagen is composed of two alpha 1 chains and one alpha 2 chain which form a heterotrimer with three domains, the amino-terminal region (7S), the carboxy-terminal noncollagenous domain (NC1), and the triple-helix region composed of glycine-X-Y repeats. The association of COL4A1 mutations with cerebral hemorrhage and porencephaly was first reported in mouse and man by Gould et al. [21]. The causative role of missense mutations affecting glycine residues within the triple helix of type IV collagen, and to a lesser degree of stop codons, was later on reported in a number of patients with various phenotypes [22, 23]. Any age can be affected from fetal life to adulthood with a highly variable expressivity (Fig. 4.2, panels a–c). In adult patients, mean age at stroke onset is 30–40 years. Deep intracerebral hemorrhage is at least twice more frequent than lacunar infarcts and can be promoted by physical efforts and anticoagulant therapy. In addition to cerebral hemorrhage, lacunar infarcts and microbleeds, porencephaly, and/or schizencephaly, neuroimaging shows subcortical white matter hypersignals and in some patients intracranial aneurysms (Fig. 4.2, panels d–h). Highly suggestive extraneurological manifestations can be observed in some adult patients including retinal arterial tortuosities and eye anterior segment dysgenesis, renal cysts, and muscle cramps (Fig. 4.2, panels i, j). These extraneurological manifestations, although inconstant, are highly suggestive

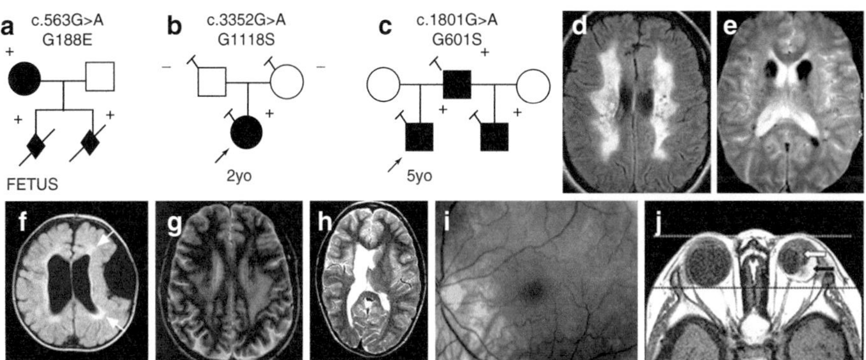

Fig. 4.2 CSVD associated with COL4A1/COL4A2 glycine mutations. Panels **a–c**: Genealogical trees of three mutated families showing the high variability in age at onset (**a–c**) from fetal life to adulthood and the de novo occurrence of some mutations (**b**). Panels **d, e**: Axial FLAIR and T2* MRI images of a 35-year-old mutated patient. Panels **f–h**: Schizencephaly in a 2-year-old patient (**f**). Confluent white matter hypersignals in a 32-year-old mutated patient (**g**). Porencephaly in a 25-year-old mutated patient (**h**). Panels **i, j**: Retinal arterial tortuosities in a 35-year-old mutated patient (**i**). Microphthalmy (**j**)

of type IV collagen mutations. Intracerebral hemorrhage can also occur during fetal and neonatal life and childhood, leading to porencephaly. Mutated children can present infantile hemiparesis, epileptic seizures, developmental delay, and microcephaly [23, 24]. The penetrance of this disease and its expressivity are highly variable even within a family.

NGS screening of genomic DNA is highly specific when it shows either a glycine missense mutation within one of the Gly-X-Y motifs of the triple helix or a stop codon. Additional screening may be needed, including analysis of the cDNA obtained by reverse transcription of mRNA extracted from skin fibroblasts to characterize the splicing effect of some mutations and quantitative techniques to search for deletions.

Missense mutations located in the NC1 domain can also be causative but their interpretation is less straightforward unless they occurred de novo.

Genetic counseling is of major importance in this condition. Presymptomatic screening and prenatal diagnosis should be offered despite the variable expressivity of this disorder and its incomplete penetrance with regard to the existence of preventive measures and the extreme severity observed in some fetuses and children. No specific treatment is yet available but, thanks to the development and the analysis of several COL4A1/COL4A2 mouse models, progress has been made in the understanding of the pathophysiological mechanisms of this disease [25, 26].

4.5.2 PADMAL

PADMAL (pontine autosomal dominant microangiopathy and leukoencephalopathy) is the acronym coined by Ding et al. in 2010 to designate an autosomal

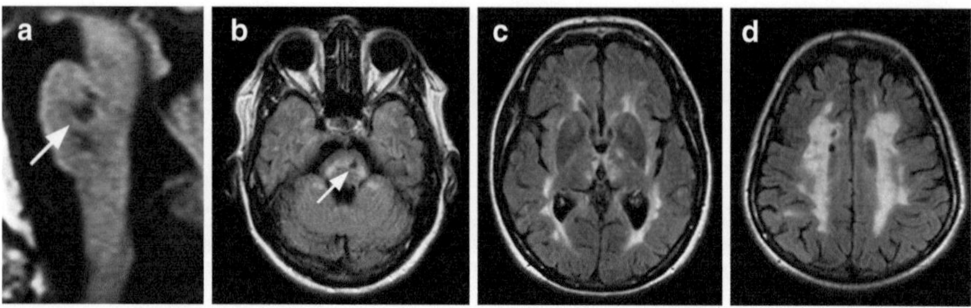

Fig. 4.3 PADMAL. (**a, b**) Sagittal and axial images showing pons infarcts (arrows) in a 54-year-old PADMAL patient. (**c, d**) Axial FLAIR images showing white matter hypersignals highly suggestive of a CSVD vascular encephalopathy in the same patient as in (**a, b**)

dominant CSVD characterized by the high occurrence of pontine infarcts in all affected members of a very large German family [27]. Verdura et al. showed that the CSVD observed in this family and several additional families showing the same clinical and MRI features (Fig. 4.3, panels a–d) was caused by point mutations located in the 3′ untranslated region (3′UTR) of COL4A1 [28]. These mutations, located within a seven-base-pair region within the COL4A1 3′ untranslated region, prevent the binding of the microRNA miR29, leading to an upregulation of COL4A1 mRNA. PADMAL's clinical features are similar to those of CADASIL with an earlier age at onset (35–45 years). Neither overt clinical cerebral hemorrhage nor extra-neurological manifestations have been observed in these patients in contrast with patients harboring COL4A1/A2 glycine mutations. Another major difference is the absence of manifestation in fetuses and children. In addition to these clinical differences, the functional consequences of PADMAL and glycine or stop codon mutations are completely different; the first ones lead to an upregulation of COL4A1 and the latter most likely to a haploinsufficiency.

Interestingly, a duplication of COL4A1/COL42 has also been associated with an adult-onset ischemic vascular leukoencephalopathy, strongly suggesting that copy-number anomalies of these genes are causative and should be searched for [29].

4.6 CARASAL

CARASAL (cathepsin A-related arteriopathy with stroke and leukoencephalopathy) is the acronym coined by Bugiani et al. to designate a very rare autosomal dominant CSVD associated with a so far unique mutation (R325C) within the serine carboxypeptidase encoded by the CTSA gene [30]. To our knowledge only 4 families segregating this mutation have been identified, including 2 Dutch families (13 affected members), 1 French family (5 clinically affected members and 9 adult asymptomatic carriers), and 1 affected case from the UK [29–32]. Hypertension, ischemic stroke, and cerebral hemorrhage have been observed repeatedly in Dutch patients, in association with a diffuse leukoencephalopathy. In contrast, a paucity

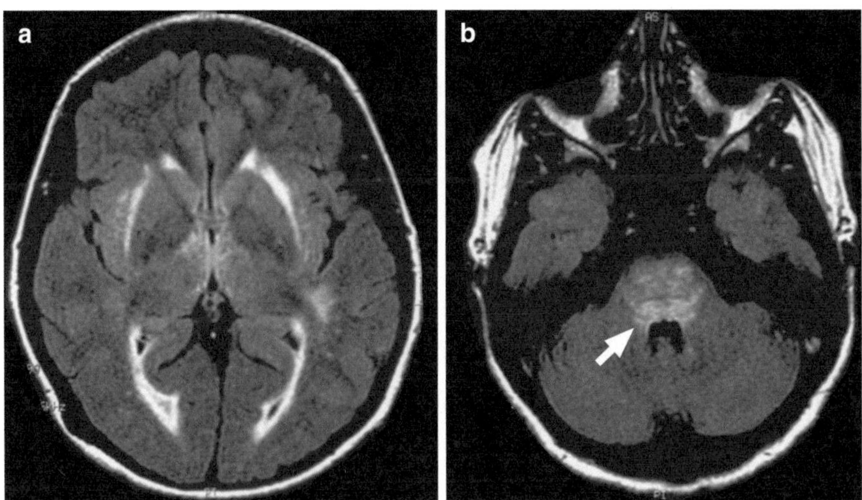

Fig. 4.4 CARASAL. (**a**) Axial FLAIR image: vascular leukoencephalopathy in a 43-year-old CARASAL patient. (**b**) Axial FLAIR image: diffuse white matter signals in the pons in the same patient

of clinical symptoms associated with an extended and highly stereotyped leukoencephalopathy is the hallmark of the phenotype observed in the French pedigree (Fig. 4.4, panels a, b). Characterization of additional families will help to delineate CTSA-associated phenotypes.

How this peculiar R325C mutation leads to a CSVD is so far unknown. Biallelic loss-of-function mutations of CTSA lead to beta-galactosialidosis, an unrelated autosomal recessive disease (OMIM 256540). However, preliminary data suggest that endothelin 1 might be involved [29].

4.7 RVCL

RVCL (retinal vasculopathy with cerebral leukoencephalopathy) is the acronym now used to designate an autosomal dominant disease previously reported under different names, cerebroretinal vasculopathy, and hereditary endotheliopathy, retinopathy, nephropathy, and stroke (HERNS). All these conditions were shown in 2007 to be caused by truncating mutations affecting the same gene (TREX1) and located in the C-terminal part of the gene [33]. Stam et al. provided a highly valuable clinicopathological and genetic characterization of this very rare disease in 11 unrelated families [34]. The two main clinical features of this microangiopathy are retinal and cerebral features but additional systemic manifestations are observed. Age at onset is around 40 years. Stroke is not a main feature of this microangiopathy which is characterized by the association of focal neurological deficits, seizures, headache, progressive cognitive impairment and/or psychiatric disturbances, and a vascular retinopathy. The association of these neurological features with a vascular retinopathy should lead to suspecting of this diagnosis. Neuroimaging is highly suggestive when there are contrast-enhancing lesions associated with edema and mass effect. White matter hypersignals sparing the gray matter as well as focal, often punctate calcifications are present. The retinal microangiopathy affects almost all patients and leads to visual impairment; fundoscopy and fluorescein angiography show various lesions including capillary obliterations, telangiectasias, and microaneurysms [33].

Despite the growing knowledge regarding the role of this exonuclease in the innate immunity pathway, the pathophysiology of this condition is still unclear and there is currently no evidence of efficacy of either antiplatelet or immunosuppressive therapy.

However, molecular screening is essential to avoid misdiagnosis such as brain tumor or vasculitis, unnecessary brain biopsies, and inadequate treatments. In addition it is needed to fully characterize this very rare and possibly underdiagnosed condition.

4.8 Perspectives

Next-generation sequencing technologies and availability of large size control databases have been instrumental for the recent identification of the genes involved in CARASAL, PADMAL, RVCL, or the autosomal dominant HTRA1-associated CSVD. Several lessons can be drawn from these data. The first one is the extreme genetic heterogeneity of CSVD. With the exception of CADASIL- and HTRA1-dominant CSVD, most of these "novel" diseases are very rare. A strong effort will therefore be needed to fully decipher the molecular basis of monogenic CSVD. Indeed, sequencing of all known CSVD genes identifies the causative gene/mutation in only 20% of patients referred for a familial CSVD (personal data) with CADASIL accounting for 10% of these patients and autosomal dominant CSVD associated with HTRA1 mutations for 2–5% of these patients.

The second one is the tremendous progress in the understanding of the pathophysiological mechanisms of CADASIL, the archetypal CSVD. Biochemical analysis of postmortem brain samples from patients and tissues from transgenic mouse models provided evidence for the mechanistic links between mutations and small vessel dysfunction and pathological alterations. Preclinical trials using NOTCH3-specific antibodies or antisense oligonucleotides are ongoing in mouse models. Although translating preclinical data into clinical trials is often challenging, it is time to prepare cohorts of patients for future clinical trials. Ongoing analysis of animal models and pathophysiological investigation of other CSVD, particularly COL4A1/COL4A2- and HTRA1-associated CSVD, have also started to provide clues towards their mechanisms, generating hope for the future.

References

1. Tan RYY, Markus HS. Monogenic causes of stroke: now and the future. J Neurol. 2015;262:2601–16.
2. Mancuso M, Arnold M, Bersano A, Burlina A, Chabriat H, Debette S, Enzinger C, Federico A, Filla A, Finsterer J, Hunt D, Lesnik Oberstein S, Tournier-Lasserve E, Markus HS. Monogenic cerebral small vessel diseases: diagnosis and therapy. Consensus Recommendations of the European Academy of Neurology. Eur J Neurol. 2020;27(6):909–27.
3. Labauge P, Denier C, Bergametti F, Tournier-Lasserve E. Genetics of cavernous angiomas. Lancet Neurol. 2007;6:237–44.
4. Joutel A, Faraci FM. Cerebral small vessel disease: insights and opportunities from mouse models of collagen IV-related small vessel disease and cerebral autosomal dominant arteriopathy with subcortical infarcts. Stroke. 2014;45(4):1215–21.
5. Seyfried SA, Tournier-Lasserve E, Derry WB. Blocking signalopathic events to treat cerebral cavernous malformations. Trends Mol Med. 2020;26(9):874–87.
6. Zeng X, Hunt A, Jin SC, Duran D, Gaillard J, Kahle KT. EphrinB2-EphB4-RASA1 signaling in human cerebrovascular development and disease. Trends Mol Med. 2019;25(4):265–86.
7. Joutel A, Corpechot C, Ducros A, Vahedi K, Chabriat H, Mouton P, et al. Notch3 mutations in CADASIL, a hereditary adult-onset condition causing stroke and dementia. Nature. 1996;383:707–10.
8. Chabriat H, Joutel A, Tournier-Lasserve E, Bousser MG. CADASIL yesterday, today and tomorrow. Eur J Neurol. 2020;27:1588–95.
9. Chabriat H, Joutel A, Dichgans M, Tournier-Lasserve E, Bousser MG. CADASIL. Lancet Neurol. 2009;8:643–53.
10. Pipucci T, Maresca A, Magini P, et al. Homozygous NOTCH3 null mutation and impaired NOTCH3 signaling in recessive early-onset arteriopathy and cavitating leukoencephalopathy. EMBO Mol Med. 2015;7:849–57.
11. Narayan SK, Gorman G, Kalaria RN, Ford GA, Chinnery PF. The minimum prevalence of CADASIL in northeast England. Neurology. 2012;78:1025–7.
12. Rutten JW, Dauwerse HG, Gravesteijn G, et al. Archetypal Notch3 mutations frequent in public exome: implications for CADASIL. Ann Clin Transl Neurol. 2016;3:844–53.
13. Rutten JW, Van Eijsden BJ, Duering M, Jouvent E, Opherk C, Pantoni L, et al. The effect of NOTCH3 pathogenic variant position on CADASIL disease severity: NOTCH3 EGFr 1–6 pathogenic variant are associated with a more severe phenotype and lower survival compared with EGFr 7–34 pathogenic variant. Genet Med. 2019;21:676–82.
14. Rutten JW, Hack RJ, Duering M, Gravesteijn G, Dauwerse JG, et al. Broad phenotype of cysteine-altering Notch3 variants in UK biobank: CADASIL to non penetrance. Neurology. 2020;95:1835–43.
15. Maeda S, Nakayama H, Isaka H, Aihara Y, Nemoto S. Familial unusual encephalopathy of Binswanger's type without hypertension. Folia Psychiatr Neurol Jpn. 1976;30:165–77.
16. Nozaki H, Nishizawa M, Onodera O. Features of cerebral autosomal recessive arteriopathy with subcortical infarcts and leukoencephalopathy. Stroke. 2014;45(11):3447–53.
17. Hara K, Shiga A, Fukutake T, Nozaki H, Miyashita A, Yokoseki A, et al. Association of HTRA1 mutations and familial ischemic cerebral small-vessel disease. N Engl J Med. 2009;360:1729–39.
18. Verdura E, Hervé D, Scharrer E, Amador MDM, Guyant-Maréchal L, Philippi A, et al. Heterozygous HTRA1 mutations are associated with autosomal dominant cerebral small vessel disease. Brain. 2015;138:2347–58.
19. Nozaki H, Kato T, Nihonmatsu M, Saito Y, Mizuta I, Noda T, et al. Distinct molecular mechanisms of HTRA1 mutants in manifesting heterozygotes with CARASIL. Neurology. 2016;86:1964–74.

20. Uemura M, Nozaki H, Kato T, et al. HTRA1 related cerebral small vessel disease: a review of the literature. Front Neurol. 2020;11:545.
21. Gould DB, Phalan FC, van Mil SE, Sundberg JP, Vahedi K, Massin P, et al. Role of COL4A1 in small-vessel disease and hemorrhagic stroke. N Engl J Med. 2006;354:1489–96.
22. Zagaglia S, Selch C, Nisevic JR, Mei D, Michalak Z, Hernandez-Hernandez L, et al. Neurologic phenotypes associated with COL4A1/2 mutations: expanding the spectrum of disease. Neurology. 2018;91(22):e2078–88.
23. Plaisier E, Gribouval O, Alamowitch S, Mougenot B, Prost C, Verpont MC, et al. COL4A1 mutations and hereditary angiopathy, nephropathy, aneurysms, and muscle cramps. N Engl J Med. 2007;357:2687–95.
24. Yoneda Y, Haginoya K, Kato M, et al. Phenotypic spectrum of COL4A1 mutations: porencephaly to schizencephaly. Ann Neurol. 2013;73:48–57.
25. Mao M, Alavi MV, Labelle-Dumais C, Gould DB. Type IV collagens and basement membrane diseases: cell biology and pathogenic mechanisms. Curr Top Membr. 2015;76:61–116.
26. Ratelade J, Klug NR, Lombardi D, et al. Reducing hypermuscularization of the transitional segment between arterioles and capillaries protects against spontaneous cerebral hemorrhage. Circulation. 2020;141:2078–94.
27. Ding XQ, Hagel C, Ringelstein EB, Buchheit S, Zeumer H, Kuhlenbäumer G, et al. MRI features of pontine autosomal dominant microangiopathy and leukoencephalopathy (PADMAL). J Neuroimaging. 2010;20:134–40.
28. Verdura E, Hervé D, Bergametti F, Jacquet C, Morvan T, Prieto-Morin C, et al. Disruption of a miR-29 binding site leading to COL4A1 upregulation causes PADMAL. Ann Neurol. 2016;80:741–53.
29. Renard D, Mine M, Pipiras E, Labauge P, Delahaye A, Benzacken B, Tournier-Lasserve E. Cerebral small-vessel disease associated with COL4A1 and COL4A2 duplications. Neurology. 2014;83(11):1029–31.
30. Bugiani M, Kevelam SH, Bakels HS, Waisfisz Q, Ceuterick-De Groote C, Niessen HWM, et al. Cathepsin A-related arteriopathy with strokes and leukoencephalopathy (CARASAL). Neurology. 2016;87:1777–86.
31. Herve D, Chabriat H, Rigal M, Dalloz M-A, Kawkabani Marchini A, De Lepeleire J, et al. A novel hereditary extensive vascular leukoencephalopathy mapping to chromosome 20q13. Neurology. 2012;79:2283–7.
32. Lynch DS, Rodrigues Brandão De Paiva A, Zhang WJ, Bugiardini E, Freua F, Tavares Lucato L, et al. Clinical and genetic characterization of leukoencephalopathies in adults. Brain. 2017;140:1204–11.
33. Richards A, Van Den Maagdenberg AMJM, Jen JC, Kavanagh D, Bertram P, Spitzer D, et al. C-terminal truncations in human 3′-5′ DNA exonuclease TREX1 cause autosomal dominant retinal vasculopathy with cerebral leukodystrophy. Nat Genet. 2007;39:1068–70.
34. Stam AH, Kothari PH, Shaikh A, Gschwendter A, Jen JC, Hodgkinson S, et al. Retinal vasculopathy with cerebral leukoencephalopathy and systemic manifestations. Brain. 2016;139:2909–22.

Pharmacodynamics and Pharmacokinetics of Stroke Therapy

5

Miguel Leal Rato, Maria José Diógenes, and Ana Sebastião

5.1 Introduction

Stroke is an umbrella designation for the acute clinical presentation of a rather heterogeneous group of cerebrovascular disorders. Among them, atherosclerotic large vessel occlusion, cardioembolic disease, and small vessel disease due to long-standing hypertension or vasculitis are examples of some of the vast diversity of causes that underlie stroke. There are two main mechanisms of cerebrovascular damage to the brain: ischemia (encompassing thrombosis, embolism, and decreased perfusion) and hemorrhage. From the diversity of causes of stroke and of the consequences for the brain tissue, one can quickly derive that there cannot be a single, common approach to stroke therapy.

Each therapeutic decision has to be tailored to either the need for emergent medical treatment (such as hypertensive emergencies in acute stroke), the setting and timing of evaluation (acute therapy assumes most strokes as similar), or the presumed mechanism of stroke (e.g., anticoagulation as secondary prevention in a patient with atrial fibrillation).

M. Leal Rato
Neurology, Department of Neurosciences and Mental Health, Hospital Santa Maria, Centro Hospitalar Universitário Lisboa Norte, Lisbon, Portugal

Instituto de Farmacologia e Neurociências, Faculdade de Medicina, Universidade de Lisboa, Lisbon, Portugal
e-mail: mlrato@medicina.ulisboa.pt

M. J. Diógenes (✉) · A. Sebastião
Instituto de Farmacologia e Neurociências, Faculdade de Medicina, Universidade de Lisboa, Lisbon, Portugal

Instituto de Medicina Molecular João Lobo Antunes, Faculdade de Medicina, Universidade de Lisboa, Lisbon, Portugal
e-mail: diogenes@medicina.ulisboa.pt; anaseb@medicina.ulisboa.pt

© Springer Nature Switzerland AG 2021
A. C. Fonseca, J. M. Ferro (eds.), *Precision Medicine in Stroke*,
https://doi.org/10.1007/978-3-030-70761-3_5

As our knowledge of stroke grows, so grows the need for more precise strategies to treat and prevent each cause. Familiarity with the pharmacodynamics and pharmacokinetics of drugs used in stroke care is therefore essential for a tailored approach to each patient. Importantly, genetic diversity and variants can also affect drug pharmacokinetics, pharmacodynamics, and clinical efficacy, establishing a rationale for the need of better knowledge in stroke pharmacogenetics.

In this chapter, we briefly review key concepts in stroke therapy and then focus on the main pharmacokinetic and pharmacodynamic aspects of commonly used drugs. In addition, we address highlights on the key concepts in precision medicine and pharmacogenetics, wherever clinically relevant.

5.2 General Principles of Stroke Therapy

Ischemic and hemorrhagic stroke therapy can be broadly divided into (hyper)acute stroke therapy and secondary preventive therapy.

In acute ischemic stroke therapy, the imperative that "time is brain" guides the approach, along with strategies to optimize collateral flow and avoid secondary brain injury [1–3]. Clinical decisions and algorithms aim to quickly identify patients with acute ischemic stroke that might benefit from thrombolytic and other acute reperfusion therapies (including non-pharmacological therapies such as mechanical thrombectomy) [1]. Acute hemorrhagic stroke has a less directed approach and the strategy is mainly supportive. Antiplatelet therapy is the default antithrombotic approach for secondary ischemic stroke prevention of most stroke etiologies, with the exception of cardioembolic stroke (e.g. atrial fibrillation) in which anticoagulation is usually indicated [1, 4, 5]. Comorbidities should also be aggressively assessed and addressed, and holistic strategies include antihypertensive therapy, cholesterol-lowering therapy, and glycemic control, among others. A summary of the pharmacological targets for stroke therapy is depicted in Fig. 5.1.

5.3 Pharmacological Acute Stroke Therapy

Intravenous (IV) thrombolysis changed stroke care from a slow-paced investigation-driven approach to an aggressive and prompt fight for acute therapy delivery. There is incontrovertible evidence that reperfusion therapies improve global and neurological outcomes in stroke patients [6–8]. The prototype drugs are fibrinolytic agents, the only ones approved for this effect, when administered up to 4.5 h from stroke symptom onset [1]. Importantly, the therapeutic window of opportunity is quickly expanding and with the help of advanced imaging techniques more and more patients, including patients with unclear time of onset, will benefit from IV thrombolytics [9–11].

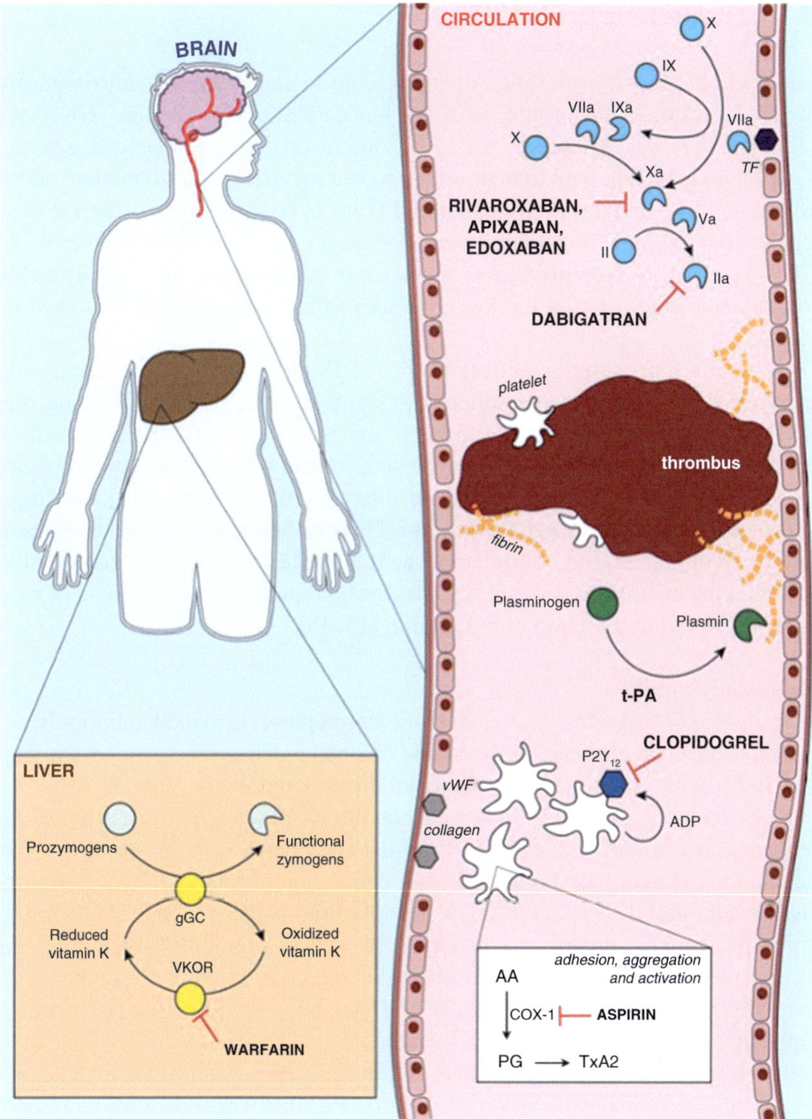

Fig. 5.1 Summary of the pharmacological targets in stroke. Stroke is a multisystemic disease with a preferential cerebrovascular presentation. Pharmacological treatment and prevention of stroke include strategies modulating aggregation and platelet function, coagulation factor synthesis in the liver, and coagulation factor activity in circulation. Other therapies (not shown in this figure) aim to control risk factors and comorbidities and include antihypertensive drugs, cholesterol-lowering drugs, primary thromboprophylaxis in the subacute setting, and glycemic control with antidiabetics in diabetic patients. Neuroprotective strategies have not yet been proven effective in a clinical setting. Abbreviations: *AA* arachidonic acid, *ADP* adenosine diphosphate, *COX-1* cyclooxygenase-1, *gGC* gamma-glutamyl carboxylase, *PG* prostaglandins, *TF* tissue factor, *t-PA* tissue plasminogen activator, *TxA₂* thromboxane A2, *VKOR* vitamin K epoxide reductase, *vWF* von Willebrand factor; coagulation factors are identified by their respective Roman numeral (II, V, VII, VIII, IX, X), and activated factors are marked with an "a" after the Roman numeral (e.g., IIa)

5.3.1 Fibrinolytic Drugs

Fibrinolytic drugs with relevance in stroke care include recombinant tissue plasminogen activator (rt-PA or alteplase) and tenecteplase (TNK, or the TNK mutant of alteplase) [1, 12]. Alteplase (rt-PA) is administered intravenously at a dose of 0.9 mg/kg body weight with total dose not exceeding 90 mg. It is given over 60 min, with 10% of dose administered as an initial bolus over 1 min [1, 6]. Lower doses of alteplase (0.6 mg/kg body weight) were evaluated in the ENCHANTED trial. This RCT did not show non-inferiority of low-dose alteplase [1, 13, 14]. Therefore, standard-dose alteplase (0.9 mg/kg) continues to be recommended over low-dose alteplase.

Briefly, the most serious adverse events of IV thrombolytics are hemorrhagic complications including asymptomatic or symptomatic intracranial hemorrhage (sICH) and systemic bleeding. A thorough revision of the eligibility and exclusion criteria for IV thrombolysis is beyond the scope of this chapter, but should be done for each patient based on a detailed and directed clinical history [1]. Orolingual angioedema occurs in between 0.9% and 5.1% of patients, may be life threatening, is typically unilateral and contralateral to the stroke, occurs more commonly in patients taking angiotensin-converting enzyme inhibitors, and is thought to be mediated by rt-PA-induced release of bradykinin [15–18].

Pharmacodynamics

The main goal of these drugs (alteplase and tenecteplase) is to induce fibrinolysis of a thrombus through cleavage of the single-chained inactive precursor plasminogen to plasmin, with consequent intravascular fibrin degradation and dissolution of blood clots (Figs. 5.1 and 5.2). In normal conditions, the serine protease tissue plasminogen activator (t-PA) is released from the endothelial cells in response to specific stimuli and then rapidly cleared from circulation or inhibited by plasminogen activator inhibitor-1 (PAI-1) [19–22]. If plasmin is generated, circulating α_2-antiplasmin rapidly inhibits it, blocking its active site for fibrin degradation. However, when plasmin is linked to fibrin, the domains to which α_2-antiplasmin is bound become occupied, and fibrin-bound plasmin becomes protected from α_2-antiplasmin. This explains the selective nature and increased catalytic action of t-PA to sites where a fibrin-rich thrombus exists [23, 24]. Plasmin is a cofactor of t-PA. Alteplase is the first recombinant t-PA (rt-PA) that was generated, and is identical to native t-PA. Tenecteplase is also a t-PA, developed from modifications of natural human t-PA complementary DNA (cDNA).

Pharmacokinetics

Alteplase (rt-PA): Pharmacokinetic data are mainly derived from acute myocardial infarction studies, and doses differ significantly from the ones used in acute ischemic stroke. In circulation, rt-PA is both free and bound to plasma proteins (including PAI-1, α2-antiplasmin, and α1-antitrypsin). From the systemic circulation, alteplase is eliminated following a two-compartment model and a first-order kinetics, with a rapid initial elimination ($t_{1/2a}$ = 3.3–6 min) and a delayed slower

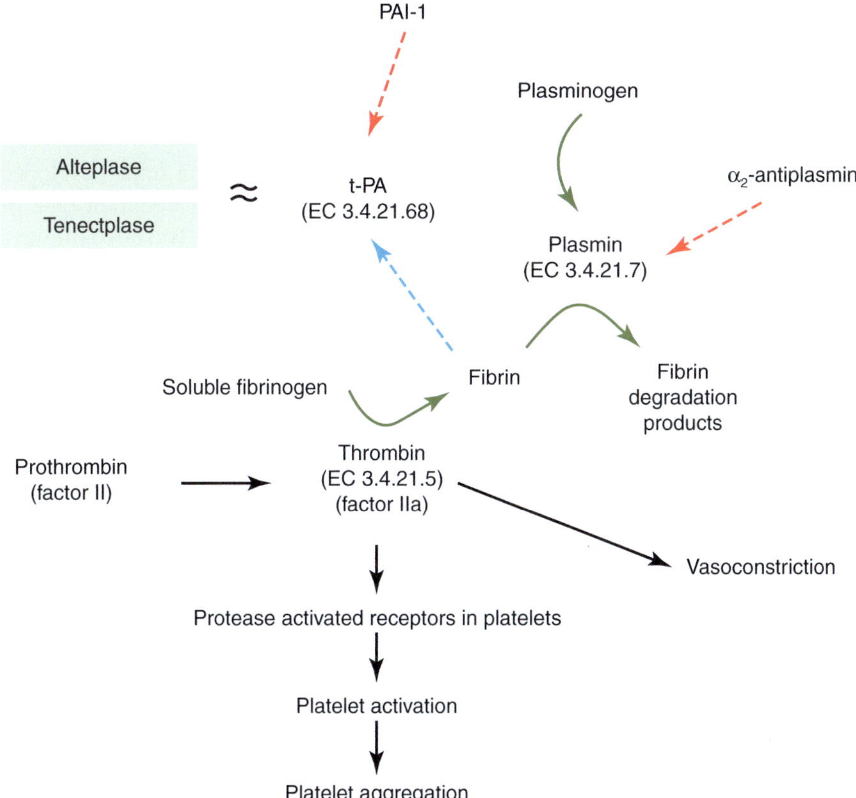

Fig. 5.2 Main pathways involved in the conversion of soluble fibrinogen to fibrin, and target for fibrinolytic drugs. Green arrows indicate enzymatic steps; dashed red arrows indicate inhibition: blue dashed arrow indicates facilitation as a cofactor of enzymatic activity. Black arrows indicate pathways that may involve more than one step. See text for details. Abbreviations: *PAI-1* plasminogen activator inhibitor-1, *t-PA* tissue plasminogen activator

elimination phase ($t_{1/2b}$ = 26–40 min) [23]. The short half-life requires a continuous infusion after bolus in order to achieve steady plasma concentrations and maximal opportunity for early recanalization. Metabolization of alteplase takes place mainly in the liver, through receptor-mediated endocytosis, and deletion of the fibronectin fingerlike and kringle 1 domains explains the reduced clearance and longer half-life of mutant forms of alteplase [23].

Tenecteplase is a mutant form of t-PA that has a longer half-life (biphasic disposition, with an initial half-life of 17–24 min and a terminal half-life of 65–132 min) [25] and hence can be given as a single bolus. It is also slightly more fibrin specific than alteplase. In a subset of stroke patients with documented occlusion of the internal carotid artery or proximal middle cerebral artery, tenecteplase (0.25 mg/kg body weight, as a single bolus, maximum 25 mg) was superior to alteplase (standard dose) [26]. Higher doses of tenecteplase (0.4 mg/kg body weight as a single bolus) had a safety and efficacy profile similar to alteplase in a population composed primarily of patients with minor neurological impairment [27]. As such, guidelines are changing to accommodate another IV thrombolytic in these specific settings [1].

Pharmacogenetics

Precision medicine in the context of IV thrombolysis is still an underdeveloped field. Two single-nucleotide polymorphisms (SNPs)—the most common type of genetic variants—located in the A2M gene (rs669) and F12 gene (rs1801020) were associated with alteplase-related hemorrhagic transformation and in-hospital death, respectively [28, 29]. As for efficacy prediction, SNPs in the IL1B gene (rs1143627 and rs16944) and in the von Willebrand factor (vWF) gene (rs1063856) were associated with early recanalization after thrombolysis [30]. In the field of biomarkers, plasma levels of cellular fibronectin (c-Fn) [31], matrix metalloproteinase-9 (MMP-9) [31], and vascular adhesion protein-1/semicarbazide-sensitive amine oxidase (VAP-1/SSAO) [32] activity may predict parenchymal hematoma after alteplase. Further studies might bring light to why there is a significant clinical interindividual variability in the efficacy and safety of IV fibrinolytics. Whether or not these polymorphisms are relevant once we account for all other hemorrhagic transformation risk factors (such as number and location of microbleeds or white matter disease) is still to be determined.

5.4 Secondary Preventive Therapy

Currently, there are no clinically used drugs that can revert neuronal death caused by infarction. After a stroke, the goal of patient care is twofold: first, directed rehabilitation must be offered and tailored to each patient, including physical therapy, occupational therapy, speech therapy, and dysphagia therapy, among others depending on the neurological sequelae; second, prevention of a recurrence must be carefully planned. Furthermore, as discussed previously, not all patients can be offered acute therapies, for safety reasons. As such, preventive measures and choice of a secondary preventive treatment must be made carefully and with a clear pharmacological goal in mind. Prevention of recurrent stroke is started as soon as the diagnosis is made for patients who did not receive IV thrombolytics, and in cases where hemorrhagic complications did not occur, from 24 h after IV thrombolytics. The choice of a preventive therapy must be revised every time clinical status changes or new information about probable stroke etiology is gathered. Not rarely, patients will start a preventive treatment and then be switched to a more suitable, more tailored one. The default option is antiplatelet therapy, and the more commonly used drugs are aspirin, clopidogrel, or a combination of both. In special cases (mainly cardioembolic strokes), anticoagulants are used, and direct oral anticoagulants are normally preferred unless a contraindication exists, when warfarin or other vitamin K antagonists are used.

5.4.1 Antiplatelet Drugs

Platelets can be conceptualized as anucleated cellular fragments. In sites of vascular lesion such as ruptured atheroma plaques, the initial hemostatic plug is formed by platelets. Platelets are initially activated through the exposure to subendothelial collagen and von Willebrand factor (vWF) (Fig. 5.1), whose primary function is binding to other proteins, in particular factor VIII, being important in platelet adhesion to wound sites [33]. This is followed by a complex cascade that ends in the release of many bioactive substances. Platelets serve as initiators and as a scaffold for coagulation pathways, and have other hemostatic functions such as promotion of local vasoconstriction. Antiplatelet drugs act through a relatively nonspecific pathophysiologic mechanism preventing platelet adhesion, activation, and aggregation, and can be used in stroke, myocardial infarction, or peripheral artery thrombosis prevention, among other disorders. There are several drugs that inhibit platelet function through different mechanisms and thus they can be used in isolation or combined resulting in an additive or even synergistic effect. The two main classes of antiplatelet drugs relevant in stroke care are cyclooxygenase-1 (COX-1) inhibitors (aspirin) and adenosine 5-diphosphate (ADP) receptor antagonists (Fig. 5.1). Their pharmacokinetic, pharmacodynamic, and pharmacogenetic characteristics are determinant of their clinical use. Dipyridamole is also sometimes used. Although glycoprotein IIb/IIIa antagonists play a role during some endovascular treatments, they do not have an established place in stroke prevention and thus will not be revised here.

5.4.1.1 Aspirin

Several studies have demonstrated aspirin's efficacy in ischemic stroke and transient ischemic attack (TIA) [34–37].

Pharmacodynamics

In the platelet, arachidonic acid is converted to prostaglandins and thromboxane A_2 (TxA_2) in a reaction catalyzed by COX-1 (EC1.14.99.1). TxA_2 induces platelet aggregation, is a potent vasoconstrictor, and acts with other platelet-released products (such as fibrinogen, ADP, and factor V) in order to further promote platelet activation. The principal mechanism of action of aspirin (or acetylsalicylic acid) is the irreversible (covalent) acetylation of serine residues in the catalytic subunits of COX-1, blocking its action (Fig. 5.1) [38, 39]. Complete inhibition of platelet COX-1 can be achieved by doses as low as 75 mg a day, and clinical effective antithrombotic doses range from 50 to 325 mg. Considering all this, administration of 50–325 mg of aspirin is recommended in patients with acute ischemic stroke within 24–48 h after onset, or 24 h after IV fibrinolytic treatments [1]. In patients with minor noncardioembolic ischemic stroke who did not receive IV thrombolytics, dual-antiplatelet therapy with aspirin and clopidogrel should be started within 24 h after stroke onset and continued for 21 days [40–42]. Despite playing a role in other inflammatory pathways, aspirin-mediated COX-1 inhibition in these doses has a selective antiplatelet effect for two leading reasons: firstly, platelets are exquisitely sensitive to the action of aspirin, being acetylated in the portal (presystemic) circulation within minutes and even with low aspirin doses, before aspirin is deacetylated by the liver and turned into the platelet-inactive salicylic acid [43]; secondly, at higher doses, endothelial COX blockade inhibits prostacyclin production, and counteracts the beneficial TxA_2 inhibition [44]. Thus, there is a differential clinical effect between a low-dose aspirin (antiplatelet effect) and high-dose aspirin (anti-inflammatory effect, through inhibition of COX-1 and COX-2). The loss of this differential action on the COX isoforms is why concomitant administration of other nonsteroidal anti-inflammatory drugs (NSAIDs), such as the nonselective reversible COX inhibitor ibuprofen, impairs the antiplatelet function of aspirin in a clinically significant way [45, 46]. Because platelets are unable to synthetize new enzymes, aspirin-mediated platelet function inhibition is limited by the turnover of the circulating platelet pool and life span of a platelet, which is around 7–10 days [47].

Pharmacokinetics

Aspirin (acetylsalicylic acid) is rapidly absorbed following oral ingestion, similar to other NSAIDs, with a peak plasma level (Cmax) reached in around 30 min (Tmax). It is extensively bound to plasma proteins (50–90%, mainly albumin), and rapidly eliminated from plasma ($t_{1/2}$ = 15–20 min). It is quickly deacetylated by spontaneous hydrolysis or esterases in the intestinal wall, red blood cells, and liver. Salicylates and their metabolites are then excreted in the urine. Salicylate clearance has a high variability between people, and is lower in women (due to reduced esterase activity and differences in hepatic metabolism) and in the elderly.

Enteric-coated formulations aim to reduce gastrointestinal side effects due to the decrease in prostaglandin-dependent gastric protection induced by COX inhibitors, and result in a delay of 3–4 h of peak plasma levels and a possible lower bioavailability, differences that might be clinically relevant [45, 48, 49]. Despite having a dose-dependent gastrointestinal side, there is no clear benefit of enteric-coated formulations due to its systemic effects [50].

Pharmacogenetics

Aspirin resistance can be defined as laboratory resistance, in which there is a failure to inhibit platelet TxA_2 formation [51–53], or as clinical resistance in which there is a failure to prevent clinical ischemic events, such as stroke [54–56]. The latter is sometimes preferably referred to as aspirin treatment failure [55, 57]. On the one hand, laboratory measures are limited by the lack of a clear cutoff between aspirin resistance and nonresistance and technical limitations. On the other hand, the clinical definition is hindered by its retrospective nature and non-specificity because of the many competing factors for aspirin treatment failure such as poor patient compliance [58, 59], inadequate dose, increased platelet turnover, long-term tachyphylaxis [60, 61], concurrent intake of other NSAIDs, and non-atherothrombotic causes of embolism, among others [55]. A thorough review of each possible cause of stroke recurrence, including aspirin resistance or pseudoresistance, has to be made when dealing with a patient with aspirin treatment failure [55, 57, 62].

Aspirin resistance is most likely multifactorial, and there is a possibly significant genetic influence in at least some patients. Epidemiological data postulates that up to one-third of the variation in laboratory tests assessing response to antiplatelet drugs is genetically determined [63]. Several polymorphisms and even haplotypes involving COX-1 and COX-2 appear to modify the antiplatelet effect of aspirin [64–67]. While some other genes involved in the thrombotic pathways have been implicated (e.g., PlA1/2 variant in the glycoprotein IIIa gene) [68, 69], their role in aspirin resistance of others remains controversial (e.g., the $P2Y_1$ ADP receptor gene) [70–72]. To this date, in spite of all the identified and proposed genes, no test has been adequately validated to predict aspirin resistance, so laboratory platelet function assays remain the only clinical tool to accurately identify resistance.

5.4.1.2 Clopidogrel

Pharmacodynamics

Platelets contain two receptors for ADP, $P2Y_1$ and $P2Y_{12}$. Both receptors are G-protein coupled receptors, and maximal platelet activation requires activation of the two receptors. When activated by ADP, the G_i-coupled $P2Y_{12}$ receptor inhibits adenylyl cyclase, lowering cellular cyclic AMP concentration, which in turn reduces cyclic AMP-dependent inhibition of platelet activation. Blockade of the $P2Y_{12}$ receptor releases its inhibitory action upon platelet activation, therefore resulting in reduced platelet activation, adhesion, and aggregation. $P2Y_{12}$ antagonists include both the prodrug thienopyridines (clopidogrel, prasugrel) that induce an irreversible inactivation of the receptor and the non-thienopyridines (ticagrelor, cangrelor) that do not require metabolic activation and bind reversibly to the receptor [73].

Clopidogrel is the most widely used $P2Y_{12}$ antagonist in stroke (Fig. 5.1). As mentioned above, it is a prodrug that irreversibly inhibits the $P2Y_{12}$ receptor. The other ADP antagonists have not yet been as extensively studied in clinical trials or did not show benefit, and thus are not used outside of very specific situations and certain endovascular procedures. As such, they will not be analyzed here. Recently, a clinical trial evaluated the use of ticagrelor in addition to aspirin in patients with mild-to-moderate acute noncardioembolic ischemic stroke [74]. Despite a reduced risk of a composite outcome of death or stroke recurrence, disability did not differ between groups and severe bleeding was more frequent with ticagrelor and aspirin than with aspirin alone.

Clopidogrel is used in stroke prevention as an alternative to aspirin. Furthermore, as mentioned above, two multicenter placebo-controlled clinical trials have established the efficacy of short-term (21–30 days) dual-antiplatelet therapy to prevent recurrent ischemic stroke in patients with minor stroke or high risk of transient ischemic attack [1, 40–42, 75]. Dual-antiplatelet therapy might also benefit patients with large atherosclerotic stroke and intracranial artery stenosis (during up to 90 days), although which patients really benefit from it and for how long is still a matter of debate [76–78]. Triple-antiplatelet therapy with dipyridamole is offset by a significant increase in hemorrhagic risk [79]. Dipyridamole inhibits platelet aggregation through several mechanisms that converge to increases in intracellular cyclic AMP, and thus to inhibition of platelet aggregation. Among these, the most relevant is its ability to inhibit phosphodiesterases and to inhibit the uptake of adenosine, thus enhancing extracellular levels of adenosine and favoring activation of adenylate cyclase-coupled membrane-located A2 (both A2A and A2B) adenosine receptors present in platelets [80].

Pharmacokinetics

Clopidogrel is rapidly absorbed after oral ingestion. On the luminal surface of the enterocyte, p-glycoprotein (p-gp; encoded by the ABCB1 gene) actively pumps clopidogrel back into the duodenum [81]. Clopidogrel then moves on to the portal circulation and the liver, where it suffers extensive first-pass metabolism (approximately 85%) by liver carboxylesterase-1 (encoded by the CES1 gene). The remaining 5–15% requires a two-step enzymatic activation in the liver: it is first converted to an inactive intermediate, 2-oxo-clopidogrel, and then transformed into the active thiol metabolite R-130964 (clop-AM) [73, 82–85]. Cytochrome P450 (CYP) 2C19 is the major enzyme responsible for the bioactivation of clopidogrel, with other CYPs (including 1A2, 2B6, 2C9, and 3A4/5) playing a less preponderant role [84, 85]. Clopidogrel has a $t_{1/2}$ of 6 h, while its active metabolite clop-AM has a much shorter $t_{1/2} = 30$ min. Both clopidogrel and clop-AM are extensively bound to plasma proteins (98% and 94%, respectively), and excretion occurs via urine and feces in similar proportion [38, 73]. Because it requires activation in the liver and because it binds irreversibly to its target, clopidogrel has both a slow onset (time to peak effect of 2–6 h) and offset of action (5–10 days). After a loading dose of 300 or 600 mg, maximum inhibition of platelet aggregation is reached within approximately 2–6 h, and is higher with the 600 mg loading dose, but not different from the 900 mg dose, suggesting a saturable mechanism [86, 87]. A maintenance dose of 75 mg a day reaches a 50% inhibition of platelet aggregation, although response varies widely across individuals [88]. Body weight, but not age or sex, influences pharmacokinetic parameters of clopidogrel [73].

As a brief note, proton pump inhibitors (PPI, such as omeprazole, lansoprazole, pantoprazole) inhibit CYP2C19 and may reduce conversion to the active metabolite of clopidogrel [89, 90]. Whether this interaction is clinically significant in the real world, is restricted to only omeprazole and not to the whole drug class, or has just an in vitro effect is still controversial, and PPI deprescription in patients with dual-antiplatelet therapy might increase bleeding adverse events [89, 91–95].

Pharmacogenetics

There is a very significant intersubject variability to the commonly used 75 mg maintenance dose of clopidogrel [88, 96], and up to 40% of the population fails to achieve an adequate response, possibly due to insufficient metabolite generation. Genes encoding CYP enzymes are polymorphic, and thus, to a certain degree, each individual has his or her own personal genetically determined profile of response to drugs. More than 33 polymorphisms have been identified in CYP2C19, and the most common in people of European descent (CYP2C19*1) allows extensive metabolism of clopidogrel to clop-AM. Some people carry a CYP2C19 reduced-function allele (CYP2C19*2) that translates into a one-third reduction of plasma exposure to clop-AM. This reduced-function allele is more common in people of Asian origin where it is present in around 30–50% of the population [97–99]. Homozygous *1/*1 carriers have higher blood concentrations of clop-AM than *1/*2 carriers, and residual platelet activity as measured by aggregometry is also decreased [98, 100, 101].

In coronary artery disease, there is a risk odds ratio of 1.96 (95% CI, 1.14–3.37) for recurrent cardiovascular events per CYP2C19*2 allele [102], and gain-of-function variants are associated with a lower risk of cardiovascular events but a higher risk of bleeding [103, 104]. This relationship is also clinically significant in stroke therapy, to the point where pre-specified subgroup analyses found no benefit of clopidogrel plus aspirin in carriers of a CYP2C19 loss-of-function allele who otherwise had indication for dual-antiplatelet therapy [105]. Several studies, including a meta-analysis of 15 studies with patients with stroke or TIA, found that carriers of CYP2C19 loss-of-function alleles (*2, *3, and *8) have a greater risk of stroke and composite vascular events when compared with noncarriers (12.0% vs. 5.8%, RR 1.92, 95% CI 1.57–2.35, $p < 0.001$) [106–109]. Patients carrying two loss-of-function alleles have a greater risk of ischemic events compared with patients with only one [107]. In response to this growing body of evidence, the FDA has issued a black-box warning on clopidogrel describing reduced effectiveness in poor metabolizers and recommending CYP2C19 testing as a complement to clinical management [1, 97, 110]. Therefore, stroke patients on clopidogrel monotherapy could potentially benefit from the knowledge of CYP2C19 genotype, as presence of the CYP2C19*2 allele could justify retrial of aspirin or a switch to another antiplatelet drug [110].

Polymorphisms in other genes have also been associated with variability of response to clopidogrel, including polymorphisms in CES1 [111, 112], ABCB1 [81, 113, 114], and $P2Y_{12}$ receptor gene [115]. The relationship between these variants is not as clear and strong, sometimes even contradictory, as with CYP2C19 loss-of-function polymorphisms.

5.4.2 Anticoagulant Drugs

Hemostasis depends on platelet activation and aggregation and on blood coagulation. The human coagulation pathways are complex networks of sequential enzyme activations that, once activated, self-perpetuate through a system of positive feedback. There is also a significant interplay with platelets that provide a surface on which clotting factors assemble and release stored coagulation factors and other bioactive substances. The end result of the coagulation cascade is a surge of prothrombin (coagulation factor II) and then thrombin (EC 3.4.21.5; coagulation factor IIa) that converts soluble fibrinogen into fibrin strands (Fig. 5.2), activates platelets, and has a positive feedback on more thrombin generation besides having strong vasoconstrictor activity. Hence, after the first hemostatic plug which is composed essentially of activated platelets that were exposed to subendothelial molecules, the coagulation system begins a cascade of events that culminate on the conversion of

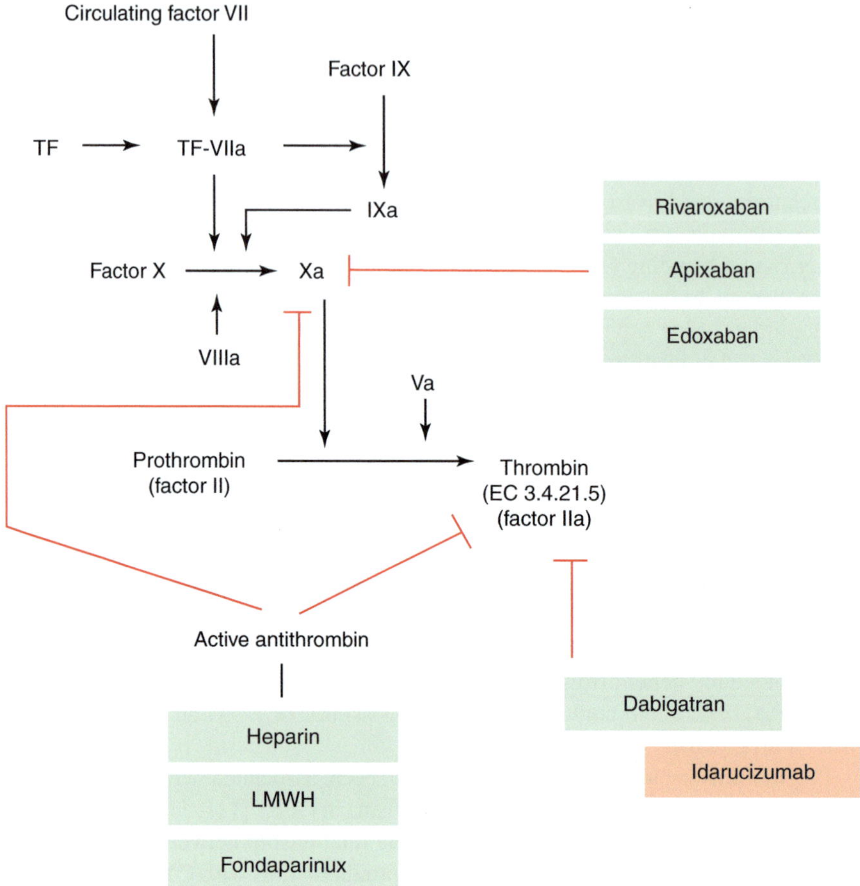

Fig. 5.3 Schematic representation of the mechanism of action of the main anticoagulant drugs (green rectangles) and of an antidote (red rectangle); red traces indicate pathway inhibition. See text for details. Abbreviations: *LMWH* low-molecular-weight heparins, *TF* tissue factor. Coagulation factors are identified by their respective Roman numeral and activated factors are marked with an "a" after the Roman numeral

fibrinogen to a stable clot of cross-linked fibrin and platelet aggregates. Classically, there are two pathways in the coagulation system. The extrinsic pathway is initiated through exposure of tissue factor (TF) when there is damage to the vessel wall. Circulating factor VIIa binds TF and the TF-factor VIIa complex activates factors X and IX (Fig. 5.3). The intrinsic pathway on the other hand is initiated in vivo when factor XII is activated to factor XIIa upon exposure to foreign devices (e.g., mechanical heart valves), cell-free DNA, neutrophil extracellular traps, or other platelet-released products. Factor XIIa then creates a sequential activation of factors XI, IX, and X (in a reaction accelerated by factors VIIIa and Ca^{2+}). Both pathways end in the activation of prothrombin (factor II) into thrombin (factor IIa) through factor

Xa-mediated cleavage of two peptide bonds on prothrombin, in the presence of Ca^{2+} and factor Va (Fig. 5.2). In reality, in vivo reactions are much more interconnected, and, in most instances, distinction between the two systems becomes more a matter of conceptual theoretical organization (Fig. 5.1).

Oral anticoagulants can be broadly divided into two major categories: vitamin K antagonists (VKAs, e.g., warfarin, acenocoumarol) and direct (formerly known as "new" or "novel") oral anticoagulants (dOACs: dabigatran, rivaroxaban, apixaban, and edoxaban). Vitamin K is involved in the carboxylation of glutamate residues in certain proteins to form gamma-carboxyglutamate (Gla) residues. Gla residues bind calcium, and are essential for the biological activity of the so-called Gla proteins. Prothrombin (factor II) and factors VII, IX, and X possess Gla residues essential for their function, hence the critical role of vitamin K in coagulation. dOACs can be further divided into direct oral thrombin inhibitors (dabigatran) or direct oral factor Xa inhibitors (rivaroxaban, apixaban, edoxaban). Other anticoagulants like the parenteral heparin, low-molecular-weight heparins, and fondaparinux act by binding to inactive antithrombin, activating it, and therefore accelerating the rate of antithrombin-mediated inhibition of various coagulation factors and enzymes as factor Xa and thrombin (Fig. 5.3). These drugs also have a place in stroke therapy, namely as thromboprophylaxis, bridging therapies, or alternatives to the oral anticoagulants.

Anticoagulants have no established use in acute stroke therapy, and they are reserved for secondary stroke prevention. They are used in patients in specific settings, namely cardioembolic causes (e.g., atrial fibrillation, prosthetic valves) or prothrombotic states (e.g., antiphospholipid syndrome). The main drawback is the risk of hemorrhagic adverse events and, particularly in stroke, the risk of hemorrhagic transformation of ischemic stroke and of symptomatic or asymptomatic intracranial hemorrhage. There is no clear consensus on when to start long-term anticoagulation therapy after an acute stroke, and evidence is scarce and errs on the side of waiting too long (especially in high-risk situations such as mechanical aorto-mitral heart valves). Depending on the size of stroke and on the baseline risk of recurrence, one can start anticoagulation between 24 h (e.g., TIAs) and 2 weeks after stroke. dOACs are usually withheld for 48 h due to the more rapid onset of anticoagulation effect [1, 116–119].

We will focus our discussion on the oral anticoagulant alternatives, as they are the most widely used long-term options in secondary prevention of stroke.

5.4.2.1 Vitamin K Antagonists
Pharmacodynamics
As briefly mentioned above, vitamin K is essential for the synthesis of the vitamin K-dependent plasma coagulation factors II, VII, IX, and X and proteins C and S. These factors become biologically activated once their glutamic acid (Glu) residues are γ-carboxylated to form the active Ca^{2+}-binding γ-carboxyglutamic acid (Gla) domain (Fig. 5.1). Transformation of the nonfunctional prozymogens (F) to functional zymogens (Fa) is mediated by γ-glutamyl carboxylase (γGC). This

carboxylation reaction needs oxygen and carbon dioxide and is coupled to the oxidation of vitamin K to its epoxide form. In order to regenerate the epoxide form and assure sustained carboxylation and synthesis of active coagulation factors, oxidized vitamin K is reduced in a reaction catalyzed by the vitamin K epoxide reductase (VKOR, encoded by the VKORC1 gene) with consumption of NADH [120–122]. Vitamin K antagonists (VKAs or coumarinics) act by blocking VKOR and thus the synthesis of new active coagulation factors [123, 124]. Of note, they have no effect on the already γ-carboxylated circulating factors, which stay active for the remainder of their half-life (ranging from 4–6 h of factor VII to 42–72 h of factor II) [122]. The naturally occurring anticoagulant proteins C and S have somewhat shorter half-lives (9 h and 60 h, respectively), which explains the increased thrombotic risk in the first days of coumarin use. In fact, the full antithrombotic effect of VKAs such as warfarin is not achieved before 4–5 days of therapy. From the several 4-hydroxycoumarin-derived VKAs including warfarin, acenocoumarol, and phenprocoumon, warfarin is the most commonly used and the prototypical drug of the class [38, 125].

Pharmacokinetics

Warfarin is an oral VKA that, at therapeutic doses, decreases by 30–70% the functional amount of each vitamin K-dependent coagulation factor. It is rapidly and extensively absorbed from the stomach and small intestine following oral administration, with an almost complete bioavailability. Approximately 99% of warfarin circulates bound to plasma proteins, especially albumin, and only the free fraction is pharmacologically active. Plasma concentrations of warfarin peak in 2–8 h, and its free fraction is highly variable among patients, independently of serum concentrations, and increases with decreased albumin concentrations [122, 126, 127]. Warfarin is administered in a racemic mixture of the two active enantiomers S- and R-warfarin, the former being 3–5-fold more potent than the latter, due to differences in receptor affinity to VKOR [122, 128]. In the liver, warfarin is metabolized in a stereoselective fashion: S-warfarin, the more potent enantiomer, is 90% oxidized by CYP2C9 to 7- and 6-hydroxywarfarin, and CYP3A4 makes only a minor contribution. On the other hand, R-warfarin is 60% oxidized by CYP1A1, 1A2, 3A4, and 2C19 to 4-, 6-, 7-, 8-, and 10-hydroxywarfarin; the remaining 40% are reduced. These metabolites are then eliminated by urinary excretion, and elimination half-lives differ for S- and R-warfarin (29 h and 45 h, respectively) [122]. Nevertheless, the biological duration of action is around 2–5 days. Although there seems to be a positive correlation between warfarin dose and concentrations of total and free racemic warfarin and its enantiomers, there does not seem to be a correlation between warfarin dose and prothrombin time [122, 127, 129]. Furthermore, the list of clinically significant warfarin drug and food interactions is astonishingly extensive [130, 131], greatly affecting therapeutic control both in a clinical trial setting and in a real-world, pragmatic, setting. The most frequent drug interactions result from inhibition or induction of the hepatic microsomal enzymes involved in warfarin metabolism, especially when interacting with CYP2C9, due to its role in metabolizing the more active S-warfarin [122, 132].

Taking all the above factors into account, dose response to warfarin is relatively unpredictable, and the therapeutic index is narrow, so the often empiric dosing must be individualized by trial and error. This is done using the international normalized ratio (INR), a corrected ratio measure of the prothrombin time. Target INR varies according to clinical indication, and normally ranges from 2 to 3 in most situations, or 2.5 to 3.5 in high-risk situations (a normal INR is around 1.0) [128, 133–135]. For efficacy of warfarin, it is important for the time in the therapeutic INR range (INR) to be high (>70%) [136]. Personalized approaches to warfarin dosing are, therefore, of great potential clinical significance.

Pharmacogenetics

Interindividual warfarin dose response is significantly influenced by polymorphisms in two genes, one involved in the metabolism of S-warfarin (CYP2C9) and the other one encoding the pharmacological target of coumarinic oral anticoagulants, VKOR (VKORC1). In fact, it is estimated that polymorphisms in these genes account for 35–50% of the variability in both initial and maintenance dose requirements of vitamin K antagonists [137–140].

CYP2C9 polymorphisms were first associated with dose requirement and adverse events in 1999 [141]. The two most important variants are the loss-of-function CYP2C9*2 (rs1799853) and CYP2C9*3 (rs1057910) alleles [142, 143]. Individuals with these variants have a reduced warfarin metabolism, need lower doses to reach target INR, and have a higher risk of overanticoagulation and bleeding [141, 143, 144]. Additional reduced-activity CYP2C9 variant alleles (CYP2C9*5, *6, *8, and *11) contribute to dose variability among African Americans [143].

Regarding the VKORC1 gene, there are two important variants: a common polymorphism (−1639G>A, rs9923231) alters a VKORC1 transcription factor-binding site, resulting in a reduced liver expression of VKOR, and so patients require lower doses and have an increased risk of bleeding events, while carriers of other rarer VKORC1 mutations are warfarin resistant and have an increased risk of ischemic events [145–148]. A third type of pharmacogenetic variant (rs2108622, CYP4F2) has also been associated with higher vitamin K levels and, hence, a need for higher warfarin doses [149].

For both CYP2C9 and VKORC1, pharmacogenetic-based dosing algorithms have been developed, but there is still some debate on exactly which SNPs and haplotypes better predict dosing needs [150–152].

5.4.2.2 Direct Oral Anticoagulants

Compared with warfarin, dOACs have a more attractive pharmacokinetic profile, fewer food and drug interactions, and shorter effect half-lives and do not usually require monitorization of anticoagulant effects as they are more predictable. dOACs are associated with a significant reduction of hemorrhagic stroke (RR 0.43, 95% CI 0.29–0.64) and death from any cause (RR 0.87, 95% CI 0.80–0.95) when compared to dose-adjusted warfarin [4]. As such, they are normally preferred for long-term secondary prevention in cardioembolic stroke or TIA in patients with atrial fibrillation, unless there is a contraindication, in which VKAs should be used [1, 4, 118, 135].

Choosing between either one of the dOACs should be made based on patients' characteristics, pharmacokinetic profile, adverse effects profile, availability of a reversal agent, and the prescriber's experience managing dOACs, as there are no trials directly comparing dOACs [153, 154].

Pharmacodynamics

In opposition to VKAs, which act indirectly through inhibition of the synthesis of coagulation factors, the dOACs inhibit either thrombin or activated factor X (Xa) (Figs. 5.1 and 5.3) [155]. The only direct thrombin inhibitor in use in stroke therapy is dabigatran [156, 157]. Regarding Xa inhibitors there are three drugs commonly used, namely rivaroxaban [158, 159], apixaban [160, 161], and edoxaban [162, 163].

Direct Thrombin Inhibitor Dabigatran

Dabigatran is given twice daily in two approved dosages, 150 or 110 mg. In its cornerstone trial [156, 157], the 150 mg dose was superior to warfarin in stroke prevention with similar rates of major hemorrhage, and the 110 mg was non-inferior to warfarin in the prevention of stroke and systemic embolism. A dosage reduction to 110 mg twice daily is needed for patients with severe renal impairment (creatinine clearance <30 mL/min/1.73m^2); there is no recommendation due to lack of data for patients with creatinine clearance <15 mL/min/1.73m^2 [164]. Dabigatran should not be used for stroke prevention in patients with mechanical heart valves [165]. Recently, a randomized clinical trial found that dabigatran at a dose of 150 mg twice daily is a safe alternative to warfarin for prevention of recurrent thromboembolic events in patients with CVT [166]. Optimal duration of oral anticoagulation with dabigatran in CVT is still under evaluation [167].

In cases of life-threatening hemorrhage, all dOACs can be at least partially reverted using nonspecific strategies of low evidence with prothrombin complex concentrate (PCC), activated PCC, or activated factor VII [155]. Dabigatran, however, has a specific antidote that can be used as a procoagulant for reversal: idarucizumab (Fig. 5.3) [168, 169]. Idarucizumab is a humanized monoclonal antibody that binds dabigatran 350 times more avidly than dabigatran binds thrombin, completely reversing the biological activity of dabigatran within minutes [170]. It does not bind thrombin, activate platelets, or convert fibrinogen to fibrin. It is given as two consecutive 2.5 g IV infusions no more than 15 min apart (total dose of 5 g) [168]. Specific reversal has many advantages, one of which is the possibility of offering treatment with IV thrombolytics in previously anticoagulated patients [171–176].

Pharmacokinetics

Dabigatran is administered as a prodrug (dabigatran etexilate) which is rapidly converted by CES and other plasma esterases to dabigatran. It binds the active site of both free and clot-bound thrombin, in a competitive and reversible way. As a consequence, dabigatran blocks thrombin-mediated conversion of fibrinogen to fibrin, positive feedback over the coagulation cascade, and, indirectly, platelet activation. Dabigatran is rapidly absorbed following oral administration with a low bioavailability (6%), low metabolism (<10%, by glucuronidation), relatively low protein-bound fraction (~35%), and high renal clearance (80–85%). Its half-life of 14–17 h is slightly longer than that of Xa inhibitors. Although no routine monitoring is usually necessary, it can be done through measurement of the diluted thrombin time; while it prolongs the activated partial thromboplastin time (aPTT), its effect on the aPTT plateaus with higher drug levels; the effect on INR is also unreliable.

Direct Activated Factor X Inhibitors
Pharmacodynamics
Direct, highly selective, Xa inhibitors include rivaroxaban, apixaban, and edoxaban (Figs. 5.1 and 5.3). A newer dOAC, betrixaban, is not yet approved for stroke prevention. Contrary to other Xa inhibitors, such as fondaparinux (Fig. 5.3), dOACs do not require cofactors to exert their anticoagulant effect. They inhibit unbound and clot-associated factor Xa, reducing thrombin generation.

All three Xa inhibitors are given in a fixed dose without need for monitoring. They prolong the prothrombin time (PT) more than the aPTT, but neither is reliable for monitoring. In some specific situations (namely in elderly and frail patients, extremely overweight subjects, impaired kidney function, or bleeding due to overdosing), anti-Xa assays may be beneficial to estimate anticoagulation activity [177], although they are not widely available.

Andexanet alfa is a modified recombinant protein derived from human Xa that acts as a decoy for Xa inhibitors reversing their anticoagulant effect [169, 178]. It completely reverses the anticoagulation activity of Xa inhibitors as measured by anti-Xa assays. It is given as a bolus and a subsequent 2-h infusion [179], which may limit its future applicability for hyperacute stroke care, compared with idarucizumab for dabigatran.

Pharmacokinetics
Rivaroxaban: It has a very high bioavailability (80–100%) owing to an almost complete absorption and lack of significant first-pass systemic metabolism, reaching a maximum plasma concentration in around 2–4 h [180, 181]. Maximum absorption occurs in the stomach, and rivaroxaban should be given with a meal to increase absorption [182]. It is transported in plasma highly bound to proteins (92–95%), mainly albumin, with a $t_{1/2} = 5$–13 h. Elimination is dual: one-third is excreted in the urine unchanged, while the remaining 66% is metabolized via hepatic CYP3A4 (and CYP2J2 to a lesser extent) and via hydrolysis. The inactive metabolites are excreted through urinary and hepatobiliary routes. In total, two-thirds of rivaroxaban's elimination are dependent on renal clearance [155, 180]. The normal unadjusted dose is 20 mg once daily; in patients with creatinine clearances between 15 and 50 mL/min/1.73m^2, dose should be adjusted to 15 mg daily; it should not be used in the setting of a lower creatinine clearance [164].

Apixaban: It has an oral bioavailability of 50% and peak plasma levels are reached in 3–4 h. Food does not affect absorption. It is slightly less plasma bound than rivaroxaban (87%), and has a $t_{1/2} = 12$ h. Elimination is renal (27%) and hepatic, through metabolization by the hepatic CYP3A4/5 (and the CYP21A2, SC8, 2C9/19, and 2J2 to a lesser extent) [155, 183]. In secondary stroke prevention, apixaban is usually given in a dose of 5 mg twice daily. The dose is reduced to 2.5 mg twice daily if two of the three following criteria are met: (1) age over 80 years; (2) body weight of 60 kg or less; and (3) serum creatinine concentrations of 1.5 mg/dL or higher. It should not be given if creatinine clearance is under 15 mL/min/1.73 m^2 [164].

Edoxaban: It has a bioavailability of 62%, and peak plasma concentrations are achieved in 1–2 h after oral administration. It is the Xa inhibitor with lowest protein-bound fraction (55%), and has a plasma $t_{1/2}$ similar to the other dOACs (6–11 h). Edoxaban has minimal hepatic metabolization, 50% is excreted unchanged in urine, and the remainder suffers hydrolysis. Mild to moderate hepatic impairment does not appear to significantly interfere with the pharmacokinetic profile [155, 184, 185]. Edoxaban is given once daily at a dose of 60 mg. Dose should be reduced to 30 mg once daily in patients with a creatinine clearance between 15 and 50 mL/min/1.73 m^2 and body weight of 60 kg or less, or in patients taking potent P-glycoprotein inhibitors (e.g., cyclosporine, quinidine, dronedarone, or rifampicin). Edoxaban should not be given with creatine clearances under 15 (lack of safety data) or over 95 mL/min/1.73 m^2 (increased risk of ischemic stroke compared to warfarin) [164].

Pharmacokinetics and Precision Medicine Considerations
As newer drugs get safer and have a more consistent efficacy, it is expected that interindividual differences, including genetic polymorphisms and drug-drug interactions, become less determinant for the general population of patients (or at least more difficult to prove to be determinant). They might have a deeper impact in special populations or in other particular subgroups of patients, especially since, contrary to VKAs, they are used in a fixed-dose regimen. For example, chronic kidney disease patients may benefit from adjusted dose schemes instead of facing contraindication due to reduced creatinine clearance.

Nonetheless, there is an interindividual variability in the blood concentration of dabigatran among patients, with possible implications in safety and efficacy [148]. In fact, a pharmacodynamic-pharmacokinetic guided approach, contrary to the fixed-dose approach that produces a variable exposure of drug in the population, might better represent and predict dOAC exposure in each patient [186]. This can be done by implementing routine dOAC drug-level determination and use of quantitative assays (diluted thrombin time for dabigatran; anti-Xa assays for rivaroxaban, apixaban, and edoxaban). These measures will probably have more impact in adjusting and personalizing drug doses in pharmacokinetic outliers [186].

As for pharmacogenetics, evidence is scarce and its widespread clinical utility still a matter of theory [187, 188]. For dabigatran, genetic variants in CES1 (rs2244613) and ABCB1 (rs4148738) were associated with trough concentrations of dabigatran etexilate and reduced hemorrhagic risk, while other variants in CES1 (rs8192935) and ABCB1 (rs1045642) were associated with peak levels and increased risk of bleeding of undetermined clinical significance [187, 189, 190]. Concerning rivaroxaban, screening for p-gp coding ABCB1 polymorphisms and certain haplotypes may be useful in reducing bleeding adverse events, although data is still preliminary; CYP3A4 gene loci and their SNPs have also been implicated in altering plasma drug levels [187, 191, 192]. Apixaban peak and trough levels might be influenced by pharmacogenetic variants in its metabolic pathways, such as in sulfotransferases (SULT1A1 and SULT1A2) responsible for metabolization of its most important metabolite (*O*-demethyl-apixaban) [187, 193]. ABCB1 variants, as in other dOACs, may also be of relevance [194]. No studies have found relevant differences across genetic variants for edoxaban [187, 188]. Notwithstanding the growing body of knowledge, pharmacogenomics of dOACs is still a relatively new and untapped field of research, and stroke-specific clinical trials are needed.

5.5 Conclusion and Perspectives for the Future

Stroke is a systemic multifactorial disease, anatomical and phenotypically diverse, with complex genetic associations. On the top of this there are clearly distinct time windows in what concerns the evolution of brain damage/brain recovery, which include in a simplistic way of describing it early excitotoxicity, followed by inflammatory events and late glial scar formation. Despite extensive basic and preclinical data promising good results, neuroprotection strategies (including inflammation modulation, excitotoxicity targeting, vasogenic or cytotoxic edema reduction) have, to this date, failed to show benefit in the setting of clinical trials. As such, at present, pharmacological or nonpharmacological treatments with putative neuroprotective actions are not recommended [1].

As stroke phenotypes are highly variable, the application of a tailored diagnosis and therapy for each patient is, as we discussed above, of high importance. The application of this type of precision medicine in a disease so anatomically and pathophysiologically diverse will remain a challenge. Ultimately, the goal would be that of achieving a status of theranostics: the complete synchronization of therapeutic strategies based on specific diagnostic data, be it either genotype or phenotype based [195–197]. As of today, there are some limitations to this goal, namely (1) lack of consistent and standardized methods between clinical trials and between a trial and a real-life setting; (2) inconsistencies and imprecisions in data collection; (3) limited external validity of trial-defined outcomes and difficulties in establishing clinically significant differences; (4) heterogeneity in the contribution of genetic factors to different stroke syndromes (higher in monogenic causes of stroke, probably more determinant in younger patients); (5) need for precise, accurate, rapid, efficient point-of-care testing before hyperacute therapies; (6) development of clinical useful biomarkers, either for prognosis or for therapeutic response prediction; and (7) perfection of imaging acquisition and evaluation, data integration, and big data analysis, among others [195, 197]. Cost-effectiveness of these strategies, specifically pharmacogenetic-based approaches, will most probably depend on context, but appears to be an attainable goal in the near future [198].

References

1. Powers WJ, Rabinstein AA, Ackerson T, Adeoye OM, Bambakidis NC, Becker K, et al. Guidelines for the early management of patients with acute ischemic stroke: 2019 update to the 2018 guidelines for the early management of acute ischemic stroke: a guideline for healthcare professionals from the American Heart Association/American Stroke. Stroke. 2019;50(12):E344–418.
2. Meretoja A, Keshtkaran M, Saver JL, Tatlisumak T, Parsons MW, Kaste M, et al. Stroke thrombolysis: save a minute, save a day. Stroke. 2014;45(4):1053–8.
3. Emberson J, Lees KR, Lyden P, Blackwell L, Albers G, Bluhmki E, et al. Effect of treatment delay, age, and stroke severity on the effects of intravenous thrombolysis with alteplase for acute ischaemic stroke: a meta-analysis of individual patient data from randomised trials. Lancet. 2014;384(9958):1929–35.
4. Klijn CJM, Paciaroni M, Berge E, Korompoki E, Kõrv J, Lal A, et al. Antithrombotic treatment for secondary prevention of stroke and other thromboembolic events in patients with stroke or transient ischemic attack and non-valvular atrial fibrillation: a European Stroke Organisation guideline. Eur Stroke J. 2019;4(3):198–223.
5. Love BB, Bendixen BH. Classification of subtype of acute ischemic stroke definitions for use in a multicenter clinical trial. Stroke. 1993;24(1):35–41.
6. The National Institute of Neurological Disorders and Stroke rt-PA Stroke Study Group. Tissue plasminogen activator for acute ischemic stroke. N Engl J Med. 1995;333(24):1581–8.
7. Hacke W, Kaste M, Bluhmki E, Brozman M, Dávalos A, Guidetti D, et al. Thrombolysis with alteplase 3 to 4.5 hours after acute ischemic stroke. N Engl J Med. 2008;359(13):1317–29.
8. Wardlaw JM, Murray V, Berge E, del Zoppo GJ. Thrombolysis for acute ischaemic stroke. Cochrane Database Syst Rev. 2014;2014(7):CD000213.
9. Thomalla G, Simonsen CZ, Boutitie F, Andersen G, Berthezene Y, Cheng B, et al. MRI-guided thrombolysis for stroke with unknown time of onset. N Engl J Med. 2018;379(7):611–22.
10. Campbell BCV, Ma H, Ringleb PA, Parsons MW, Churilov L, Bendszus M, et al. Extending thrombolysis to 4·5–9 h and wake-up stroke using perfusion imaging: a systematic review and meta-analysis of individual patient data. Lancet. 2019;394(10193):139–47.
11. Ford GA, Ahmed N, Azevedo E, Grond M, Larrue V, Lindsberg PJ, et al. Intravenous alteplase for stroke in those older than 80 years old. Stroke. 2010;41(11):2568–74.
12. Meretoja A, Tatlisumak T. Thrombolytic therapy in acute ischemic stroke—basic concepts. Curr Vasc Pharmacol. 2006;4(1):31–44.
13. Liu H, Zheng H, Cao Y, Pan Y, Wang D, Zhang R, et al. Low- versus standard-dose intravenous tissue-type plasminogen activator for acute ischemic stroke: an updated meta-analysis. J Stroke Cerebrovasc Dis. 2018;27(4):988–97.
14. Anderson CS, Robinson T, Lindley RI, Arima H, Lavados PM, Lee TH, et al. Low-dose versus standard-dose intravenous alteplase in acute ischemic stroke. N Engl J Med. 2016;374(24):2313–23.
15. Hill MD, Lye T, Moss H, Barber PA, Demchuk AM, Newcommon NJ, et al. Hemi-orolingual angioedema and ACE inhibition after alteplase treatment of stroke. Neurology. 2003;60(9):1525–7.
16. Lin SY, Tang SC, Tsai LK, Yeh SJ, Hsiao YJ, Chen YW, et al. Orolingual angioedema after alteplase therapy of acute ischaemic stroke: incidence and risk of prior angiotensin-converting enzyme inhibitor use. Eur J Neurol. 2014;21(10):1285–91.
17. Hurford R, Rezvani S, Kreimei M, Herbert A, Vail A, Parry-Jones AR, et al. Incidence, predictors and clinical characteristics of orolingual angio-oedema complicating thrombolysis with tissue plasminogen activator for ischaemic stroke. J Neurol Neurosurg Psychiatry. 2015;86(5):520–3.
18. Fröhlich K, MacHa K, Gerner ST, Bobinger T, Schmidt M, Dörfler A, et al. Angioedema in stroke patients with thrombolysis: a lesion mapping study. Stroke. 2019;50(7):1682–7.

19. Emeis JJ, van den Eijnden-Schrauwen Y, van den Hoogen CM, de Priester W, Westmuckett A, Lupu F. An endothelial storage granule for tissue-type plasminogen activator. J Cell Biol. 1997;139(1):245–56.
20. Bivard A, Lin L, Parsonsb MW. Review of stroke thrombolytics. J Stroke. 2013;15(2):90.
21. Rijken DC, Lijnen HR. New insights into the molecular mechanisms of the fibrinolytic system. J Thromb Haemost. 2009;7(1):4–13.
22. Hoylaerts M, Rijken DC, Lijnen HR, Collen D. Kinetics of the activation of plasminogen by human tissue plasminogen activator. Role of fibrin. J Biol Chem. 1982;257:2912–9.
23. Acheampong P, Ford GA. Pharmacokinetics of alteplase in the treatment of ischaemic stroke. Expert Opin Drug Metab Toxicol. 2012;8(2):271–81.
24. Verheijen JH, Caspers MP, Chang GT, de Munk GA, Pouwels PH, Enger-Valk BE. Involvement of finger domain and kringle 2 domain of tissue-type plasminogen activator in fibrin binding and stimulation of activity by fibrin. EMBO J. 1986;5(13):3525–30.
25. Tanswell P, Modi N, Combs D, Danays T. Pharmacokinetics and pharmacodynamics of tenecteplase in fibrinolytic therapy of acute myocardial infarction. Clin Pharmacokinet. 2002;41(15):1229–45.
26. Campbell BCV, Mitchell PJ, Churilov L, Yassi N, Kleinig TJ, Yan B, et al. Tenecteplase versus alteplase before endovascular thrombectomy (EXTEND-IA TNK): a multicenter, randomized, controlled study. Int J Stroke. 2018;13(3):328–34.
27. Logallo N, Novotny V, Assmus J, Kvistad CE, Alteheld L, Rønning OM, et al. Tenecteplase versus alteplase for management of acute ischaemic stroke (NOR-TEST): a phase 3, randomised, open-label, blinded endpoint trial. Lancet Neurol. 2017;16(10):781–8.
28. Del Río-Espínola A, Fernández-Cadenas I, Giralt D, Quiroga A, Gutiérrez-Agulló M, Quintana M, et al. A predictive clinical-genetic model of tissue plasminogen activator response in acute ischemic stroke. Ann Neurol. 2012;72(5):716–29.
29. Falcone GJ, Malik R, Dichgans M, Rosand J. Current concepts and clinical applications of stroke genetics. Lancet Neurol. 2014;13(4):405–18.
30. Fernández-Cadenas I, Del Río-Espínola A, Giralt D, Domingues-Montanari S, Quiroga A, Mendióroz M, et al. IL1B and VWF variants are associated with fibrinolytic early recanalization in patients with ischemic stroke. Stroke. 2012;43(10):2659–65.
31. Castellanos M, Sobrino T, Millán M, García M, Arenillas J, Nombela F, et al. Serum cellular fibronectin and matrix metalloproteinase-9 as screening biomarkers for the prediction of parenchymal hematoma after thrombolytic therapy in acute ischemic stroke: a multicenter confirmatory study. Stroke. 2007;38(6):1855–9.
32. Hernandez-Guillamon M, Garcia-Bonilla L, Solé M, Sosti V, Parés M, Campos M, et al. Plasma VAP-1/SSAO activity predicts intracranial hemorrhages and adverse neurological outcome after tissue plasminogen activator treatment in stroke. Stroke. 2010;41(7):1528–35.
33. Sadler JE. Biochemistry and genetics of von Willebrand factor. Annu Rev Biochem. 1998;67(1):395–424.
34. International Stroke Trial Collaborative Group. The International Stroke Trial (IST): a randomised trial of aspirin, subcutaneous heparin, both, or neither among 19435 patients with acute ischaemic stroke. International Stroke Trial Collaborative Group. Lancet. 1997;349(9065):1569–81.
35. CAST (Chinese Acute Stroke Trial) Collaborative Group. CAST: randomised placebo-controlled trial of early aspirin use in 20,000 patients with acute ischaemic stroke. Lancet 1997;349:1641–9.
36. UK-TIA Study Group. The United Kingdom transient ischaemic attack (UK-TIA) aspirin trial: final results UK-TIA Study group. J Neurol Neurosurg Psychiatry. 1991;54:1044–54.
37. Hart RG, Benavente O, McBride R, Pearce LA. Antithrombotic therapy to prevent stroke in patients with atrial fibrillation. Ann Intern Med. 1999;131(7):492.
38. Apostolakis S, Lip GY, Shantsila E. Pharmacokinetic considerations for antithrombotic therapies in stroke. Expert Opin Drug Metab Toxicol. 2013;9(10):1335–47.

39. Roth GJ, Calverley DC. Aspirin, platelets, and thrombosis: theory and practice. Blood. 1994;83(4):885–98.
40. Wang Y, Wang Y, Zhao X, Liu L, Wang D, Wang C, et al. Clopidogrel with aspirin in acute minor stroke or transient ischemic attack. N Engl J Med. 2013;369(1):11–9.
41. Claiborne Johnston S, Donald Easton J, Farrant M, Barsan W, Conwit RA, Elm JJ, et al. Clopidogrel and aspirin in acute ischemic stroke and high-risk TIA. N Engl J Med. 2018;379(3):215–25.
42. Pan Y, Elm JJ, Li H, Easton JD, Wang Y, Farrant M, et al. Outcomes associated with clopidogrel-aspirin use in minor stroke or transient ischemic attack: a pooled analysis of clopidogrel in high-risk patients with acute non-disabling cerebrovascular events (CHANCE) and platelet-oriented inhibition in new TIA and minor ischemic stroke (POINT) trials. JAMA Neurol. 2019;76(12):1466–73.
43. Pedersen AK, FitzGerald GA. Dose-related kinetics of aspirin. Presystemic acetylation of platelet cyclooxygenase. N Engl J Med. 1984;311(19):1206–11.
44. Cheng Y, Austin SC, Rocca B, Koller BH, Coffman TM, Grosser T, et al. Role of prostacyclin in the cardiovascular response to thromboxane A2. Science. 2002;296(5567):539–41.
45. Catella-Lawson F, Reilly MP, Kapoor SC, Cucchiara AJ, DeMarco S, Tournier B, et al. Cyclooxygenase inhibitors and the antiplatelet effects of aspirin. N Engl J Med. 2001;345(25):1809–17.
46. Li X, Fries S, Li R, Lawson JA, Propert KJ, Diamond SL, et al. Differential impairment of aspirin-dependent platelet cyclooxygenase acetylation by nonsteroidal anti-inflammatory drugs. Proc Natl Acad Sci U S A. 2014;111(47):16830–5.
47. Patrono C, Ciabattoni G, Patrignani P, Pugliese F, Filabozzi P, Catella F, et al. Clinical pharmacology of platelet cyclooxygenase inhibition. Circulation. 1985;72(6):1177–84.
48. Cox D, Maree AO, Dooley M, Conroy R, Byrne MF, Fitzgerald DJ. Effect of enteric coating on antiplatelet activity of low-dose aspirin in healthy volunteers. Stroke. 2006;37(8):2153–8.
49. Peace A, Mccall M, Tedesco T, Kenny D, Conroy RM, Foley D, et al. The role of weight and enteric coating on aspirin response in cardiovascular patients. J Thromb Haemost. 2010;8(10):2323–5.
50. Kelly JP, Kaufman DW, Jurgelon JM, Sheehan J, Koff RS, Shapiro S. Risk of aspirin-associated major upper-gastrointestinal bleeding with enteric-coated or buffered product. Lancet. 1996;348(9039):1413–6.
51. Rand ML, Leung R, Packham MA. Platelet function assays. Transfus Apher Sci. 2003;28(3):307–17.
52. Harrison P. Progress in the assessment of platelet function. Br J Haematol. 2000;1111(3):733–44.
53. Michelson AD. Platelet function testing in cardiovascular diseases. Circulation. 2004;110(19):e489–93.
54. Bhatt DL, Topol EJ. Scientific and therapeutic advances in antiplatelet therapy. Nat Rev Drug Discov. 2003;2(1):15–28.
55. Hankey GJ, Eikelboom JW. Aspirin resistance. Lancet. 2006;367(9510):606–17.
56. Patrono C. Aspirin resistance: definition, mechanisms and clinical read-outs. J Thromb Haemost. 2003;1(8):1710–3.
57. Topçuoglu MA, Arsava EM, Ay H. Antiplatelet resistance in stroke. Expert Rev Neurother. 2011;11(2):251–63.
58. De Schryver ELLM, Van Gijn J, Kappelle LJ, Koudstaal PJ, Algra A. Non-adherence to aspirin or oral anticoagulants in secondary prevention after ischaemic stroke. J Neurol. 2005;252(11):1316–21.
59. Al AlShaikh S, Quinn T, Dunn W, Walters M, Dawson J. Predictive factors of non-adherence to secondary preventative medication after stroke or transient ischaemic attack: a systematic review and meta-analyses. Eur Stroke J. 2016;1(2):65–75.
60. Helgason CM, Bolin KM, Hoff JA, Winkler SR, Mangat A, Tortorice KL, et al. Development of aspirin resistance in persons with previous ischemic stroke. Stroke. 1994;25(12):2331–6.

61. Pulcinelli FM, Pignatelli P, Celestini A, Riondino S, Gazzaniga PP, Violi F. Inhibition of platelet aggregation by aspirin progressively decreases in long-term treated patients. J Am Coll Cardiol. 2004;43(6):979–84.

62. Krasopoulos G, Brister SJ, Beattie WS, Buchanan MR. Aspirin "resistance" and risk of cardiovascular morbidity: systematic review and meta-analysis. BMJ. 2008;336(7637):195–8.

63. O'Donnell CJ, Larson MG, Feng D, Sutherland PA, Lindpaintner K, Myers RH, et al. Genetic and environmental contributions to platelet aggregation. Circulation. 2001;103(25):3051–6.

64. Halushka MK, Walker LP, Halushka PV. Genetic variation in cyclooxygenase 1: effects on response to aspirin. Clin Pharmacol Ther. 2003;73(1):122–30.

65. Cambria-Kiely JA, Gandhi PJ. Aspirin resistance and genetic polymorphisms. J Thromb Thrombolysis. 2002;14(1):51–8.

66. Li Q, Chen BL, Ozmedir V, Ji W, Mao YM, Wang LC, et al. Frequency of genetic polymorphisms of COX1, GPIIIa and P2Y1 in a Chinese population and association with attenuated response to aspirin. Pharmacogenomics. 2007;8(6):577–86.

67. Maree AO, Curtin RJ, Chubb A, Dolan C, Cox D, O'Brien J, et al. Cyclooxygenase-1 haplotype modulates platelet response to aspirin. J Thromb Haemost. 2005;3(10):2340–5.

68. Andrioli G, Minuz P, Solero P, Pincelli S, Ortolani R, Lussignoli S, et al. Defective platelet response to arachidonic acid and thromboxane A2 in subjects with PlA2 polymorphism of beta3 subunit (glycoprotein IIIa). Br J Haematol. 2000;110(4):911–8.

69. Michelson AD, Furman MI, Goldschmidt-Clermont P, Mascelli MA, Hendrix C, Coleman L, et al. Platelet GP IIIa Pl A polymorphisms display different sensitivities to agonists. Circulation. 2000;101(9):1013–8.

70. Jefferson BK, Foster JH, McCarthy JJ, Ginsburg G, Parker A, Kottke-Marchant K, et al. Aspirin resistance and a single gene. Am J Cardiol. 2005;95(6):805–8.

71. Goodman T, Ferro A, Sharma P. Pharmacogenetics of aspirin resistance: a comprehensive systematic review. Br J Clin Pharmacol. 2008;66(2):222–32.

72. Meschia JF. Pharmacogenetics and stroke. Stroke. 2009;40(11):3641–5.

73. Schilling U, Dingemanse J, Ufer M. Pharmacokinetics and pharmacodynamics of approved and investigational P2Y12 receptor antagonists. Clin Pharmacokinet. 2020;59(5):545–66.

74. Johnston SC, Amarenco P, Denison H, Evans SR, Himmelmann A, James S, et al. Ticagrelor and aspirin or aspirin alone in acute ischemic stroke or TIA. N Engl J Med. 2020;383(3):207–17.

75. Prasad K, Siemieniuk R, Hao Q, Guyatt G, O'Donnell M, Lytvyn L, et al. Dual antiplatelet therapy with aspirin and clopidogrel for acute high risk transient ischaemic attack and minor ischaemic stroke: a clinical practice guideline. BMJ. 2018;363:k5130.

76. Kim D, Park JM, Kang K, Cho YJ, Hong KS, Lee KB, et al. Dual versus mono antiplatelet therapy in large atherosclerotic stroke: a retrospective analysis of the Nationwide Multicenter Stroke Registry. Stroke. 2019;50(5):1184–92.

77. Liu L, Wong KSL, Leng X, Pu Y, Wang Y, Jing J, et al. Dual antiplatelet therapy in stroke and ICAS. Neurology. 2015;85(13):1154–62.

78. Chimowitz MI, Lynn MJ, Derdeyn CP, Turan TN, Fiorella D, Lane BF, et al. Stenting versus aggressive medical therapy for intracranial arterial stenosis. N Engl J Med. 2011;365(11):993–1003.

79. Bath PM, Woodhouse LJ, Appleton JP, Beridze M, Christensen H, Dineen RA, et al. Antiplatelet therapy with aspirin, clopidogrel, and dipyridamole versus clopidogrel alone or aspirin and dipyridamole in patients with acute cerebral ischaemia (TARDIS): a randomised, open-label, phase 3 superiority trial. Lancet. 2018;391(10123):850–9.

80. Johnston-Cox HA, Ravid K. Adenosine and blood platelets. Purinergic Signal. 2011;7:357–65.

81. Taubert D, von Beckerath N, Grimberg G, Lazar A, Jung N, Goeser T, et al. Impact of P-glycoprotein on clopidogrel absorption. Clin Pharmacol Ther. 2006;80(5):486–501.

82. Savi P, Herbert JM, Pflieger AM, Dol F, Delebassee D, Combalbert J, et al. Importance of hepatic metabolism in the antiaggregating activity of the thienopyridine clopidogrel. Biochem Pharmacol. 1992;44(3):527–32.

83. Savi P, Pereillo JM, Uzabiaga MF, Combalbert J, Picard C, Maffrand JP, et al. Identification and biological activity of the active metabolite of clopidogrel. Thromb Haemost. 2000;84(5):891–6.

84. Kazui M, Nishiya Y, Ishizuka T, Hagihara K, Farid NA, Okazaki O, et al. Identification of the human cytochrome P450 enzymes involved in the two oxidative steps in the bioactivation of clopidogrel to its pharmacologically active metabolite. Drug Metab Dispos. 2010;38(1):92–9.

85. Farid NA, Kurihara A, Wrighton SA. Review: metabolism and disposition of the thienopyridine antiplatelet drugs ticlopidine, clopidogrel, and prasugrel in humans. J Clin Pharmacol. 2010;50(2):126–42.

86. Von Beckerath N, Taubert D, Pogatsa-Murray G, Schömig E, Kastrati A, Schömig A. Absorption, metabolization, and antiplatelet effects of 300-, 600-, and 900-mg loading doses of clopidogrel: results of the ISAR-CHOICE (intracoronary stenting and antithrombotic regimen: choose between 3 high oral doses for immediate clopidogrel effect) trial. Circulation. 2005;112(19):2946–50.

87. Li YG, Ni L, Brandt JT, Small DS, Payne CD, Ernest CS, et al. Inhibition of platelet aggregation with prasugrel and clopidogrel: an integrated analysis in 846 subjects. Platelets. 2009;20(5):316–27.

88. Frelinger AL, Bhatt DL, Lee RD, Mulford DJ, Wu J, Nudurupati S, et al. Clopidogrel pharmacokinetics and pharmacodynamics vary widely despite exclusion or control of polymorphisms (CYP2C19, ABCB1, PON1), noncompliance, diet, smoking, co-medications (including proton pump inhibitors), and pre-existent variability in platelet function. J Am Coll Cardiol. 2013;61(8):872–9.

89. O'Donoghue ML, Braunwald E, Antman EM, Murphy SA, Bates ER, Rozenman Y, et al. Pharmacodynamic effect and clinical efficacy of clopidogrel and prasugrel with or without a proton-pump inhibitor: an analysis of two randomised trials. Lancet. 2009;374(9694):989–97.

90. Li X-Q, Andersson TB, Ahlström M, Weidolf L. Comparison of inhibitory effects of the proton pump-inhibiting drugs omeprazole, esomeprazole, lansoprazole, pantoprazole, and rabeprazole on human cytochrome P450 activities. Drug Metab Dispos. 2004;32(8):821–7.

91. Neubauer H, Engelhardt A, Krüger JC, Lask S, Börgel J, Mügge A, et al. Pantoprazole does not influence the antiplatelet effect of clopidogrel-A whole blood aggregometry study after coronary stenting. J Cardiovasc Pharmacol. 2010;56(1):91–7.

92. Kwok CS, Loke YK. Meta-analysis: the effects of proton pump inhibitors on cardiovascular events and mortality in patients receiving clopidogrel. Aliment Pharmacol Ther. 2010;31(8):810–23.

93. Bhatt DL, Cryer BL, Contant CF, Cohen M, Lanas A, Schnitzer TJ, et al. Clopidogrel with or without omeprazole in coronary artery disease. N Engl J Med. 2010;363(20):1909–17.

94. Laine L, Hennekens C. Proton pump inhibitor and clopidogrel interaction: fact or fiction. Am J Gastroenterol. 2010;105(1):34–41.

95. Lanas A, García-Rodríguez LA, Arroyo MT, Bujanda L, Gomollón F, Forné M, et al. Effect of antisecretory drugs and nitrates on the risk of ulcer bleeding associated with nonsteroidal anti-inflammatory drugs, antiplatelet agents, and anticoagulants. Am J Gastroenterol. 2007;102(3):507–15.

96. Oliphant CS, Trevarrow BJ, Dobesh PP. Clopidogrel response variability: review of the literature and practical considerations. J Pharm Pract. 2016;29(1):26–34.

97. Ellis KJ, Stouffer GA, McLeod HL, Lee CR. Clopidogrel pharmacogenomics and risk of inadequate platelet inhibition: US FDA recommendations. Pharmacogenomics. 2009;10(11):1799–817.

98. Mega JL, Close SL, Wiviott SD, Shen L, Hockett RD, Brandt JT, et al. Cytochrome P-450 polymorphisms and response to clopidogrel. N Engl J Med. 2009;360(4):354–62.

99. Martis S, Peter I, Hulot JS, Kornreich R, Desnick RJ, Scott SA. Multi-ethnic distribution of clinically relevant CYP2C genotypes and haplotypes. Pharmacogenomics J. 2013;13(4):369–77.

100. Shuldiner AR, O'Connell JR, Bliden KP, Ghandi A, Ryan K, Horenstein RB, et al. Association of cytochrome P450 2C19 genotype with the antiplatelet effect and clinical efficacy of clopidogrel therapy. JAMA. 2009;302(8):849–58. Available from: www.jama.com.

101. Hulot JS, Bura A, Villard E, Azizi M, Remones V, Goyenvalle C, et al. Cytochrome P450 2C19 loss-of-function polymorphism is a major determinant of clopidogrel responsiveness in healthy subjects. Blood. 2006;108(7):2244–7.
102. Sofi F, Giusti B, Marcucci R, Gori AM, Abbate R, Gensini GF. Cytochrome P450 2C19 2 polymorphism and cardiovascular recurrences in patients taking clopidogrel: a meta-analysis. Pharmacogenomics J. 2011;11(3):199–206.
103. Zabalza M, Subirana I, Sala J, Lluis-Ganella C, Lucas G, Tomás M, et al. Meta-analyses of the association between cytochrome CYP2C19 loss- and gain-of-function polymorphisms and cardiovascular outcomes in patients with coronary artery disease treated with clopidogrel. Heart. 2012;98(2):100–8.
104. Tiroch KA, Sibbing D, Koch W, Roosen-Runge T, Mehilli J, Schömig A, et al. Protective effect of the CYP2C19*17 polymorphism with increased activation of clopidogrel on cardiovascular events. Am Heart J. 2010;160(3):506–12.
105. Wang Y, Zhao X, Lin J, Li H, Johnston SC, Lin Y, et al. Association between CYP2C19 loss-of-function allele status and efficacy of clopidogrel for risk reduction among patients with minor stroke or transient ischemic attack. JAMA. 2016;316(1):70.
106. Pan Y, Chen W, Xu Y, Yi X, Han Y, Yang Q, et al. Genetic polymorphisms and clopidogrel efficacy for acute ischemic stroke or transient ischemic attack. Circulation. 2017;135(1):21–33.
107. Qiu LN, Sun Y, Wang L, Han RF, Xia XS, Liu J, et al. Influence of CYP2C19 polymorphisms on platelet reactivity and clinical outcomes in ischemic stroke patients treated with clopidogrel. Eur J Pharmacol. 2015;747:29–35.
108. Jia DM, Chen ZB, Zhang MJ, Yang WJ, Jin JL, Xia YQ, et al. CYP2C19 polymorphisms and antiplatelet effects of clopidogrel in acute ischemic stroke in China. Stroke. 2013;44(6):1717–9.
109. Sun W, Li Y, Li J, Zhang Z, Zhu W, Liu W, et al. Variant recurrent risk among stroke patients with different CYP2C19 phenotypes and treated with clopidogrel. Platelets. 2015;26(6):558–62.
110. Anderson CD, Biffi A, Greenberg SM, Rosand J. Personalized approaches to clopidogrel therapy: are we there yet? Stroke. 2010;41(12):2997–3002.
111. Neuvonen M, Tarkiainen EK, Tornio A, Hirvensalo P, Tapaninen T, Paile-Hyvärinen M, et al. Effects of genetic variants on carboxylesterase 1 gene expression, and clopidogrel pharmacokinetics and antiplatelet effects. Basic Clin Pharmacol Toxicol. 2018;122(3):341–5.
112. Lewis JP, Horenstein RB, Ryan K, O'Connell JR, Gibson Q, Mitchell BD, et al. The functional G143E variant of carboxylesterase 1 is associated with increased clopidogrel active metabolite levels and greater clopidogrel response. Pharmacogenet Genomics. 2013;23(1):1–8.
113. Wang X, Shen C, Wang B, Huang X, Hu Z, Li J. Genetic polymorphisms of CYP2C19*2 and ABCB1 C3435T affect the pharmacokinetic and pharmacodynamic responses to clopidogrel in 401 patients with acute coronary syndrome. Gene. 2015;558(2):200–7.
114. Su J, Xu J, Li X, Zhang H, Hu J, Fang R, et al. ABCB1 C3435T polymorphism and response to clopidogrel treatment in coronary artery disease (CAD) patients: a meta-analysis. PLoS One. 2012;7(10):e46366.
115. Cui G, Zhang S, Zou J, Chen Y, Chen H. P2Y12 receptor gene polymorphism and the risk of resistance to clopidogrel: a meta-analysis and review of the literature. Adv Clin Exp Med. 2017;26(2):343–9.
116. Seiffge DJ, Werring DJ, Paciaroni M, Dawson J, Warach S, Milling TJ, et al. Timing of anticoagulation after recent ischaemic stroke in patients with atrial fibrillation. Lancet Neurol. 2019;18(1):117–26.
117. Paciaroni M, Agnelli G, Corea F, Ageno W, Alberti A, Lanari A, et al. Early hemorrhagic transformation of brain infarction: rate, predictive factors, and influence on clinical outcome: results of a prospective multicenter study. Stroke. 2008;39(8):2249–56.
118. Heidbuchel H, Verhamme P, Alings M, Antz M, Hacke W, Oldgren J, et al. EHRA practical guide on the use of new oral anticoagulants in patients with non-valvular atrial fibrillation: executive summary. Eur Heart J. 2013;34(27):2094–106.

119. Munn D, Abdul-Rahim AH, Fischer U, Werring DJ, Robinson TG, Dawson J. A survey of opinion: when to start oral anticoagulants in patients with acute ischaemic stroke and atrial fibrillation? Eur Stroke J. 2018;3(4):355–60.
120. Whitlon DS, Sadowski JA, Suttie JW. Mechanism of coumarin action: significance of vitamin K epoxide reductase inhibition. Biochemistry. 1978;17(8):1371–7.
121. Holford NHG. Clinical pharmacokinetics and pharmacodynamics of warfarin. Clin Pharmacokinet. 1986;11(6):483–504.
122. Wittkowsky AK. Warfarin and other coumarin derivatives: pharmacokinetics, pharmacodynamics, and drug interactions. Semin Vasc Med. 2003;3(3):221–30.
123. Fasco MJ, Hildebrandt EF, Suttie JW. Evidence that warfarin anticoagulant action involves two distinct reductase activities. J Biol Chem. 1982;257(19):11210–2.
124. Malhotras OP, Nesheimo ME, Manntl KG. The kinetics of activation of normal and y-carboxyglutamic acid-deficient prothrombins. J Biol Chem. 1985;260(1):279–87.
125. Apostolakis S, Lip GY, Lane DA, Shantsila E. The quest for new anticoagulants: from clinical development to clinical practice. Cardiovasc Ther. 2011;29(6):e12–22.
126. Yacobi A, Udall JA, Levy G. Serum protein binding as a determinant of warfarin body clearance and anticoagulant effect. Clin Pharmacol Ther. 1976;19(5 Pt 1):552–8.
127. Routledge P, Chapman P, Davies D, Rawlins M. Pharmacokinetics and pharmacodynamics of warfarin at steady state. Br J Clin Pharmacol. 1979;8(3):243–7.
128. Hirsh J, Fuster V, Ansell J, Halperin JL. American Heart Association/American College of Cardiology Foundation guide to warfarin therapy. J Am Coll Cardiol. 2003;41(9):1633–52.
129. Chan E, McLachlan A, Pegg M, MacKay A, Cole R, Rowland M. Disposition of warfarin enantiomers and metabolites in patients during multiple dosing with rac-warfarin [see comments]. Br J Clin Pharmacol. 1994;37(6):563–9.
130. Wells PS, Holbrook AM, Crowther NR, Hirsh J. Interactions of warfarin with drugs and food. Ann Intern Med. 1994;121(9):676–83.
131. Freedman MD, Olatidoye AG. Clinically significant drug interactions with the oral anticoagulants. Drug Saf. 1994;10(5):381–94.
132. Wittkowsky AK. Drug interactions update: drugs, herbs, and oral anticoagulation. J Thromb Thrombolysis. 2001;12(1):67–71.
133. Kirchhof P, Benussi S, Kotecha D, Ahlsson A, Atar D, Casadei B, et al. 2016 ESC guidelines for the management of atrial fibrillation developed in collaboration with EACTS. Eur Heart J. 2016;37(38):2893–962.
134. January CT, Wann LS, Alpert JS, Calkins H, Cigarroa JE, Cleveland JC, et al. 2014 AHA/ACC/HRS guideline for the management of patients with atrial fibrillation: a report of the American College of Cardiology/American Heart Association Task Force on Practice Guidelines and the Heart Rhythm Society. J Am Coll Cardiol. 2014;64(21):e1–76.
135. January CT, Wann LS, Calkins H, Chen LY, Cigarroa JE, Cleveland JC, et al. 2019 AHA/ACC/HRS focused update of the 2014 AHA/ACC/HRS guideline for the management of patients with atrial fibrillation: a report of the American College of Cardiology/American Heart Association Task Force on Clinical Practice Guidelines and the Heart Rhythm Society in Collaboration with the Society of Thoracic Surgeons. Circulation. 2019;140(2):e125–51.
136. Schmitt L, Speckman J, Ansell J. Quality assessment of anticoagulation dose management: comparative evaluation of measures of time-in-therapeutic range. J Thromb Thrombolysis. 2003;15(3):213–6.
137. Bodin L, Verstuyft C, Tregouet DA, Robert A, Dubert L, Funck-Brentano C, et al. Cytochrome P450 2C9 (CYP2C9) and vitamin K epoxide reductase (VKORC1) genotypes as determinants of acenocoumarol sensitivity. Blood. 2005;106(1):135–40.
138. Schalekamp T, Brassé BP, Roijers JFM, Van Meegen E, Van Der Meer FJM, Van Wijk EM, et al. VKORC1 and CYP2C9 genotypes and phenprocoumon anticoagulation status: interaction between both genotypes affects dose requirement. Clin Pharmacol Ther. 2007;81(2):185–93.
139. Wadelius M, Chen LY, Lindh JD, Eriksson N, Ghori MJR, Bumpstead S, et al. The largest prospective warfarin-treated cohort supports genetic forecasting. Blood. 2009;113(4):784–92.

140. Manolopoulos VG, Ragia G, Tavridou A. Pharmacogenetics of coumarinic oral anticoagulants. Pharmacogenomics. 2010;11(4):493–6.
141. Aithal GP, Day CP, Kesteven PJL, Daly AK. Association of polymorphisms in the cytochrome P450 CYP2C9 with warfarin dose requirement and risk of bleeding complications. Lancet. 1999;353(9154):717–9.
142. Lee CR, Goldstein JA, Pieper JA. Cytochrome P450 2C9 polymorphisms: a comprehensive review of the in-vitro and human data. Pharmacogenetics. 2002;12(3):251–63.
143. Johnson JA, Gong L, Whirl-Carrillo M, Gage BF, Scott SA, Stein CM, et al. Clinical pharmacogenetics implementation consortium guidelines for CYP2C9 and VKORC1 genotypes and warfarin dosing. Clin Pharmacol Ther. 2011;90(4):625–9.
144. Limdi NA, Arnett DK, Goldstein JA, Beasley TM, McGwin G, Adler BK, et al. Influence of CYP2C9 and VKORC1 on warfarin dose, anticoagulation attainment and maintenance among European-Americans and African-Americans. Pharmacogenomics. 2008;9(5):511–26.
145. Rieder MJ, Reiner AP, Gage BF, Nickerson DA, Eby CS, McLeod HL, et al. Effect of VKORC1 haplotypes on transcriptional regulation and warfarin dose. N Engl J Med. 2005;352(22):2285–93.
146. Yuan HY, Chen JJ, Lee MTM, Wung JC, Chen YF, Charng MJ, et al. A novel functional VKORC1 promoter polymorphism is associated with inter-individual and inter-ethnic differences in warfarin sensitivity. Hum Mol Genet. 2005;14(13):1745–51.
147. Watzka M, Geisen C, Bevans CG, Sittinger K, Spohn G, Rost S, et al. Thirteen novel VKORC1 mutations associated with oral anticoagulant resistance: insights into improved patient diagnosis and treatment. J Thromb Haemost. 2011;9(1):109–18.
148. Ross S, Paré G. Pharmacogenetics of stroke. Stroke. 2018;49(10):2541–8.
149. McDonald MG, Rieder MJ, Nakano M, Hsia CK, Rettie AE. CYP4F2 is a vitamin K1 oxidase: an explanation for altered warfarin dose in carriers of the V433M variant. Mol Pharmacol. 2009;75(6):1337–46.
150. Sconce EA, Khan TI, Wynne HA, Avery P, Monkhouse L, King BP, et al. The impact of CYP2C9 and VKORC1 genetic polymorphism and patient characteristics upon warfarin dose requirements: proposal for a new dosing regimen. Blood. 2005;106(7):2329–33.
151. Gage BF, Eby C, Johnson JA, Deych E, Rieder MJ, Ridker PM, et al. Use of pharmacogenetic and clinical factors to predict the therapeutic dose of warfarin. Clin Pharmacol Ther. 2008;84(3):326–31.
152. Limdi NA, Wadelius M, Cavallari L, Eriksson N, Crawford DC, Lee MTM, et al. Warfarin pharmacogenetics: a single VKORC1 polymorphism is predictive of dose across 3 racial groups. Blood. 2010;115(18):3827–34.
153. López-López JA, Sterne JAC, Thom HHZ, Higgins JPT, Hingorani AD, Okoli GN, et al. Oral anticoagulants for prevention of stroke in atrial fibrillation: systematic review, network meta-analysis, and cost effectiveness analysis. BMJ. 2017;359(j5058):1–13.
154. Camm AJ, Fox KAA, Peterson E. Challenges in comparing the non-vitamin K antagonist oral anticoagulants for atrial fibrillation-related stroke prevention. Europace. 2018;20(1):1–11.
155. Gómez-Outes A, Suárez-Gea ML, Lecumberri R, Terleira-Fernández AI, Vargas-Castrillón E. Direct-acting oral anticoagulants: pharmacology, indications, management, and future perspectives. Eur J Haematol. 2015;95(5):389–404.
156. Connolly SJ, Ezekowitz MD, Yusuf S, Eikelboom J, Oldgren J, Parekh A, et al. Dabigatran versus warfarin in patients with atrial fibrillation. N Engl J Med. 2009;361(12):1139–51.
157. Diener H-C, Connolly SJ, Ezekowitz MD, Wallentin L, Reilly PA, Yang S, et al. Dabigatran compared with warfarin in patients with atrial fibrillation and previous transient ischaemic attack or stroke: a subgroup analysis of the RE-LY trial. Lancet Neurol. 2010;9(12):1157–63.
158. Patel MR, Mahaffey KW, Garg J, Pan G, Singer DE, Hacke W, et al. Rivaroxaban versus warfarin in nonvalvular atrial fibrillation. N Engl J Med. 2011;365(10):883–91.
159. Hankey GJ, Patel MR, Stevens SR, Becker RC, Breithardt G, Carolei A, et al. Rivaroxaban compared with warfarin in patients with atrial fibrillation and previous stroke or transient ischaemic attack: a subgroup analysis of ROCKET AF. Lancet Neurol. 2012;11(4):315–22.

160. Granger CB, Alexander JH, McMurray JJV, Lopes RD, Hylek EM, Hanna M, et al. Apixaban versus warfarin in patients with atrial fibrillation. N Engl J Med. 2011;365(11):981–92.
161. Easton JD, Lopes RD, Bahit MC, Wojdyla DM, Granger CB, Wallentin L, et al. Apixaban compared with warfarin in patients with atrial fibrillation and previous stroke or transient ischaemic attack: a subgroup analysis of the ARISTOTLE trial. Lancet Neurol. 2012;11(6):503–11.
162. Giugliano RP, Ruff CT, Braunwald E, Murphy SA, Wiviott SD, Halperin JL, et al. Edoxaban versus warfarin in patients with atrial fibrillation. N Engl J Med. 2013;369(22):2093–104.
163. Rost NS, Giugliano RP, Ruff CT, Murphy SA, Crompton AE, Norden AD, et al. Outcomes with edoxaban versus warfarin in patients with previous cerebrovascular events: findings from ENGAGE AF-TIMI 48 (effective anticoagulation with factor Xa next generation in atrial fibrillation-thrombolysis in myocardial infarction 48). Stroke. 2016;47(8):2075–82.
164. Steffel J, Verhamme P, Potpara TS, Albaladejo P, Antz M, Desteghe L, et al. The 2018 European Heart Rhythm Association Practical Guide on the use of non-vitamin K antagonist oral anticoagulants in patients with atrial fibrillation: executive summary. Europace. 2018;20(8):1231–42.
165. Eikelboom JW, Connolly SJ, Brueckmann M, Granger CB, Kappetein AP, Mack MJ, et al. Dabigatran versus warfarin in patients with mechanical heart valves. N Engl J Med. 2013;369(13):1206–14.
166. Ferro JM, Coutinho JM, Dentali F, Kobayashi A, Alasheev A, Canhão P, et al. Safety and efficacy of dabigatran etexilate vs. dose-adjusted warfarin in patients with cerebral venous thrombosis: a randomized clinical trial. JAMA Neurol. 2019;76(12):1457–65.
167. Miranda B, Aaron S, Arauz A, Barinagarrementeria F, Borhani-Haghighi A, Carvalho M, et al. The benefit of EXtending oral antiCOAgulation treatment (EXCOA) after acute cerebral vein thrombosis (CVT): EXCOA-CVT cluster randomized trial protocol. Int J Stroke. 2018;13(7):771–4.
168. Pollack CV, Reilly PA, Eikelboom J, Glund S, Verhamme P, Bernstein RA, et al. Idarucizumab for dabigatran reversal. N Engl J Med. 2015;373(6):511–20.
169. Dobesh PP, Bhatt SH, Trujillo TC, Glaubius K. Antidotes for reversal of direct oral anticoagulants. Pharmacol Ther. 2019;204:107405.
170. Eikelboom JW, Quinlan DJ, Van Ryn J, Weitz JI. Idarucizumab the antidote for reversal of dabigatran. Circulation. 2015;132(25):2412–22.
171. Tse DM, Young L, Ranta A, Barber PA. Intravenous alteplase and endovascular clot retrieval following reversal of dabigatran with idarucizumab. J Neurol Neurosurg Psychiatry. 2018;89(5):549–50.
172. Zhao H, Coote S, Pesavento L, Jones B, Rodrigues E, Ng JL, et al. Prehospital idarucizumab prior to intravenous thrombolysis in a mobile stroke unit. Int J Stroke. 2019;14(3):265–9.
173. Barber PA, Wu TY, Ranta A. Stroke reperfusion therapy following dabigatran reversal with idarucizumab in a national cohort. Neurology. 2020;94(19):e1968–72.
174. Beharry J, Waters MJ, Drew R, Fink JN, Wilson D, Campbell BCV, et al. Dabigatran reversal before intravenous tenecteplase in acute ischemic stroke. Stroke. 2020;51:1616–9.
175. Diener HC, Bernstein R, Butcher K, Campbell B, Cloud G, Davalos A, et al. Thrombolysis and thrombectomy in patients treated with dabigatran with acute ischemic stroke: expert opinion. Int J Stroke. 2017;12(1):9–12.
176. Seiffge DJ, Polymeris AA, Fladt J, Lyrer PA, Engelter ST, De Marchis GM. Management of patients with stroke treated with direct oral anticoagulants. J Neurol. 2018;265(12):3022–33.
177. Wieland E, Shipkova M. Pharmacokinetic and pharmacodynamic drug monitoring of direct-acting oral anticoagulants. Ther Drug Monit. 2019;41(2):180–91.
178. Lu G, Deguzman FR, Hollenbach SJ, Karbarz MJ, Abe K, Lee G, et al. A specific antidote for reversal of anticoagulation by direct and indirect inhibitors of coagulation factor Xa. Nat Med. 2013;19(4):446–51.
179. Connolly SJ, Milling TJ, Eikelboom JW, Michael Gibson C, Curnutte JT, Gold A, et al. Andexanet alfa for acute major bleeding associated with factor Xa inhibitors. N Engl J Med. 2016;375(12):1131–41.

180. Mueck W, Stampfuss J, Kubitza D, Becka M. Clinical pharmacokinetic and pharmacodynamic profile of rivaroxaban. Clin Pharmacokinet. 2014;53(1):1–16.
181. Kubitza D, Becka M, Voith B, Zuehlsdorf M, Wensing G. Safety, pharmacodynamics, and pharmacokinetics of single doses of BAY 59-7939, an oral, direct factor Xa inhibitor. Clin Pharmacol Ther. 2005;78(4):412–21.
182. Stampfuss J, Kubitza D, Becka M, Mueck W. The effect of food on the absorption and pharmacokinetics of rivaroxaban. Int J Clin Pharmacol Ther. 2013;51(7):549–61.
183. Byon W, Garonzik S, Boyd RA, Frost CE. Apixaban: a clinical pharmacokinetic and pharmacodynamic review. Clin Pharmacokinet. 2019;58(10):1265–79.
184. Stacy ZA, Call WB, Hartmann AP, Peters GL, Richter SK. Edoxaban: a comprehensive review of the pharmacology and clinical data for the management of atrial fibrillation and venous thromboembolism. Cardiol Ther. 2016;5(1):1–18.
185. Parasrampuria DA, Truitt KE. Pharmacokinetics and pharmacodynamics of edoxaban, a non-vitamin K antagonist oral anticoagulant that inhibits clotting factor Xa. Clin Pharmacokinet. 2016;55(6):641–55.
186. Chan N, Sager PT, Lawrence J, Ortel T, Reilly P, Berkowitz S, et al. Is there a role for pharmacokinetic/pharmacodynamic-guided dosing for novel oral anticoagulants? Am Heart J. 2018;199:59–67.
187. Kanuri SH, Kreutz RP. Pharmacogenomics of novel direct oral anticoagulants: newly identified genes and genetic variants. J Pers Med. 2019;9(1):7.
188. Kampouraki E, Kamali F. Pharmacogenetics of anticoagulants used for stroke prevention in patients with atrial fibrillation. Expert Opin Drug Metab Toxicol. 2019;15(6):449–58.
189. Paré G, Eriksson N, Lehr T, Connolly S, Eikelboom J, Ezekowitz MD, et al. Genetic determinants of dabigatran plasma levels and their relation to bleeding. Circulation. 2013;127(13):1404–12.
190. Sychev DA, Levanov AN, Shelekhova TV, Bochkov PO, Denisenko NP, Ryzhikova KA, et al. The impact of ABCB1 (rs1045642 and rs4148738) and CES1 (rs2244613) gene polymorphisms on dabigatran equilibrium peak concentration in patients after total knee arthroplasty. Pharmgenomics Pers Med. 2018;11:127–37.
191. Ing Lorenzini K, Daali Y, Fontana P, Desmeules J, Samer C. Rivaroxaban-induced hemorrhage associated with ABCB1 genetic defect. Front Pharmacol. 2016;7:494.
192. Gouin-Thibault I, Delavenne X, Blanchard A, Siguret V, Salem JE, Narjoz C, et al. Interindividual variability in dabigatran and rivaroxaban exposure: contribution of ABCB1 genetic polymorphisms and interaction with clarithromycin. J Thromb Haemost. 2017;15(2):273–83.
193. Nagar S, Walther S, Blanchard RL. Sulfotransferase (SULT) 1A1 polymorphic variants *1, *2, and *3 are associated with altered enzymatic activity, cellular phenotype, and protein degradation. Mol Pharmacol. 2006;69(6):2084–92.
194. Kryukov AV, Sychev DA, Andreev DA, Ryzhikova KA, Grishina EA, Ryabova AV, et al. Influence of ABCB1 and CYP3A5 gene polymorphisms on pharmacokinetics of apixaban in patients with atrial fibrillation and acute stroke. Pharmgenomics Pers Med. 2018;11:43–9.
195. Hinman JD, Rost NS, Leung TW, Montaner J, Muir KW, Brown S, et al. Principles of precision medicine in stroke. J Neurol Neurosurg Psychiatry. 2017;88(1):54–61.
196. Rostanski SK, Marshall RS. Precision medicine for ischemic stroke. JAMA Neurol. 2016;73(7):773.
197. Lin Y, Li Z, Liu C, Wang Y. Towards precision medicine in ischemic stroke and transient ischemic attack. Front Biosci. 2018;23(7):1338–59.
198. Verbelen M, Weale ME, Lewis CM. Cost-effectiveness of pharmacogenetic-guided treatment: are we there yet? Pharmacogenomics J. 2017;17(5):395–402.

Current Applications of Precision Medicine in Stroke: Acute Stroke Imaging

6

Luisa Biscoito

Abbreviations

ACA	Anterior cerebral artery
ADC	Apparent diffusion coefficient
AF	Atrial fibrillation
AIS	Acute ischemic stroke
ATP	Adenosine triphosphate
BBB	Blood-brain barrier
CAD	Carotid artery disease
CBF	Cerebral blood flow
CBV	Cerebral blood volume
COVID	Coronavirus disease
CT	Computerized tomography
CTA	Computerized tomography angiography
CTA-SI	Computerized tomography angiography-source images
DAPT	Dual-antiplatelet treatment
DWI	Diffusion-weighted imaging
ECA	External carotid artery
ECASS	European Cooperative Acute Stroke Study
EVT	Endovascular treatment
FLAIR	Fluid-attenuated inversion recovery
ICA	Internal carotid artery
ICH	Intracranial hemorrhage
LVO	Large vessel occlusion
MCA	Middle cerebral artery
MPR	Multiplanar volume reformat

L. Biscoito (✉)
Interventional/Neuroradiology Department, University Hospital Santa Maria, Lisbon, Portugal

© Springer Nature Switzerland AG 2021
A. C. Fonseca, J. M. Ferro (eds.), *Precision Medicine in Stroke*,
https://doi.org/10.1007/978-3-030-70761-3_6

MR	Magnetic resonance
mRS	Modified Rankin scale
mTICI	Modified treatment in cerebral infarction
MTT	Mean transit time
NCCT	Noncontrast computerized tomography
NIHSS	National Institutes of Health Stroke Scale
NINDS	National Institute of Neurological Disorders and Stroke
PCA	Posterior cerebral artery
PWI	Perfusion-weighted imaging
RCT	Randomized clinical trials
SWI	Susceptibility-weighted imaging
tPA	Tissue plasminogen activator
VA	Vertebral artery
VEGF	Vascular endothelial growth factor

6.1 Introduction

Ischemic stroke contributes heavily to the global burden of disease. It represents more than 80% of all strokes and happens when there is a blockage to the blood supply and subsequently a significant decrease in the cerebral blood flow to the brain.

For many years the healthcare community developed multiple scientific studies to better understand the causes of stroke and its pathophysiology and improve image diagnosis to better support adequate treatment.

In the 1980s, the first studies demonstrated that management of patients with acute stroke in stroke units had better outcomes [1].

It was in the 1990s, with intravenous fibrinolysis, that a qualitative leap in treatment was achieved with a remarkable improvement in the outcome of patients suffering from an ischemic stroke [2]. However, not all the patients meet the criteria that permit such treatment and the efficacity of IV fibrinolysis in ischemic stroke with large vessel occlusion (LVO) remains below the expectation [3].

More recently, in 2015, five randomized clinical trials heralded a change in the way ischemic stroke will be treated as standard [4–8]. The results proved that in certain selected patients with ischemic stroke due to large vessel occlusion, thrombectomy will lead to a better outcome compared to patients who did not receive thrombectomy. A real revolution has taken place in the treatment of ischemic stroke with LVO and thrombectomy become the standard treatment in ischemic stroke with large vessel occlusion.

The evolution in ischemic stroke treatment is closely related to the evolution in imaging since diagnosis through CT, MR, and angiography represents a crucial point to achieve the diagnosis itself and select patients that might be treated. Imaging became one of the major criteria to select patients for treatment [9].

Nevertheless, there are patients who do not fully meet the inclusion criteria of the guidelines but who still benefit from treatment and other patients which, despite meeting the selecting criteria, do not have the expected final result.

A number of individual factors are likely to be involved and the treatment result could be optimized if a tailored treatment according to individual characteristics of the patient (genetic, biological) could be performed. This is the role of precision medicine (tailored diagnosis and therapy for each individual patient based on the principle that subpopulations of patients exist that have different susceptibility to a disease and to treatment) applied to stroke [10].

This individual susceptibility is multifactorial depending on genetic, environment, and lifestyle factors. Genetic inheritance leading to biological effects is not dependent on the individual. Environment factors depend in a certain way on humankind and lifestyle is dependent on the individual. Nonetheless, individuals do not react in the same way when exposed to the same aggressors.

From a precision medicine point of view, which tailors diagnosis and treatment for each individual patient, it is important to collect clinical, biological, and imaging data, so that appropriate analysis can be done and applied to individualized decision-making. We depart from a collective projection that has individual repercussions.

Applying the concept of precision medicine to imaging in stroke refers to finding the most adequate imaging modality to then allow the best treatment option taking into account individual susceptibility for the disease.

If this "individualized" treatment were accomplished, it could allow patients to receive the benefit of treatment with the smallest possible risk. It could also extend the treatment to wider populations so they could benefit from treatment and save costs from futile maneuvers. With better rationalization of costs more patients can be treated.

Imaging has a central and irreplaceable role in the characterization of different etiological types of stroke and also in assigning specific treatments to each individual. Imaging is mandatory in stroke evaluation and extracting the maximum information means more precision can be applied to each patient and so determine the best treatment option.

In this chapter we present the current diagnostic imaging tools, matching of patients to the best treatment options, and the imaging tools used for mechanical reperfusion treatment.

6.2 Imaging and Diagnosis

6.2.1 Etiology

Identifying the cause of stroke is extremely important. There are five major causes of ischemic stroke according to the TOAST classification: Large artery disease is the most common stroke etiology in the world. It includes intra (ICAD) and extracranial disease (ECAD). These two locations correspond to different treatment strategies. Cardiac embolisms account for 15–30%. Aptly named "lacunar strokes" are small areas of infarct within the perforator territory and account for 15–20%. Uncommon causes (dissection, vasculitis) make up the remainder etiologies.

Imaging tools like CT/CTA and MR/MRA add essential information to differentiate the etiologic groups of ischemic stroke by categorizing different patterns of parenchyma involvement and angioarchitecture changes.

In acute treatment of ischemic stroke there are two main groups of patients that should be considered: those that have intracranial large vessel occlusions (LVO) (Fig. 6.1) and those that have not (Fig. 6.2), independently from etiology. These two groups of patients are of importance to identify since treatment differs (see treatment section).

Ischemic stroke with LVO accounts for around one-third of acute ischemic strokes [11] and may be due to several causes: embolic (cardiac, extracranial atherosclerosis (Fig. 6.3), dissection (Fig. 6.4), web (Fig. 6.5)) and local artery disease (atherosclerotic stenosis, dissection, vasculitis).

In embolic strokes, the origin of the clot may give a clue about its composition and this may influence the kind of device that will be used in thrombectomy to retrieve the clot. By imaging clot analysis some information can be extrapolated [12, 13].

In local artery disease, vessel analysis by MR may contribute to understanding the occlusion or vessel stenosis and underlying disease. However, this technique is not feasible in the acute phase.

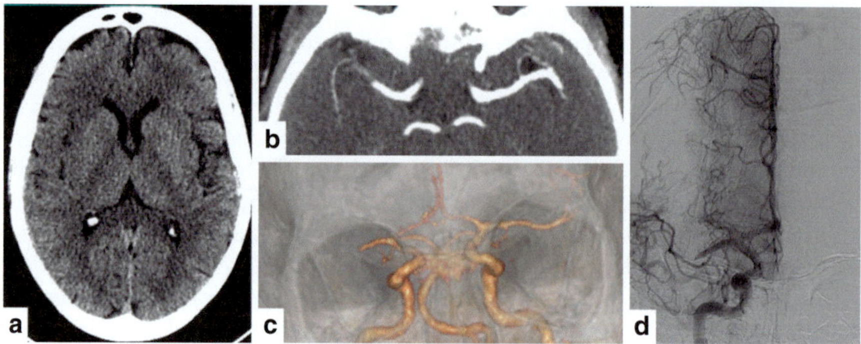

Fig. 6.1 Ischemic stroke with large vessel occlusion. Right insular ribbon hypoatennuation in NCCT (**a**). CTA filling defect in right MCA (**b**, **c**). Distal right MCA occlusion in DSA (**d**)

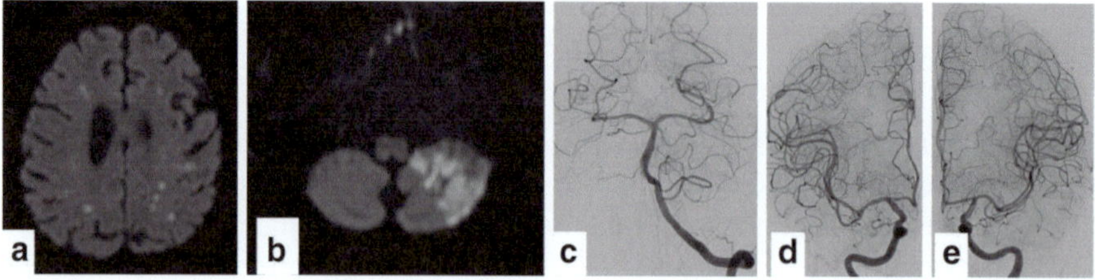

Fig. 6.2 Multiple acute ischemic stroke without large vessel occlusion. Several bright small lesions in DWI in white matter in brain hemispheres (**a**) and a larger one in left cerebellum hemisphere (**b**). Normal left vertebral and bilateral internal carotid DSA (**c–e**)

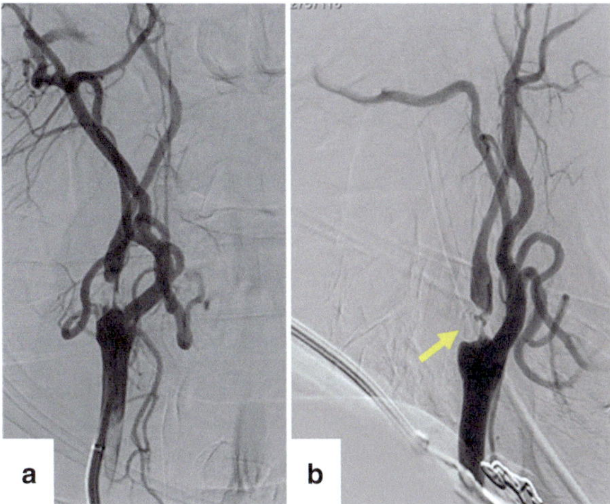

Fig. 6.3 Steno-occlusive disease with pre-obliterative right bulbar internal carotid plaque (yellow arrow). AP view (**a**). Lateral view (**b**)

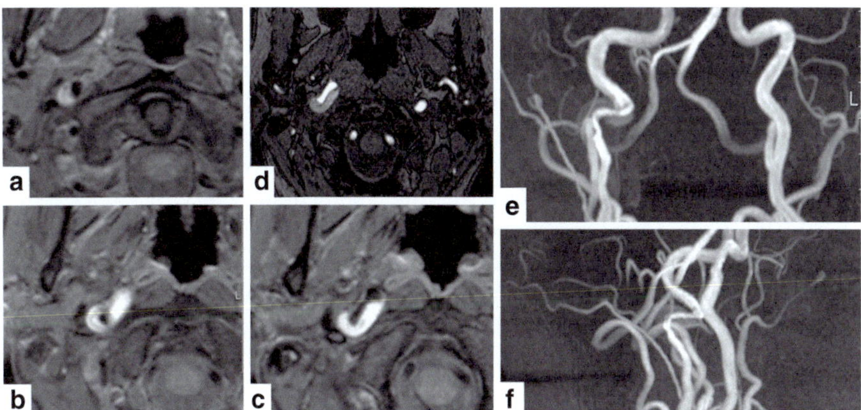

Fig. 6.4 Right internal carotid artery dissection. TIWI fat-saturated image demonstrates intramural hematoma (**a–c**). MRA TOF shows periarterial hypersignal (**d**) and vessel irregularity with lumen narrow (**e, f**)

6.2.2 Pathophysiology

Ischemic stroke happens when for some reason there is an obstruction of blood supply to the brain. As CBF (volume of blood that moves through a given unit of brain per unit time) and oxygen supply are reduced, adenosine triphosphate (ATP) will drop in ischemic tissue leading to energy-dependent membrane pump failure, increased glutamate release, and finally brain edema. If flow is not restored this is followed by blood-brain barrier (BBB) disruption resulting in an increased

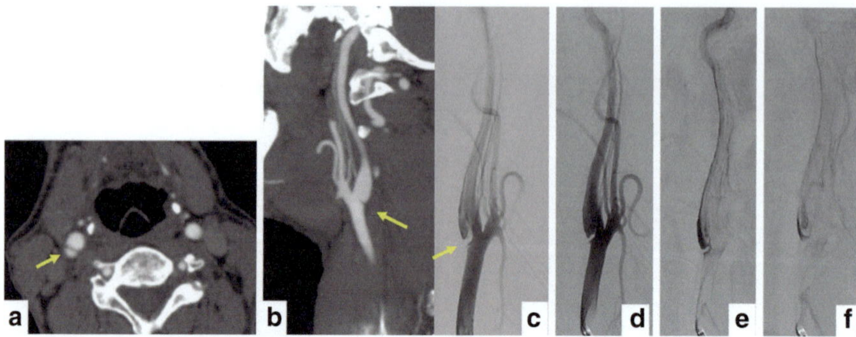

Fig. 6.5 Carotid artery web in a patient with LVO ischemic stroke (yellow arrow). Axial CTA shows a thin-line structure in the carotid artery lumen (**a**). Sag MIP CTA shows a linear indentation at the basis of posterior wall of bulb projecting superiorly (**b**). DSA with a thin 'shelf-like' filling defect and contrast stasis immediately distal to the web (**c–f**)

inflammatory response and neuronal death. Neurological impairment occurs when CBF drops below around 20 mL/100 g/min but this does not cause irreversibility damage as neuronal cells can tolerate CBF below 10 mL/100 g/min for a maximum of around 30 min; after this if no reperfusion is achieved neuronal cell death follows. For the ischemic core, that means irreversible cell death begins within minutes in areas of maximally reduced blood flow [14]. Different amounts of core reflect inter-individual differences such as collateral blood supply, rather than different time intervals between onset of symptoms and imaging studies. Thus, there is a highly variable core and this is a prognostic determinant in clinical outcome [15].

Neuronal cells can survive as under-perfused brain tissue with CBF values above 18 mL/100 mg/min for long periods of time (ischemic brain tissue with electric failure but no neuronal death). The area of the brain in this state is known as the penumbra [16]. Neuronal groups have different susceptibility to ischemic injury. Oligodendrocytes are more vulnerable than astroglial or endothelial cells. The white matter is more resistant to ischemia than gray matter so white matter has a longer time window; nevertheless infarcts of white matter cause severe disability.

Ischemic but not infarcted tissue can last for hours even days and tends to decrease with time [17]. The penumbra state is a dynamic process that depends on multiple factors; one of the more important is collateral circulation.

The size of the core and the penumbra in LVO stroke will depend on blood flow provided by collateral circulation.

Imaging contribution in acute ischemic stroke has evolved from an anatomical point of view to an anatomical and physiological concept that permits better identification of those patients that could benefit from reperfusion techniques.

Pathophysiology states in stroke are the target of precision medicine era regarding the treatment effect by measuring the prognostic value of different scenarios. Outlining subgroups at baseline pathophysiology by anatomical and functional selection may contribute to improving our aptitude to better choose the right treatment in order to obtain the best individualized treatment effect, rather than applying one treatment to a different, heterogeneous group of patients that probably will not benefit in the same way.

CT and MR are the two main imaging methods used for diagnosis and planning therapy in ischemic stroke. Depending on the availability and experience of the imaging department, the imaging investigation is done by one method or another. In some specific situations, CT may be followed by an MR. Each of them, CT and MR, have strengths, weaknesses, and limitations that are detailed below.

CT is easy to perform, fast, less costly, and widely available and has no absolute contraindications. However, there is some radiation exposure and it is difficult to interpret in patients with chronic ischemic disease and posterior fossa infarcts.

MR allows easy identification of an infarct by DWI and has no radiation exposure; however it needs more time, is more expensive, is less available, has some contraindications like metalwork and older pacemakers, and is not feasible in claustrophobic and uncooperative patients without anesthesia. MR has better resolution in posterior fossa than CT, making it the preferable method in such cases to visualize the infarcted area.

There are mainly four questions that should be answered by imaging methods in patients with suspicion of a stroke:
– Is the stroke hemorrhagic or ischemic?
– How extensive is the core (infarcted area)?
– Is there a large vessel occlusion?
– Is there still any tissue to be rescued (penumbra area)?

6.2.3 The Core

6.2.3.1 In CT

Noncontrast CT (NCCT) can rapidly exclude intracranial hemorrhage (ICH) (Fig. 6.6) or a stroke mimic.

In acute ischemic stroke, CT can either be negative or show early signs of infarct. CT scans measure X-ray beam attenuation through a region of interest. The attenuation is measured in HU (Hounsfield units) and is directly proportional to tissue density. For every 1% increase in water content, X-ray attenuation decreases 3–5% and that corresponds to a drop of 2.5 HU on CT.

Cytotoxic edema is not detected by CT since there is not a true increase in tissue water but a change of water in compartments (from extracellular to intracellular space). Hypoattenuation reflects the ionic edema that follows cytotoxic edema due to failure of ion pumps from inadequate ATP supply. In ionic edema, there is an uptake of water molecules from the intravascular to the extracellular space with a normal BBB [18]. Hypoattenuated regions on CT are likely to correspond to irreversibly infarcted tissue—core. Even if reperfusion is achieved this tissue that forms the core will not return to normal. This may be confirmed at CT scan control follow-up.

Sensitivity values for NCCT in detecting acute stroke vary in literature as they are dependent on the CT scanner's generation. In one study NCCT has 57% sensitivity for acute ischemic stroke [19]. This may be improved by using narrow window width to accentuate the contrast between normal and edematous tissue (up to 71%). It requires

Fig. 6.6 NCCT—spontaneous hyperattenuation in right thalamus and frontal horn which corresponds to acute hemorrhage with rupture to the ventricle

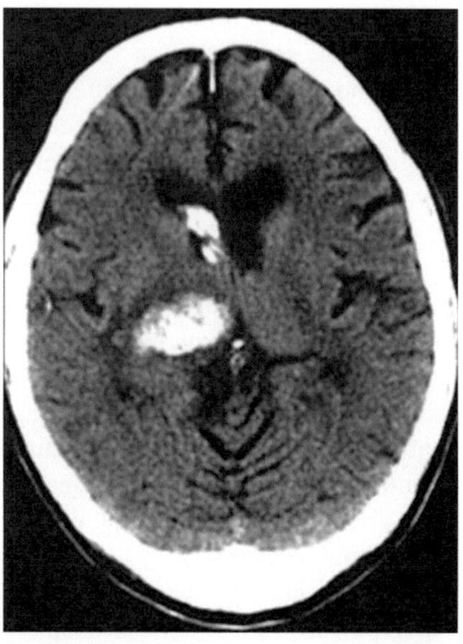

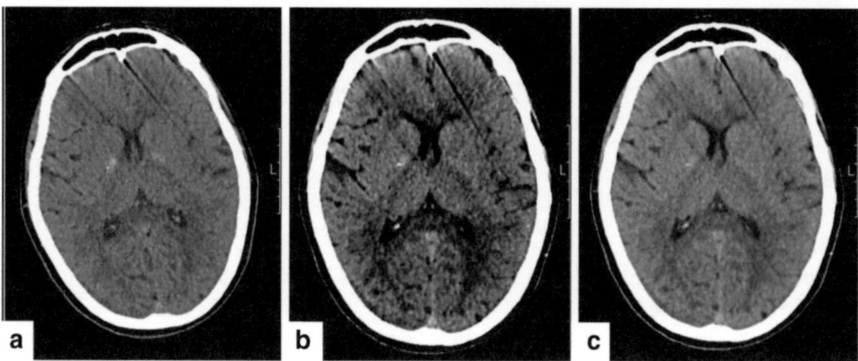

Fig. 6.7 Normal axial cut NCCT. Same cut with different white/gray matter interface contrast. Motion artifacts. Acquisition thin-cut images (**a**), narrow window and level settings (**b**), standard NCCT settings (**c**)

thick reconstruction images (4–6 mm) to guarantee an acceptable signal-to-noise ratio (SNR) and a level and window parameters that permit differentiation between gray and white matter (Fig. 6.7).

The **early signs of infarct** that can be found in the first 3–6 h after stroke onset are (Fig. 6.8):

- Loss of white/gray matter differentiation in cerebral cortical mantle in a vascular territory
- Loss of white/gray matter differentiation in basal ganglia
- Loss of the insular ribbon
- Cortical sulcal effacement

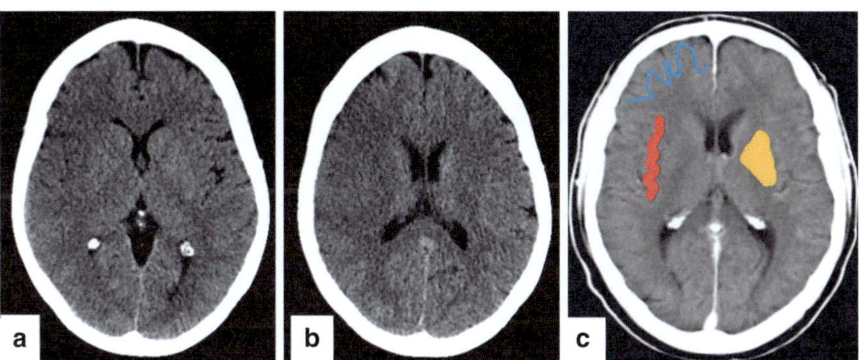

Fig. 6.8 Right MCA acute ischemic stroke. Early signs of ischemic stroke. Loss of insular ribbon (red), loss of white/gray matter differentiation in cortex (blue) and lentiform nucleus (yellow) (**a–c**)

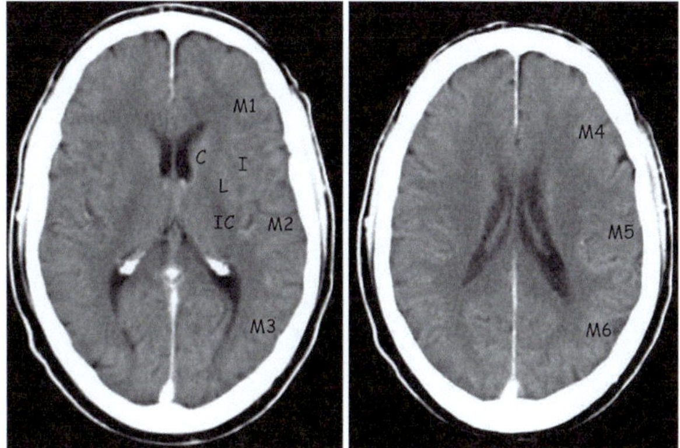

Fig. 6.9 ASPECTS. C—caudate; L—lentiform; IC—internal capsule; I—insulae; M1—anterior inferior frontal MCA cortex; M2—temporal lobe MCA cortex lateral to insular ribbon; M3—posterior temporal MCA cortex; M4, M5, and M6—anterior, lateral, and posterior MCA cortices above M1, M2, and M3

These changes can be semi-quantified with the ASPECTS (Alberta Stroke Program Early CT score) (Fig. 6.9) [20]. This score was developed to standardize detection and reports of the extent of hypoattenuation. ASPECTS analyzes two regions of MCA territory: the basal ganglia level and the supraganglionic level. Hypoattenuation should be visible in at least two consecutive cuts to ensure that it is truly abnormal and not an artifact. With a score of 10 points distributed by cortical (7) and deep (3) locations 1 point is subtracted from 10 for each region involved.

Three groups of ASPECTS may be considered regarding outcome: good (8–10) (Fig. 6.10a), moderate (5–7) (Fig. 6.10b), and bad (0–4) (Fig. 6.10c) according to results: good outcome (mRS 0–2) of 46%, 38.6%, and 5% and mortality of 19%, 28.9%, and 55%, respectively [21].

There are some limitations to this score: poor scan quality of image acquisition and old patients with leukoaraiosis may make interpretation difficult (Fig. 6.11); it

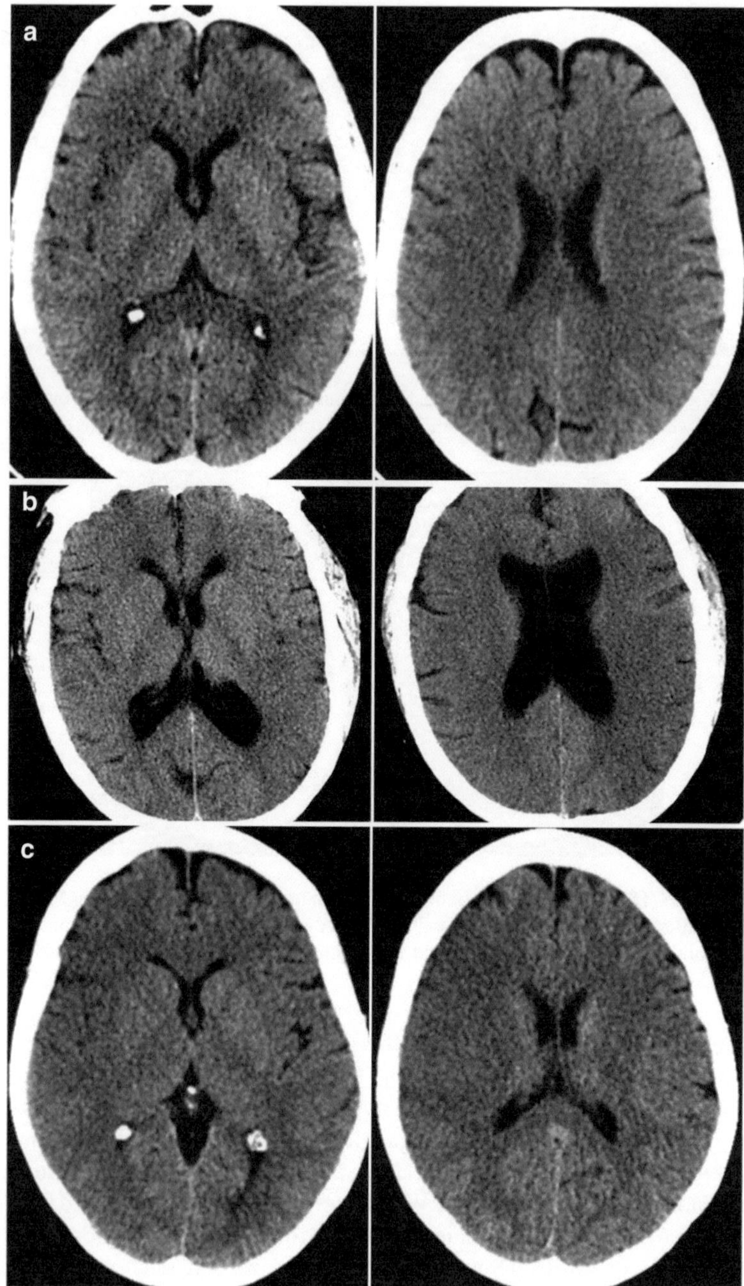

Fig. 6.10 (**a**) ASPECTS 9. Insular ribbon hypodensity on right hemisphere. (**b**) ASPECTS 5. M2, M3, M4, M5, M6 hypodensity on left hemisphere. (**c**) ASPECTS 3. L, I, M1, M2, M3, M4, M5 hypodensity on right hemisphere

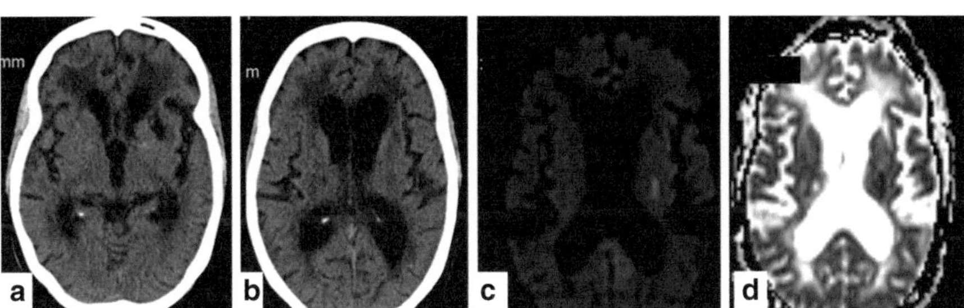

Fig. 6.11 Small acute infarct in a patient with leukoaraiosis. NCCT multiple hypodense lesions in white matter of corona radiata (**a**, **b**), DWI (**c**), and ADC (**d**) demonstrate small bright lesion on DWI and hypo on ADC in left supra-capsular white matter

is a score to be used in middle cerebral artery (MCA) infarcts; it does not take into account the different neurological weight of different locations (e.g.: an M3 or M5 has the same value as the caudate head); and it does not consider white matter infarct volume. White matter is more resistant to ischemia than gray matter but white matter infarcts cause severe disability due to damage to connecting fiber tracts (projection, association, commissural) passing through.

6.2.3.2 In MR

The core is represented by increased signal in diffusion-weighted imaging (DWI) which reflects the beginning of the transfer of water from extracellular to intracellular compartments secondary to ionic pump failure with a loss of ionic gradients (cytotoxic edema). Restriction in diffusion is observed as early as a few minutes (sensitivity from 88% to 100% and specificity from 86% to 100%) and apparent diffusion coefficient (ADC) progressively drops [22].

The DWI lesion at first represents tissue that is evolving to infarct, the final volume of which will depend on whether the surrounding tissue evolves or not from ischemia to infarct. Reversion of hypersignal in DWI is not frequent, and is usually partial and in regions where ADC values are not exceptionally low (Fig. 6.12). It may happen if reperfusion is quickly achieved. It may correspond to tissue with cytotoxic edema that did not evolve to ionic edema. In this situation, the lesion volume on DWI corresponds to areas of core plus areas still in penumbra. The degree of ADC decrease correlates with severity of perfusion deficits [23]. An ADC between 600 and 625 × 10^{-6} mm^2/s may correlate with infarct tissue—core (sensitivity 69% and specificity 78%) [24]. After a period of time, if no reperfusion occurs the bright signal on DWI will be the area of infarct.

The ADC values continue to decrease till 1–4 days when DWI is markedly hyperintense. The ADC returns to baseline at 1–2 weeks when DWI is mildly hyperintense. After this time, ADC becomes hyperintense due to increased extracellular water, tissue cavitation, and gliosis.

FLAIR sequence cannot detect early infarct because it requires a large increase of water in tissues to become hyperintense. Usually it becomes progressively positive (hyperintense after 4–4.5 h). With FLAIR it is possible to estimate the age of infarct in stroke with known and unknown time of onset (Fig. 6.13). It also provides diagnostic value in detecting hemorrhage.

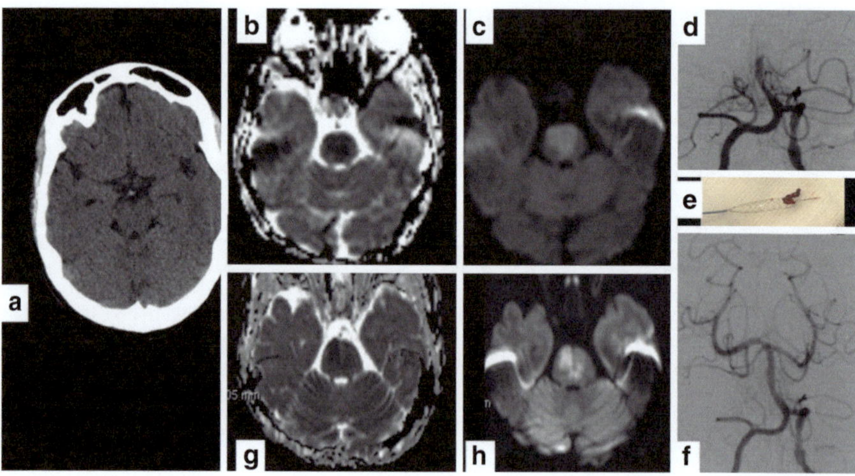

Fig. 6.12 34-Year-old woman with sudden loss of consciousness and progress to tetraparesis with total recovery 1 week after thrombectomy. Foramen ovale persistence was found. In NCCT the parenchyma is normal and hyperdensity in basilar artery is seen (**a**). DWI/ADC before thrombectomy demonstrates central pontine acute lesion (**b**, **c**). Occlusion of superior third of basilar artery (**d**). Stent retriever with clot (**e**). Total repermeabilization of basilar artery (**f**). DWI/ADC after thrombectomy shows partial reversion of hypersignal on DWI and hypo on ADC (**g**, **h**)

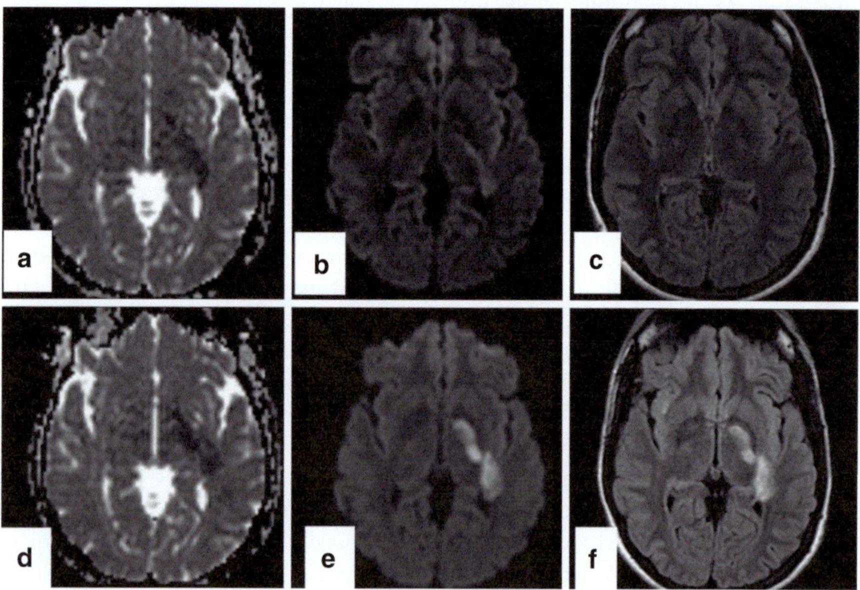

Fig. 6.13 Hyperacute ischemic stroke of left choroidal territory in a patient with unknown time of onset. Moderate bright signal in DWI and hyposignal on ADC in posterior limb of internal capsule with normal FLAIR correspond to an infarct less than 4–4.5 h (**a–c**). Twenty-four-hour follow-up demonstrates lesion on DWI, ADC, and FLAIR (**d–f**)

Gradient echo sequences (GRE) are used to detect hemorrhage (Fig. 6.14) concomitant with DWI and FLAIR (Fig. 6.15). GRE contributes also to detection of an intravascular clot.

Either in CT or in MR, evaluation of the core is an approximate measure mainly because there is no total consensus on the definition of core and there is a lack of validity parameters. Some authors propose the term severely ischemic tissue with uncertain viability (SIT-uv) instead of ischemic core [25].

6.2.4 The Clot

The location and extension of vessel occlusion may be characterized by clot analysis image. Clot components differ according to the underlying cause of stroke (atherosclerotic, cardiac). The clot may have a higher quantity of platelets or more red blood cells and fibrin, among other substances.

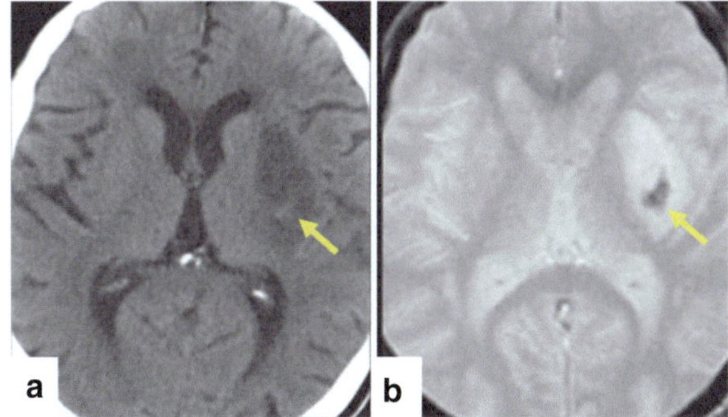

Fig. 6.14 Small hemorrhagic transformation in acute ischemic stroke of left nucleo-capsular region. NCCT (**a**). GRE (**b**)

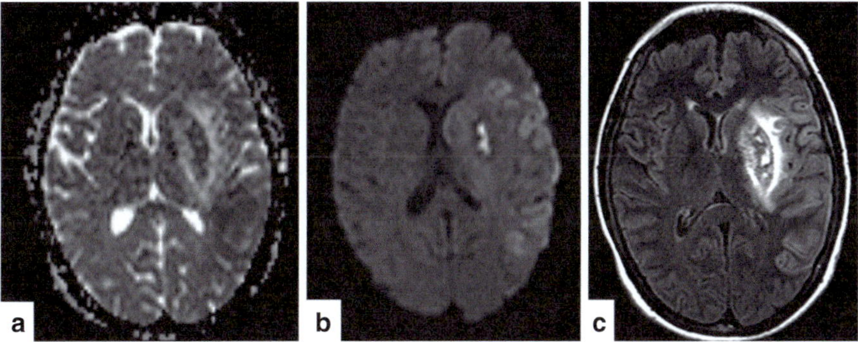

Fig. 6.15 Subacute ischemic infarct in left hemisphere with hemorrhagic transformation in lentiform nucleus. Normalizing DWI and ADC signal in cortex with hyperintensity in FLAIR. Small hemorrhagic transformation in lentiform nucleus—hypersignal in FLAIR (**c**) and DWI (**b**) and hyposignal in ADC (**a**)

For the time being, location of the thrombus is the only parameter that is considered in the majority of stroke treatment procedures. Recanalization with rt-PA has better results with distal rather than proximal occlusions [26].

Nevertheless, thrombus length, clot attenuation in CT, and clot burden score (CBS) [27] may be analyzed and knowing this additional information might have some influence in thrombolysis and thrombectomy decisions that later reflect in functional outcome.

CBS is a semiquantitative method to measure clot extension in the anterior circulation on CTA. It is scored on a scale from 0 to 10, knowing that a 10 score is absence of any filling defect on CTA and 0 indicates no contrast filling of all major intracranial ipsilateral arteries. Two points are subtracted for each segment that is not filling on CTA in M1 or supraclinoid ICA segment; one point is subtracted for each M2, A1, or infraclinoid ICA segment. A lower CBS means it is more likely to have a larger final infarct, hemorrhagic transformation, and a less independent functional outcome.

Distal clot locations, shorter clots, and a higher clot burden score all correlate with better functional outcome [28]. Red cell-rich thrombus is associated with better recanalization and a shorter procedure time [29]. Yet there is a lot of heterogeneity in thrombus content, and two extreme patterns of clot may be considered: platelet-rich clot (white clot) that formed in areas of high shear stress such as arterial systems, and red blood cell-rich clot (red clot) trapped in fibrin formed in low-pressure system such as cardiac atria or venous systems. But all clot compositions exist as a continuum and a secondary component that results from stasis around the occlusion site may contaminate the original clot composition.

Clot length seems to have an impact on recanalization with intravenous thrombolysis. Clots bigger than 8 mm have almost no potential for recanalization [30], but there is no evidence that this influences the success of recanalization by an endovascular approach. Even so, larger clots may be more difficult to extract and might be associated with no recanalization or more passes needed.

Research regarding the influence of clot composition and length on the selection of endovascular devices for thrombectomy is needed so first-pass recanalization and better outcome results are achieved [12].

In CT, hyperdense MCA signal (HMCAS) seen on unenhanced CT means part of the artery is denser than other parts of the vessel or its counterpart, not attributable to calcification. This was first described in 1990 [31] and is present in 40–60% of patients with occlusion of the MCA (Fig. 6.16). Absence of this signal does not exclude thrombotic occlusion (Fig. 6.17). It has high specificity but low sensitivity (47%). It should be measured in thin cuts (<2.5 mm) with three (rather than one) volumes of interest. The hyperdensity signal correlates with red blood cell quantity. There is no strict correlation between clot density and revascularization success in acute ischemic stroke [32].

In MR, the clot is seen as hyperintense in FLAIR and hypointense in magnetic susceptibility sequences with blooming effect in GRE or SWI. The underlining

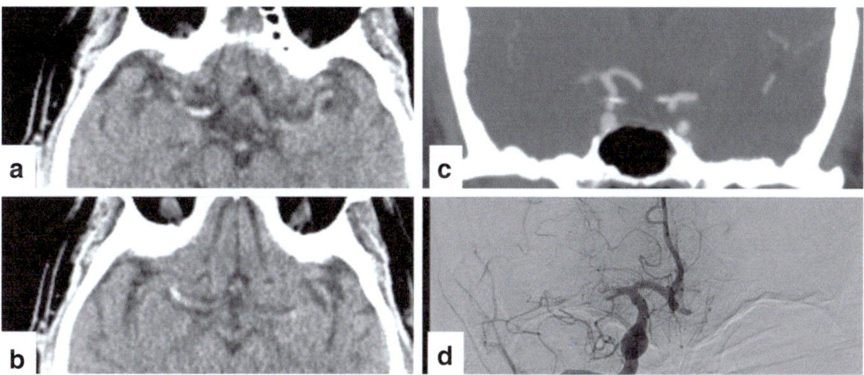

Fig. 6.16 Right MCA clot in M1 segment hyperdense in NCCT with more than 8 mm. Axial thin-cut NCCT—hyperdense sign in M1 segment (**a**, **b**). Coronal MIP CTA with filling defect since the proximal one-third M1 (**c**). DSA shows occlusive clot in M1 segment (**d**)

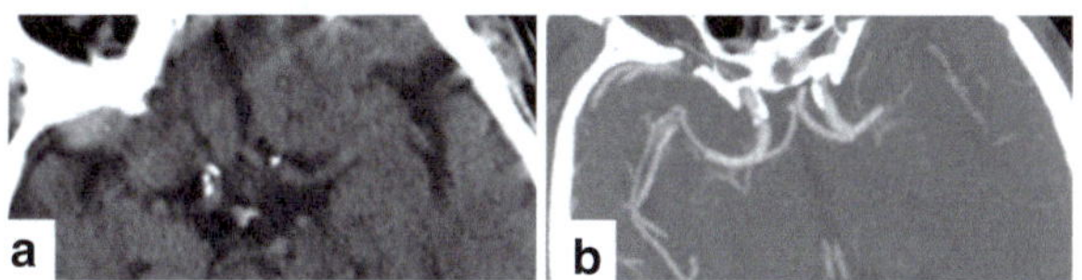

Fig. 6.17 Left MCA clot in M1 segment. Axial NCCT—clot is isodense (**a**). Axial MIP CTA with filling defect in distal 2/3 of M1 segment confirm occlusion (**b**)

concept is that paramagnetic deoxyhemoglobin trapped in red blood cells causes signal loss. Higher blooming effect signifies a greater red cell component and probability of originating from a cardiac source. This may have implications in therapeutic decisions regarding fibrinolysis, reperfusion, and prognostic value.

Studies did point out that susceptibility vessel sign (SVS) seen in GRE or SWI was associated with better recanalization [33].

Regarding the length of the clot, SVS may identify the proximal and distal end of the clot which is comparable to contrast gap in CTA or loss of signal in MRA. GRE shows a blooming effect that can extend beyond the real size of the thrombus. SWI is more accurate because it has less artifacts.

6.2.5 The Vessel Occlusion

CTA and MRA are now part of the standard diagnostic protocol.

The main objective of early vessel imaging is to determine as quickly as possible if there is a LVO that is amenable to thrombectomy.

The majority of imaging exams for any stroke triage planning are done by CT. It is faster, less costly, widely available, well tolerated, and less sensitive to motion artifacts than MRI.

Rather than studying only the intracranial circulation the study should also include the supra-aortic vessels. The CT scan acquisition should be from the aortic arch to vertex. This allows visualization of supra-aortic vessel origins, carotid bifurcations, and intracranial circulation and so reveals the status of large cervical vessels looking for atherosclerotic disease and dissection but also the intracranial occlusion site and collateral circulation pattern.

Performing cervical vessel studies is crucial to plan thrombectomy. A vessel abnormality can be seen, such as a tandem lesion, dissection, or tortuosity, that may make the access difficult (Fig. 6.18). Looking for such details permits a better plan for access (if femoral or radial) and informs if carotid stenting is needed.

Vascular imaging from an aortic arch to vertex saves time in procedure, increases safety, and optimizes the choice of device in thrombectomy. Intracranially, location of occlusion and morphology of the vessels will also dictate the choice of the device that will be used. Other vascular pathologies such as aneurysms (Figs. 6.19 and 6.20) and AVMs should be identified if present.

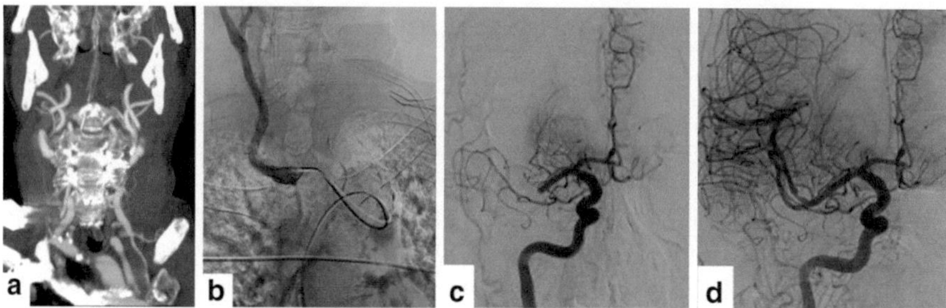

Fig. 6.18 78-Year-old woman with acute ischemic stroke with NIHSS 19, ASPECTS 6, and occlusion of right M1 segment. Cor MIP CTA from an aortic arch demonstrates tortuous supra-aortic vessel origin (**a**). Catheterization of right carotid artery with "Simmons" catheter (**b**) to perform angiography and progress to thrombectomy with recanalization of the vessel (**c, d**)

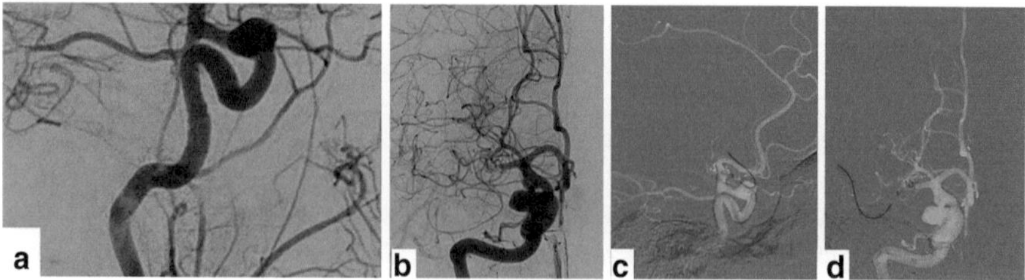

Fig. 6.19 Patient with ischemic stroke due to occlusion of right M1. Simultaneous nonrupture right carotid aneurysm. DSA lateral and AP view—occlusion of middle segment of M1 and carotid aneurysm pointing lateral (**a, b**). Thrombectomy by aspiration technique in M1 (**c, d**)

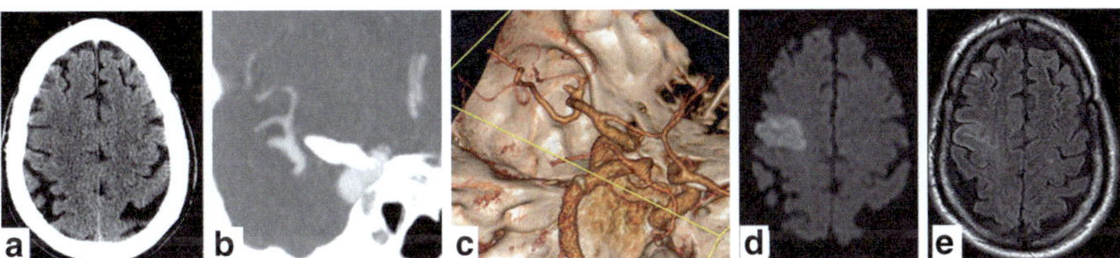

Fig. 6.20 Patient with left hemiparesis due to acute ischemic stroke without LVO and small berry aneurysm in right MCA bifurcation. Normal NCCT (**a**). Coronal MIP CTA with small aneurysm that should not be confounded with vessel occlusion (**b**). VR CTA small aneurysm point lateral with neck between the two M2 branches (**c**). Bright signal in DWI (**d**) with incipient hypersignal in FLAIR (**e**)

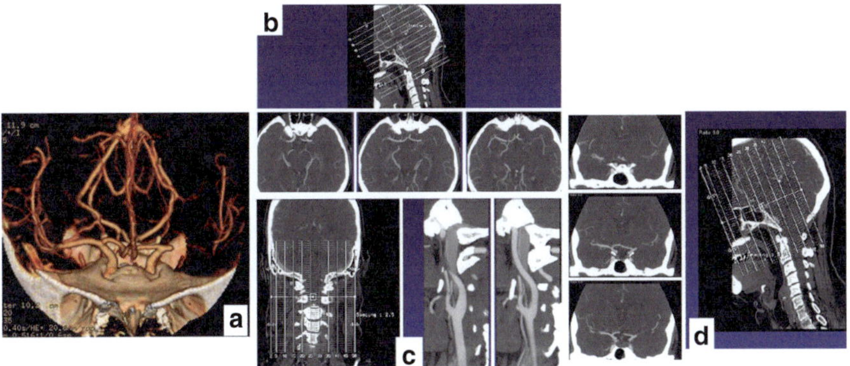

Fig. 6.21 Patient with occlusion of left M1 segment. CTA protocol. VR (**a**), axial MIP (**b**), sag MIP (**c**), cor MIP (**d**)

6.2.5.1 CTA

CTA is a thin-cut volumetric acquisition performed with a timed bolus of iodine contrast to enhance supra-aortic vessels and intracranial circulation in an arterial time, only with a tiny venous enhancement. Acquisition is performed from the aortic arch till vertex.

Evaluation of source images (CTA-SI) is done and multiplanar maximum intensity projection (MIP) with axial, coronal, and sagittal is reformatted usually with a 3 mm slab thickness with 0.5 cm overlap post-processed or thicker with 20 mm slice width. Volume rendering (VR) is also performed (Fig. 6.21). Multiple projection reconstructions (MPR) with the possibility to perform straight, oblique, curved plans are particularly useful to depict atherosclerotic plaques and intimal flaps.

The whole brain should be evaluated in CTA-SI with a narrow window to provide a "perfusion blood volume map" effect. The contrast fills the normal microvasculature but not the one in the infarcted region which is visualized as hypoattenuated parenchyma. This region is very well correlated with DWI hyperintense lesion and the low CBV seen in CT perfusion. CTA-SI is a stronger predictor of clinical outcome than the initial NIHSS score and may predict infarct volume and clinical outcome [34].

CTA identifies exactly the occlusion location by a segmental filling defect in the artery.

CTA has high sensitivity for LVO and specificity (98.4% and 98.1%) in proximal large vessels [35] with the possibility to easily identify the top of carotid "T" or "L" occlusions and more distal occlusions in the MCA or other intracranial vessels. Correlation of hyperattenuation vessel segment in NCCT (either in cervical or intracranial) if it exists with the filling defect in CTA should be done. Contrast filling in vessels distal to the occlusion represents collateral circulation.

Pseudo-occlusion of internal carotid or vertebrobasilar arteries from top of carotid or top of basilar thrombosis occlusion should not be confounded with true occlusion since they can mimic cervical occlusion due to a delay in contrast progression. For cervical vessels, CTA can depict dissection (Figs. 6.22 and 6.23) that is important to differentiate from pseudo-occlusion (Fig. 6.24).

Carotid bifurcation atherosclerotic disease can be identified with calcified plaques and plaque ulceration as also vulnerable plaque with noncalcified core. In those cases, curved MPR may be useful (Fig. 6.25).

CTA should be performed as a routine in stroke workup in all patients presenting with acute ischemic stroke within 24 h of last known well baseline NIHSS as it improves patient management and clinical outcome by increasing adequate treatment selection [36].

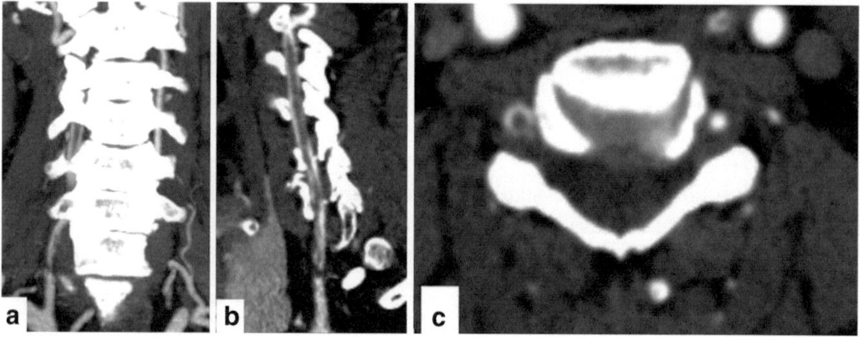

Fig. 6.22 Right vertebral dissection in the initial segment with focal stenosis and intraluminal distal clot in cervical vertebral. Cor MIP (**a**) and sag MIP CTA (**b**) with columnar centro-luminal filling defect. Axial MIP CTA with "donut" sign (**c**)

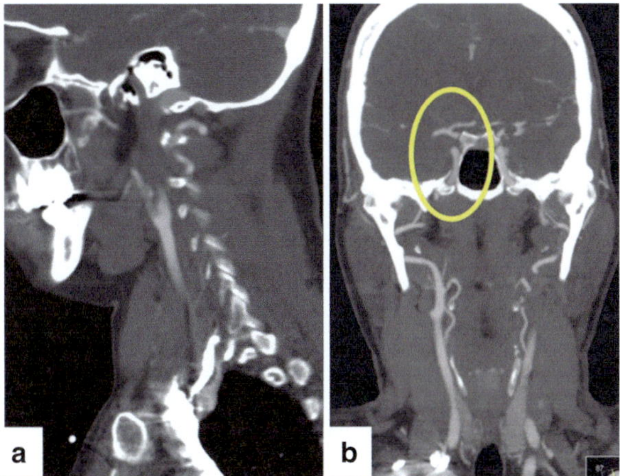

Fig. 6.23 Internal carotid artery dissection occlusive with filling of petrous, cavernous, and supra-clinoid segment by anastomosis with external carotid artery. This image differentiates from pseudo-occlusion by a distal clot in ICA. Sag MIP CTA—Distal to bulb an occlusion of the vessel with a flame-shaped end (**a**). Cor MIP CTA—normal filling of distal segments by collateral flow (**b**)

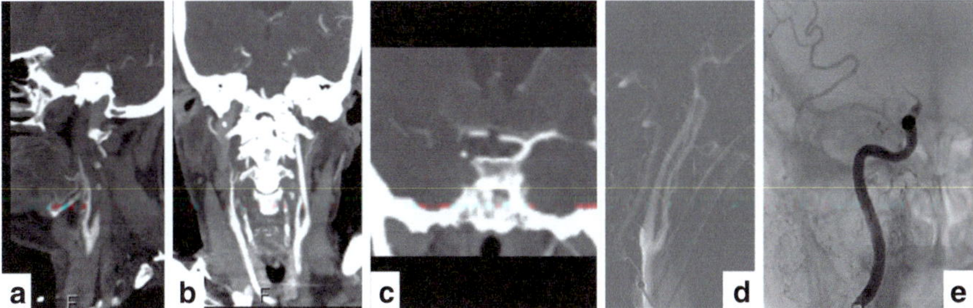

Fig. 6.24 Pseudo-occlusion right ICA due to a thrombus in distal ICA. Sag and cor MIP CTA—suprabulbar ICA is not filling with contrast and has a flame-shaped termination (**a**, **b**). Cavernous and supraclinoid segments of ICA are not filling with contrast (**c**). DSA shows normal morphology of cervical ICA (**d**). DSA—occlusion of distal ICA due to a clot (e)

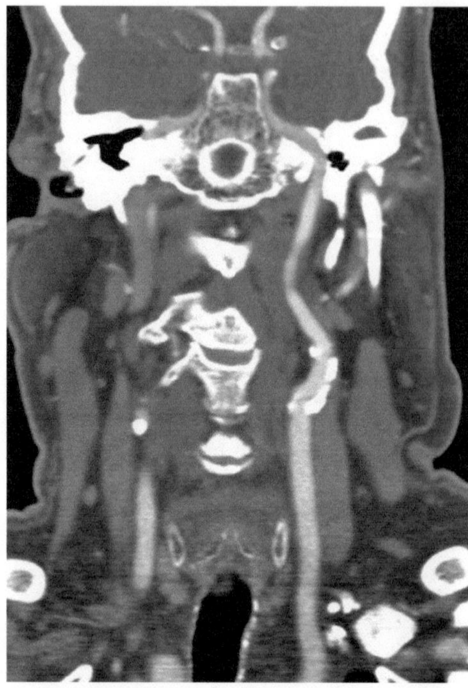

Fig. 6.25 Steno-occlusive disease of carotid. Curved cor MIP CTA—bulbar carotid plaque calcified nonocclusive

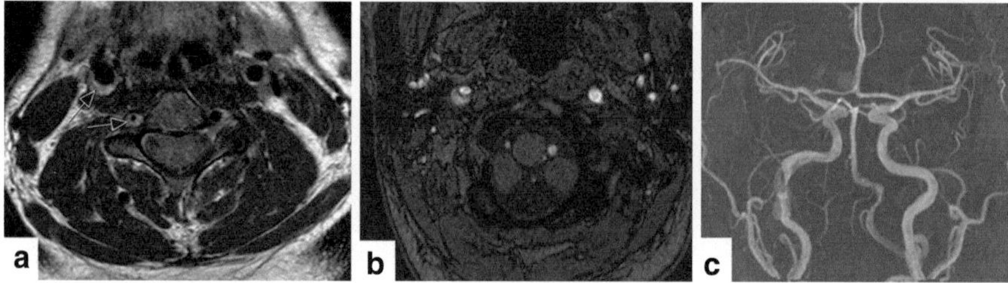

Fig. 6.26 Right internal carotid artery dissection. Axial T1WI—hyperintense signal at the periphery of right ICA (in crescent) consistent with intramural hematoma and at the periphery of vertebral artery (in ring) consistent with slow flow in hypoplastic artery (arrows) (**a**). Another case with right internal carotid dissection. Axial source image from 3D TOF with periarterial hyperintense signal in ICA which surrounds the narrow arterial lumen (in crescent) (**b**). Cor MIP MRA—narrow vessel segment surrounded by "tattoo" of mural hematoma (**c**)

6.2.5.2 MRA

The imaging techniques used in patients with acute ischemic stroke should point to the lesser time-consuming modalities, knowing that some patients are unstable and uncooperative.

Time-of-flight (TOF) MRA is a gradient echo sequence that has been used in routine stroke protocols to evaluate the status on intracranial and cervical arteries (Fig. 6.26). Disadvantages are the long acquisition time (6–7 min), and the fact that it is sensitive to movement and may overestimate arterial stenosis if slow or turbulent flow exists because the vessel contrast or flow-related enhancement is proportional to the speed of blood in the vessels.

More recently with CE-MRA (contrast-enhanced MRA) technique, images of head and neck can be obtained with less spatial resolution compared to TOF technique but with the advantage of being quicker and more tolerable for uncooperative patients [37]. It has the disadvantage that gadolinium is needed, and it cannot be repeated if needed till circulating gadolinium is cleared. In elderly patients with comorbidities and impairment of renal function that will probably need a thrombectomy in which more dye will be used (iodine) it may be a concern. Within a short time (less than 2 min) information about aortic arch, supra-aortic vessels, and intracranial vasculature is achieved. It is a technique less sensitive to turbulence and does not have signal loss due to saturation effects. These are the reasons why CE-MRA is preferred to TOF to evaluate patients with acute stroke.

6.2.6 The Collaterals

Collateral circulation is physiological and consists of specialized endogenous vessels present in tissues that protect against ischemic injury. The increased interest on collaterals is due to the capacity to restrict the growth of ischemic penumbra.

There is a personalized collateral pattern which results from a genetic background-dependent variation in collaterals and from acquired factors (like age, blood pressure, diabetes, smoking, cardiac disease, high uric acid level, dehydration). Duration of ischemia also seems to play a role but for the time being little is known about it [38].

Native collateral (preexisting) by sort of number and diameter play a critical role in the final expression of infarct tissue. Native pial collateral circulation (collaterogenesis) begins in the embryonic state and dictates the amount of collaterals in adulthood. Genetic background seems to be a major factor [39].

Collaterals are arterio-arteriolar connections (anastomosis) at the borders of main arterial routes which maintain the vascularization in a territory distal to an occlusion by reverse flow. The amount of this reverse flow by the collateral system is dependent on being an acute or progressive occlusion (collateral remodeling), site of occlusion, and some less understood process. It is known that two patients with the same location of vessel occlusion, same age, and same time of symptom onset may have different core/penumbra imaging and this is due to such a personalized system of collaterals

Collateral remodeling is stimulated by fluid shear stress, resulting in extension of increased collateral flow that depends on native collaterals and metabolic/molecular factors that mediate arteriogenesis. It is a dynamic process that starts when an occlusion or significant stenosis develops, as a response to provide perfusion and avoid infarct.

Regarding collaterals in brain system two main pathways are considered: extra and intracranial [40].

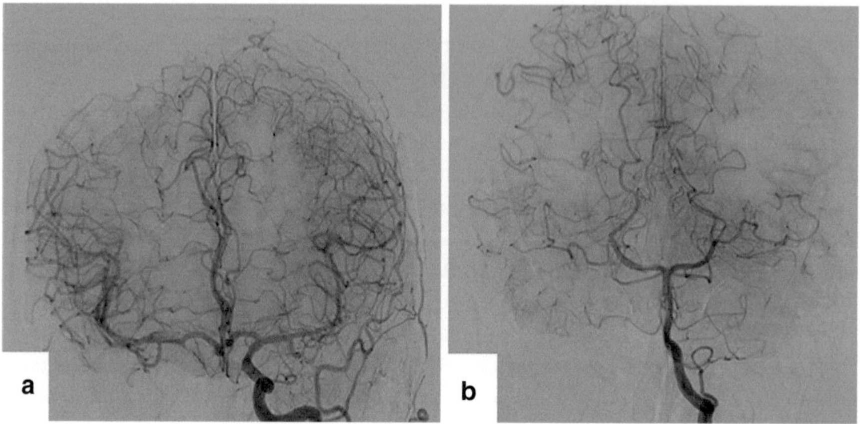

Fig. 6.27 Right internal carotid occlusion with collateral circulation. Through anterior communicating artery (**a**) and through cortico-pial anastomosis MCA-PCA (**b**)

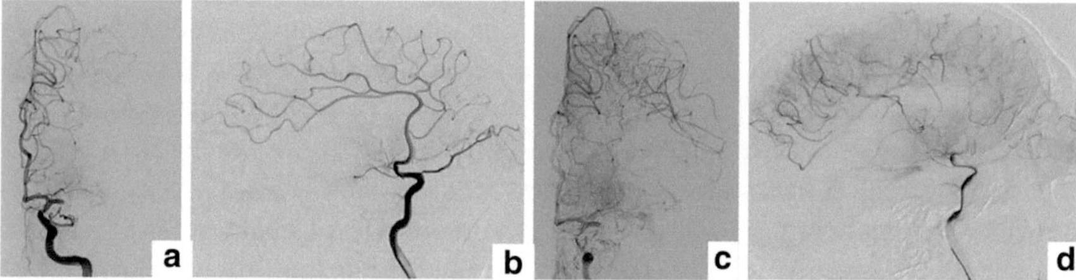

Fig. 6.28 78-Year-old patient with left hemisphere symptoms with NIHSS 26 with onset 8 h before angiogram for thrombectomy. Left MCA occlusion with retrograde flow in MCA vessels by anastomosis with ACA. DSA AP and lateral view—early arterial image (**a**, **b**) and late arterial image (**c**, **d**)

Extracranial consists of physiologic anastomosis between ECA and ICA and VA that open and develop particularly in chronic progressive steno-occlusive disease by a pressure gradient mechanism.

Intracranial can be primary collaterals (components of the circle of Willis) and secondary collaterals (leptomeningeal anastomosis) (Fig. 6.27). In primary collaterals there is an absence of the anterior communicating artery in 1%, hypoplastic anterior communicating artery in 10%, and lack or hypoplasia of posterior communicating artery in 30% [41]. Persistence of primary collateral pathways does not mean effectiveness during LVO.

The secondary collaterals (leptomeningeal anastomosis) are an important route of retrograde flow when a proximal occlusion occurs, connecting main territory arteries (ACA, MCA, PCA). On the pial surface, these anastomoses of small distal cortical vessels (50–40μ) are important connections when acute occlusion occurs (Figs. 6.28 and 6.29).

Fig. 6.29 Detail from 6.28 (**c**) image—corticopial anastomosis ACA-MCA in late phase

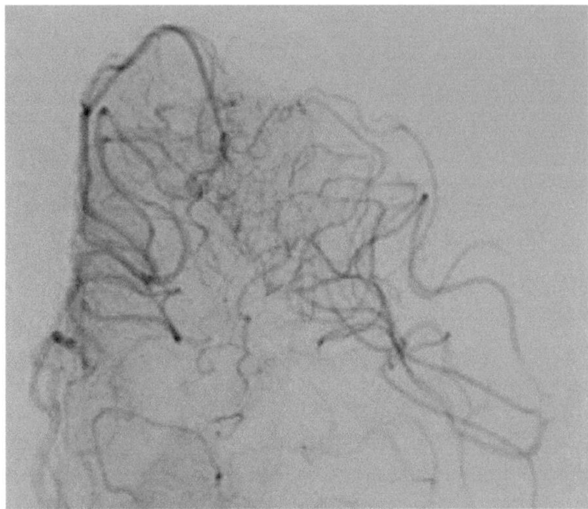

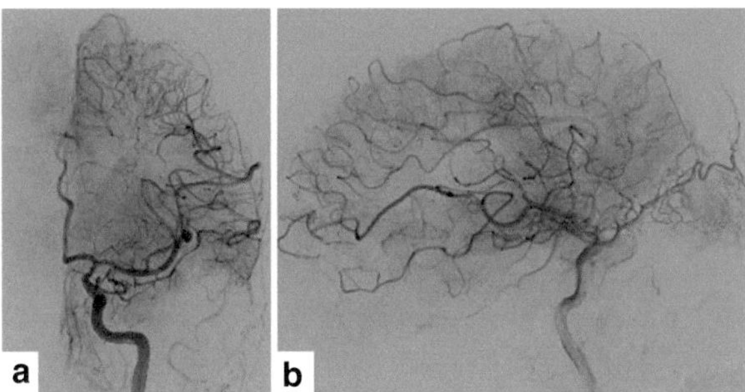

Fig. 6.30 Same patient as in Fig. 6.28. After thrombectomy with TICI 2b recanalization AP and lateral views (**a, b**) show anterograde flow in MCA and reduction in retrograde flow compared to prethrombectomy

Development of new vessels in response to occlusion also exists—arteriogenesis triggered by vascular endothelial growth factors and pressure gradient. Such a phenomenon occurs in chronic ischemia.

In LVO occlusion, around 20–30% have a poor pial collateral score, with more risk to develop larger infarcts in less time [42]. Those are known as the "fast progressors." In those, time is absolutely crucial because they do not have collateral reserves. For this reason, evaluation of collateral score is of more and more paramount importance to targeted treatment planning and prognostic value. It is important to quantify the relationship between collateralization grade and infarct core.

The balance between collateral circulation (retrograde flow) and anterograde flow will dictate the evolution of the ischemic territory (Figs. 6.30 and 6.31).

Evaluation of collaterals prior to recanalization procedure gives a perspective of clinical outcome and how important fast treatment is. Stroke symptoms are a

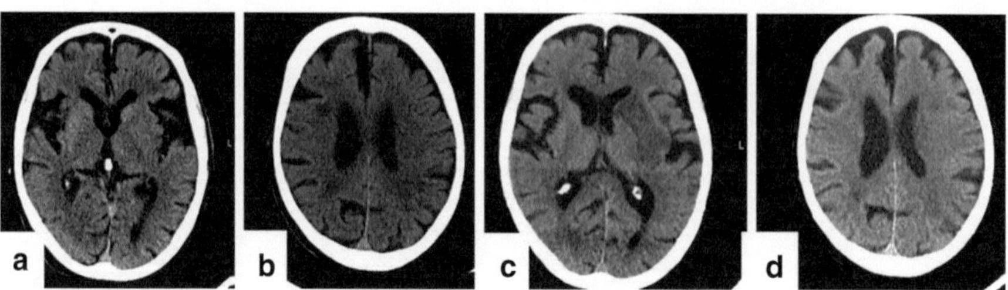

Fig. 6.31 Same patient as in Figs. 6.29 and 6.30 and this figure. NCCT 7 h after symptom onset—ASPECTS 8 (**a, b**). Twenty-four-hour follow-up (**c, d**)—lenticulo-capsulo-caudate infarct. No cortical infarct

manifestation of collateral flow failure. Collaterals are an independent factor that is associated with clinical outcome in acute ischemic stroke patients [43]. They may predict final infarct size and clinical outcome.

Each patient has their own collateral profile that will influence the way ischemic behavior will evolve to infarct or not. Imaging access is of paramount importance to guide decision-making in precision medicine of acute ischemic stroke.

Physiology is more relevant than time alone in acute ischemic stroke, because of collateral flow that increases microvasculature perfusion and so increases ischemic tolerance. The concept has evolved from "time is brain" alone to "time is brain and physiology is brain."

Good collaterals delay loss of penumbral tissue and reperfusion can occur by recanalization of the occluded vessel or by collateral flow. Some patients with LVO may experience a transitory improvement in deficits due to collateral circulation sustenance and a late clinical deterioration when collaterals fail and LVO still persists. These patients with good collaterals are the "slow progressors." They will benefit from thrombectomy even at a late time window (Fig. 6.32).

Patients with poor collaterals are associated with poor outcome and increased incidence of hemorrhagic transformation. In patients with poor collaterals, the hyperperfusion after recanalization indicates a higher hemorrhagic transformation risk (Fig. 6.33). Collateral flow reflects the risk of infarct growth. Patients with poor collaterals have poor clinical outcome if no recanalization is rapidly achieved and are namely the "fast progressors."

A "malignant profile" is called when there are no collaterals in an ischemic stroke with LVO [44]. Imaging may rapidly identify these patients that are severely affected by lack of collaterals in which time is critical and thrombectomy emergent. These patients may develop large infarcts even with successful thrombectomy as time is scarce and they do not have any tolerance to ischemia. They should be under surveillance and they may benefit from early craniectomy (Fig. 6.34).

The best method to evaluate collaterals is still controversial and the methods that exist are qualitative or semiquantitative and highly dependent on the reader.

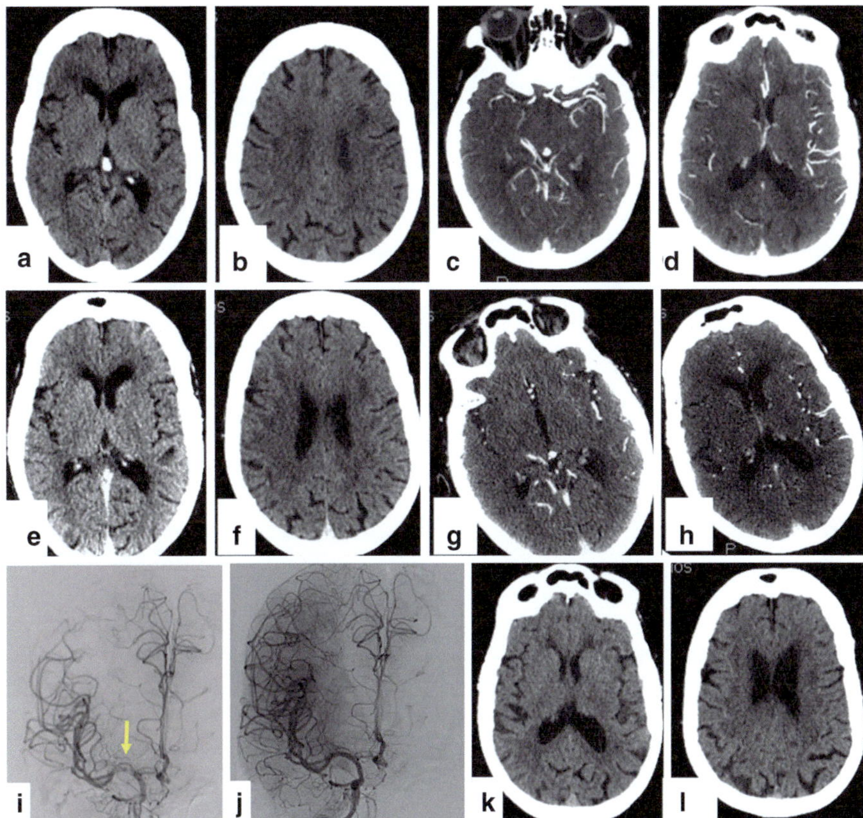

Fig. 6.32 82-Year-old woman, with blood hyperpressure and dyslipidemia with wake-up right hemisphere stroke last seen well 9 h before and NIHSS 18. Improve to NIHSS 5 and then aggravate to NIHSS 12. First CT/CTA done at 11 h from last seen well (**a–d**)—doubtful hypodensity in insula ribbon and lentiform nucleus; leukoaraiosis. Moderate collateral circulation. Right M1 filling defect. Repeat TC/CTA 2 h later when aggravate from neurologic deficit (**e–h**)—same result. Decided to perform thrombectomy with complete recanalization (**i, j**). NCCT 24-h follow-up without acute ischemic lesions (**k, l**)

In MR, collateral flow is visualized as hyperintensity in FLAIR in vessels distal to the occlusion site. This hypersignal corresponds to slow flow in leptomeningeal collaterals (Fig. 6.35) [45].

In CT, single-phase CTA is widely available and has higher sensitivity than NCCT; however it tends to overestimate collateral supply since it is a snapshot. Whole brain should be evaluated in CTA-SI with a narrow window to provide a "perfusion blood volume map" effect in a single-phase technique.

Multiphase CTA is more accurate since it captures a snapshot in different contrast injection phases but has a greater radiation dose. CTA-SI is more sensitive and specific than NCCT to evaluate infarct tissue as areas of hypoattenuation. However,

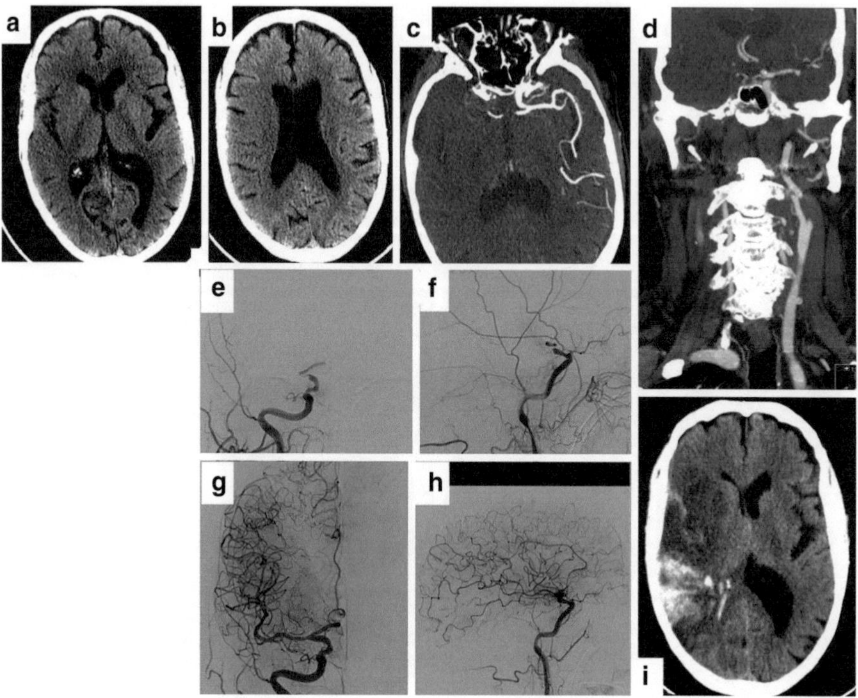

Fig. 6.33 82-Year-old man with sudden symptoms of right cerebral hemisphere, NIHSS 17. CT/CTA 2.5 h after onset of symptoms ASPECTS 3–4 (**a**, **b**), no collateral circulation (**c**), "T" carotid occlusion (**d**). Did tPA. "Drip and ship" transportation with thrombectomy within 4 h from symptom onset (**e**, **f**). First aspiration result with total recanalization (**g**, **h**). NCCT 24-h follow-up with hemorrhagic transformation (**i**)

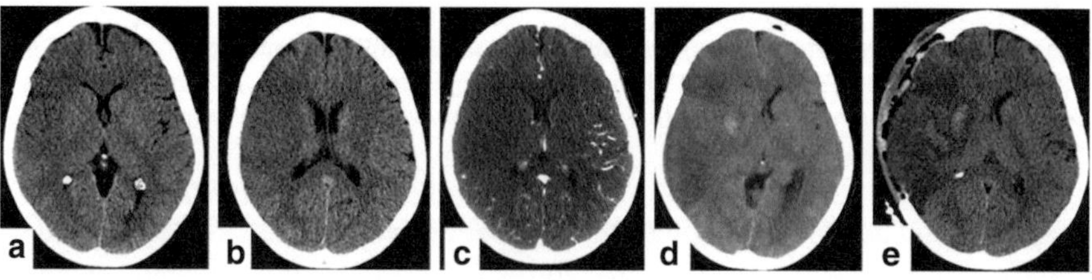

Fig. 6.34 46-Year-old woman with occlusive right carotid dissection with low ASPECTS (**a**, **b**), poor collateral circulation (**c**), and unsuccessful recanalization. Developed mass effect with parenchymal herniation with craniectomy needed (**d**, **e**)

these images tend to overestimate the infarct area if scan acquisition is too early and only arteries are depicted.

For a better evaluation of collaterals on CTA-SI, acquisition should be on the arterial phase with a discreet venous contamination; if not it may overestimate the lack of collaterals (Fig. 6.36).

Multiple collateral grading scores exist to evaluate collaterals based on different imaging modalities such as CTA, MRI, and digital angiography. The ASITN/SIR, ASPECTS, Tan scale, and the score of Christoforidis et al. and Miteff et al. are some examples.

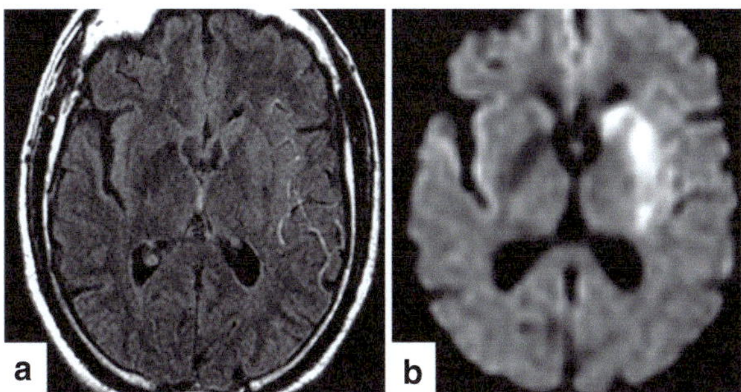

Fig. 6.35 Patient with left hyperacute ischemic stroke with collateral circulation. FLAIR (**a**) shows hyperintensity vessels that correspond to slow flow. No parenchymal lesion. DWI (**b**) shows bright signal in ribbon insula, basal ganglia, and capsule

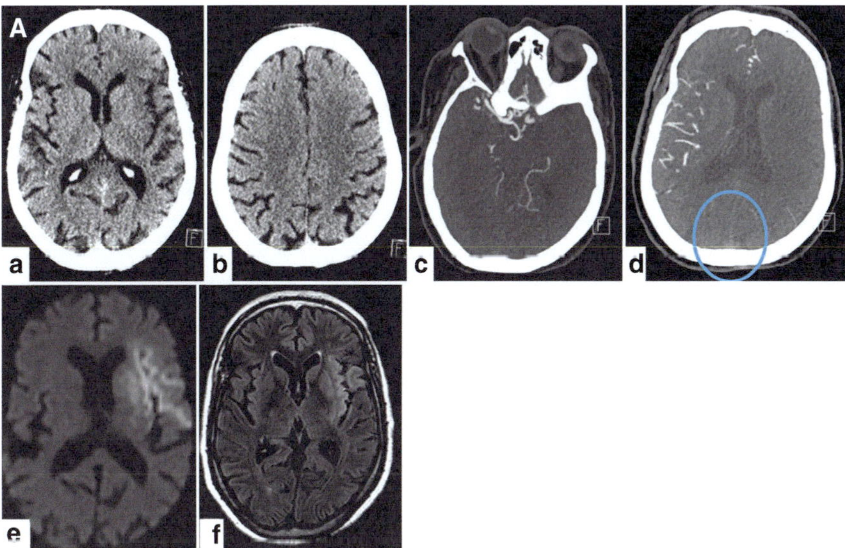

Fig. 6.36 (**A**) 85-Year-old woman with wake-up stroke from left hemisphere, NIHSS 18. NCCT (**a**, **b**)—ASPECTS 7. CTA (**c**, **d**) identifies poor collaterals but it is overestimate because the acquisition scanner time was precocious—no venous sinus contrast (blue circle). MR was performed. DWI (**e**) shows acute ischemic stroke with ASPECTS 7 and FLAIR (**f**) with a hyperintensity region smaller than DWI (mismatch). (**B**) Left internal carotid "T'" occlusion (**a**). Thrombectomy by aspiration technique with complete recanalization (**b**, **c**). Twenty-four-hour NCCT with fronto-insular and lenticulo-capsulate infarct (**d**, **e**). This result is related with collaterals that support the territory of MCA

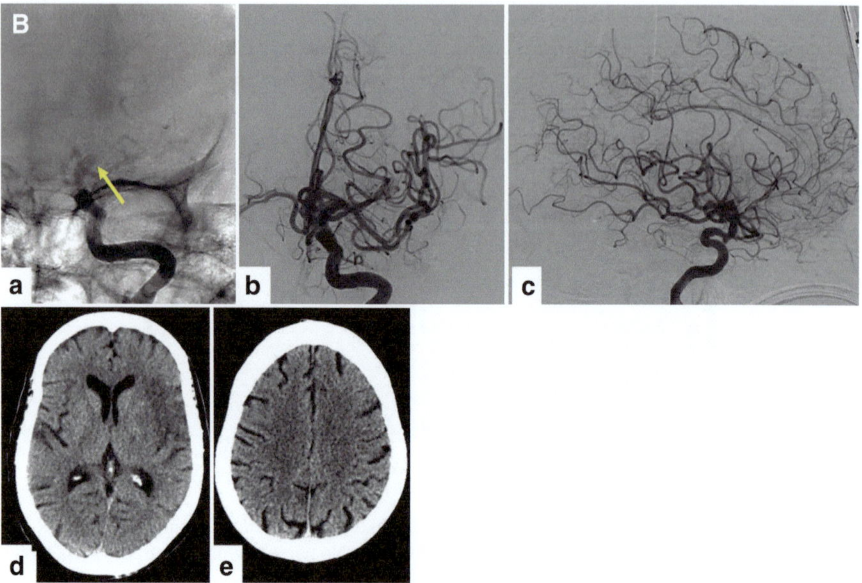

Fig. 6.36 (continued)

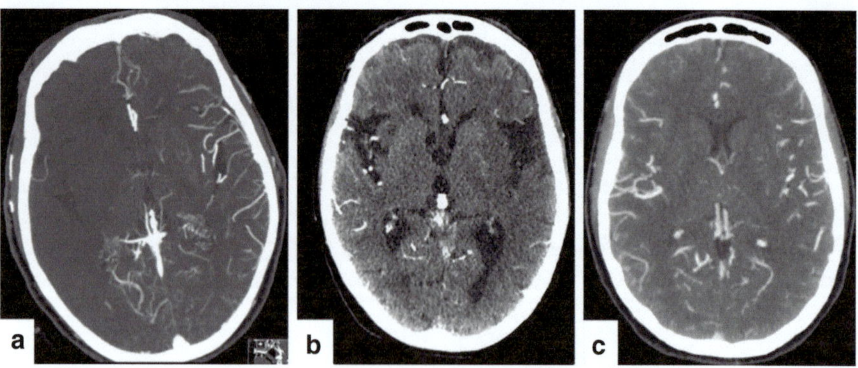

Fig. 6.37 Collateral circulation evaluation. Poor (**a**). Moderate (**b**). Good (**c**)

We consider here the Tan collateral grading scale [46] that considers four levels of collateral circulation: 0 = no visible collateral vessels to the ischemic site; 1 = less than 50% of the occluded MCA territory; 2 = more than 50% of the occluded MCA territory but less than 100%; and 3 = normal antegrade flow. There are three major grades: poor, moderate, and good (Fig. 6.37).

Perfusion in CT or MR may evaluate collaterals. Delayed MTT indicates ischemic penumbra tissue with adequate collateral supply. CBF varies with metabolic demands of the brain and is maintained by autoregulation features that seem to be mediated at several levels involving neurons, neuropil, and cerebral blood vessels. Following occlusion of an artery, pressure in distal branches falls rapidly, and after that collaterals open and provide flow in a gradient pressure trying to maintain CBV and CBF in the occluded territory.

Angiography is considered the gold standard to evaluate collaterals, but it is an invasive technique and does not inform the decision-making process of AIS.

6.2.6.1 Venous Collaterals

Venous outflow provides indirect measurement of tissue perfusion. Venous collaterals supply blood flow drainage that is compromised by arterial vessel occlusion; this reflects in less contrast venous filling in CTA or digital angiography. Quantification of venous collateral outflow provides information about prognosis and outcome in acute ischemic stroke since it relies on impaired perfusion of microvasculature (Fig. 6.38).

The impact of venous outflow on the prognosis of acute stroke considering specific venous drainage is important. Cortical venous drainage (superficial middle cerebral vein, vein of Trolard, vein of Labbé, basal vein) predicts clinical outcome (PRECISE score) [47].

Diminished contrast enhancement in the internal cerebral vein on the side of the artery occlusion represents a poor outcome [48]. Asymmetry of the deep medullary venous system with prominence on the affected side in SWI sequence is due to the high

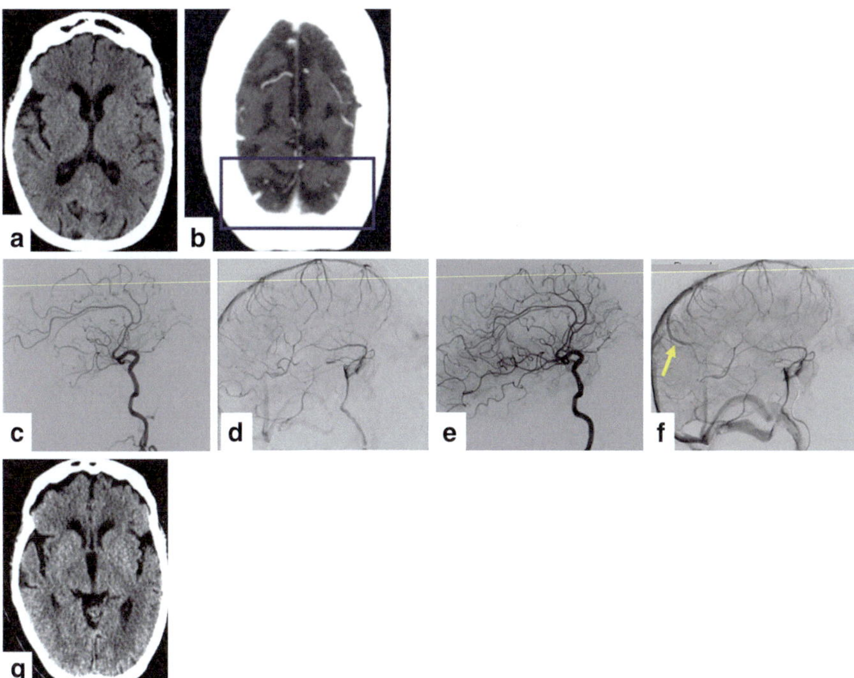

Fig. 6.38 82-Year-old woman with sudden onset of right hemiparesis, dysarthria with ASPECTS 10 (**a**), and CTA with inferior left M2 branch. Cortical veins asymmetric due to less density on left side (**b**). Angiogram before thrombectomy (**c**, **d**) shows occlusion of M2 territory and missing cortical parietal vein. After thrombectomy (**e**, **f**) total recanalization of M2 branch and cortical parietal vein is filling with normal drainage. NCCT 24-h follow-up without infarct (**g**)

sensitivity of this sequence to the increased level of deoxyhemoglobin caused by the reduced flow. This sign correlates with poor collaterals and extent of infarct growth [49].

In the future, as more experience is acquired, venous collaterals may play a role in decision making.

6.2.7 Is There Tissue to Save?

6.2.7.1 Perfusion Evaluation

Ischemic stroke is a dynamic process that results mainly from a balance between artery occlusion and collateral flow from which will result a favorable or unfavorable clinical outcome.

Perfusion imaging measures changes at tissue-microvasculature level and it not only increases information about diagnosis but may also be helpful on treatment decisions and prognosis. However, there is significant variability in parameter maps due to different software and equipment available that tend to vanish with modern automated software and better equipment. This variability is a disadvantage since differences in core and penumbra calculation may influence patient selection for recanalization techniques [50].

As penumbra imaging is measured as a snapshot in a dynamic process it may overestimate the core. If it is performed too early after symptom onset it can also overestimate the core. Also delayed tissue impregnation of contrast may be influenced by comorbidities of the patient such as poor cardiac output, AF, arrhythmias, and cervical carotid stenosis changing the true perfusion parameters.

The proposal of PWI in acute stroke is mainly to answer two questions: if there is a core what is the size of the core (tissue that is infarcted) and if there is still any potentially rescuable tissue—penumbra. This has relevance mainly in patients with unknown time since onset of stroke or stroke with time window onset more than 6 h.

Core and penumbra tissue are dysfunctional and responsible for the clinical symptoms but "penumbra symptoms" will regress if recanalization is achieved. The measured NIHSS corresponds to core plus penumbra.

An easy method to evaluate penumbra/core is clinical/DWI mismatch accepting that neurological examination (NIHSS) is an indicator of reduced perfusion and DWI is an indicator of core [51].

PWI permits individualized stroke treatments based on brain tissue condition rather than time condition only. Therefore, performing perfusion evaluation has a preferential role in those patients with late time window onset which an adequate selection of who still may benefit from thrombectomy and who does not is crucial. Not only for late selection but also as a prognostic variable, perfusion has a role, targeting those patients with very low CBV that are at high risk of hemorrhagic transformation. It may be useful in trying to avoid complications and to share with relatives the outcome of the patient.

PWI analyzes hemodynamic conditions at tissue-microvasculature level by a variety of parameters which include CBF, CBV, and MTT maps knowing that these parameters may reflect the probability of infarction in the absence of reperfusion (Fig. 6.39).

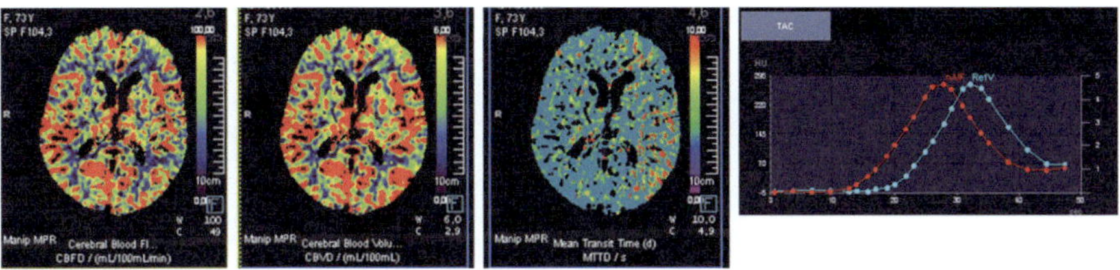

Fig. 6.39 CT perfusion maps—CBF, CBV, MTT. Arterial and venous curves

CBF is defined as the volume of blood through a unit volume of brain in a unit time (measured as mL/100 g/min). CBF is usually not considered quantitative but normalized to a presumed normal reference region of the brain, expressed proportionately (e.g.: CBF <30% means that it is >70% depressed compared to the reference region).

CBV is defined as the volume of blood in a unit volume of brain (measured as mL/100 g) and it represents impregnation of contrast in brain tissue/capillaries in a part of the brain.

CBV and CBF have been used to measure the core as they represent the quantity of contrast arrival in a region and this amount is decreased in hypoperfused tissues. The penumbra is the volume of tissue contained in the mismatch CBF/CBV and the region with a CBV <2.0 mL/100 g threshold represents the core.

MTT is defined as the average time it takes for blood to pass through a brain region from arterial inflow to venous outflow. It is measured in seconds and is related both to CBF and CBV. MTT = CBV/CBF. MTT identifies all areas that demonstrate delay in contrast arrival time. This includes core, penumbra, and benign oligemia. Benign oligemia does not have significant hypoperfusion. MTT can be overestimated if there is severe extracranial disease with stenosis or delayed intracranial flow due to atrial fibrillation or low ejection fraction [52, 53].

Tmax is defined as the delay of contrast from the proximal vessel to the tissue. Usually, the parameter Tmax >6 s mostly identifies the salvageable penumbra (used in DEFUSE study). Low TTP thresholds tend to include also benign oligemic tissue and "increase" false mismatch.

Normal perfusion parameters in gray matter are MTT = 4 s, CBV = 60 mL/100 g/min, and CBV 4 mL/100 g and in white matter MTT = 4 s, CBF = 25 mL/100 g/min, and CBV 2 mL/100 g, knowing that gray matter is more vulnerable to ischemia than white matter.

The "core" is usually defined by a decrease in CBV and CBF and the penumbra by an increase in the MTT, and TTP with CBV between normal values. Core has low CBF and increased MTT as does penumbra. CBV differs as core has low CBV and penumbra has normal or increased CBV [54]. If only CBF is used it tends to overestimate the core as penumbra also has low CBF. CBV should always be evaluated. The mismatch that corresponds to tissue potentially salvageable is the difference between both CBF and CBV.

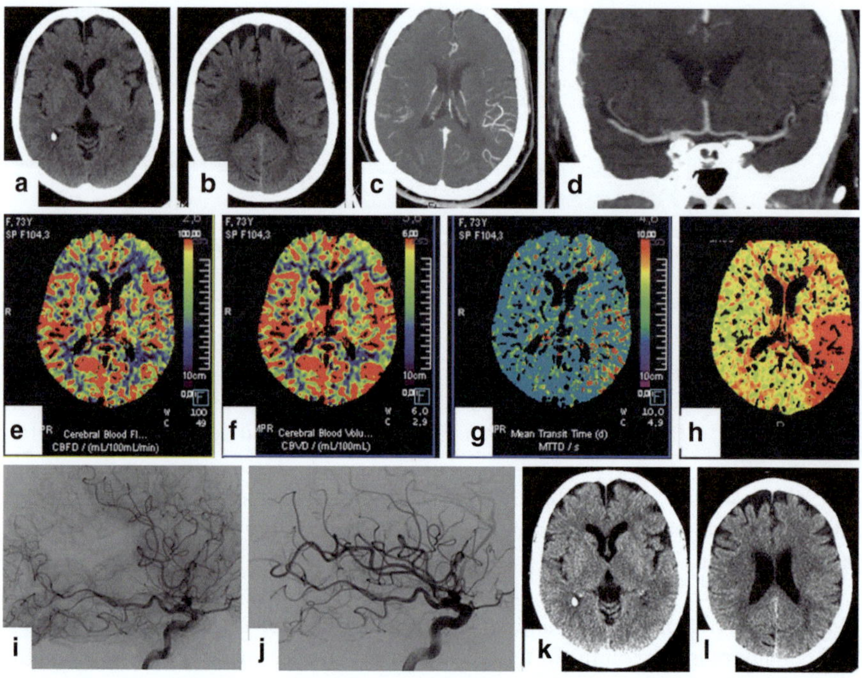

Fig. 6.40 73-Year-old woman with left hemisphere symptoms with onset at 9:00 h. Admitted to hospital at 20 h, NIHSS 12, ASPECTS 10 (**a**, **b**), CTA with occlusion of inferior M2 branch with good collateral circulation (**c**, **d**). CTP shows mismatch at left temporoparietal region (**e–h**). At 22:00 h thrombectomy with total recanalization (**i**, **j**). NCCT 24-h follow-up without infarct (**k**, **l**)

In ischemic tissue, perfusion is impaired but this does not mean an irreversible scenario. This is the penumbra area, the tissue that can be rescued if vessel recanalization is achieved (Fig. 6.40).

6.2.7.2 Perfusion Can Be Done in CT or in MR

In CTP there is a continuous image acquisition in a specific volume of brain tissue during the intravenous injection of a certain volume of iodine contrast. This volume of brain tissue depends on the generation of the scanner that is being used. More recent scanners allow evaluation of larger brain volume.

Perfusion on CT is easily available, cheap, and fast but uses ionizing radiation; it has limited brain coverage and is not sensitive in the posterior fossa.

In MR most of the clinical protocols use contrast agent (gadolinium) techniques but it can also be done with agents that are already present in the blood—arterial spin labeling—(ASL) technique. There are advantages like less cost, no gadolinium, acquisition can be repeated, and it may produce absolute measurement of CBF. As disadvantages it generates less spatial resolution and is more time consuming. This is the reason why in most centers that use MR perfusion, the technique used is with dynamic susceptibility exogenous contrast imaging. PWI is a semi-quantitative method that analyzes the decrease of signal intensity in a certain area of brain tissue after IV injection of contrast that results from the paramagnetic effect of the contrast on T2*.

6.2.8 Protocols

Acute stroke imaging protocols need to be concise and assertive without delaying fibrinolysis or thrombectomy. They should exclude hemorrhage and provide data about the core, site of vessel occlusion, tissue viability, and collaterals (Table 6.1).

In CT with the new-generation technology available, multimodal CT permits acquisition of CTA and perfusion. The protocol in **CT is NCCT, CTA (from aortic arch till vertex), and CTP (if within 6–24 h after symptom onset)** (Table 6.2).

MR is more sensitive to detect acute ischemia and more precise for core volume detection than CT and there is no radiation. However, longer time acquisition is needed and it is more sensitive to movement artifacts in uncooperative patients. Its availability is limited, and the need for GAD injection makes CT by far the first-choice technique in most of the stroke investigation centers. The protocol in **MR is DWI, FLAIR, GRE, MRA (from aortic arch till vertex), and MR perfusion (if within 6–24 h after symptom onset)** (Table 6.3).

Table 6.1 Summary of what is needed for decision-making in acute ischemic stroke

	CT	MR
Is the stroke hemorrhagic or ischemic?	NCCT	DWI, GRE
How extensive is the core (infarcted area)?	NCCT CTA-SI	DWI
Is there a large vessel occlusion?	CTA	MRA
Is there still any tissue to be rescued (penumbra area)?	CTP	FLAIR MRP (DWI/PWI)

Table 6.2 CT protocol for acute ischemic stroke

NCCT (reconstruct images with 4–6 mm)	Exclude hemorrhage ASPECTS Old infarcts
CTA (from aortic arch to vertex)	Extracranial disease LVO site occlusion Clot composition Collateral circulation (by S-images) Confirm the core (by S-images)
CTP (in late time window onset)	Confirm stroke Identify tissue at risk (mismatch)

Table 6.3 MR protocol for acute ischemic stroke

DWI/ADC	May be positive after a few minutes. Rarely reversible Identify infarct tissue
FLAIR	Negative in first 4.5 h Vessels hypersignal (slow flow)—collateral circulation
GRE	Hemorrhage Identify clot
MRA	Extracranial vessels LVO
MRP (in late time window onset)	Tissue at risk (core/penumbra) Collateral circulation (increase MTT with normal CBV or CBF)

6.3　Imaging and Treatment

6.3.1　New Era Began

The new imaging techniques ignited the development of new treatments for AIS as patients that may benefit from treatment are better and faster identified on image-based selection.

For a long period of time, patients with acute ischemic stroke were treated by supportive and conservative measures.

In the 1980s and early 1990s observational studies of intra-arterial and intravenous fibrinolysis emerged, followed by RCTs such as NINDS and ECASS with intravenous fibrinolysis, changing forever the way ischemic stroke will be treated going forward. Intravenous thrombolysis was approved as a standard therapeutic in selected patients up to 3 h after stroke symptom onset, in the USA in 1996 and later on in Europe in 2002, since it improved the outcome at 90 days by reducing stroke-related disability and mortality. In 2008, in Europe the extension of the time interval till 4.5 h after stroke symptom onset was approved based on the results of ECASS III [55].

With the advent of intravenous thrombolysis in the 1990s a qualitative leap toward active treatment emerged. This treatment, done in selected patients, demonstrated better outcomes at 90 days than no treatment. Nevertheless, it was soon verified that, in patients with large vessel occlusion, thrombolysis was not so effective [26].

In the 1990s RCTs of intra-arterial selective thrombolysis (Proact II) started but treatment was not approved in the USA. Since the 1980s there have been isolated cases or small case series published about the rescue of thrombus in brain arteries with different tools.

Innovation and investment in new endovascular devices capable of navigating in a safe manner distal enough to reach and take out the clot in intracranial arteries were promoted. Through "snares" and "Merci" devices a long trial was carried out until the stent retrievers era. Nowadays, different stent retrievers with various frames and scaffolds are available.

RCTs were done with these new devices (stent retrievers) and in 2015 results from the "big 5" trials (MR CLEAN, SWIFT PRIME, ESCAPE, EXTEND, REVASCAT) [4–8] were published and heralded the change in treatment of ischemic stroke with LVO. Later in 2018 results from two more RCTs (DAWN and DEFUSE 3) confirmed that an extended time window for treatment was possible in some selected cases [56, 57].

This new treatment would change the outcome of stroke patients that otherwise had such a high morbimortality. Results of thrombectomy were superior to medical treatment alone with a number needed to treat of 2.6 for an improvement in the mRS of 1 point at 90 days and a low complication rate [58]. Thrombectomy became the standard method of treatment in LVO ischemic stroke.

This huge change in treatment forced the health community to adapt measures to deal with the spread of thrombectomy to all eligible patients. There was a necessity to create new stroke centers with neurointerventional teams capable of commencing endovascular treatment as soon as needed. Endovascular teams need trained doctors in the field with standard programs and practice as a learning curve should be achieved so the ability to do well can be mirrored in results [59].

Implementation of fast transportation is urgent and is still a main concern requiring significant investment. Depending on geography, local organization, and availability of comprehensive stroke centers, two strategies of transportation may be considered: "mothership" in which the patient is transported directly to a comprehensive stroke center or "drip and ship" in which the patient is transported first to a primary hospital where imaging is performed and eventually thrombolysis is initiated before further transport to a comprehensive stroke center. The ideal situation is when the patient is conveyed directly to a comprehensive stroke center, imaging is performed, and treatment is carried out, but if the patient is far distant from such a center, it is reasonable to go to a primary hospital, perform imaging and thrombolysis if applicable, and then be sent to a comprehensive stroke center. In this way the patient may benefit from the effect of thrombolysis [60].

Thrombectomy is a cost-effective therapy compared with standard care including thrombolysis even if the cost of thrombectomy is higher. As it reduces disability and dependency it saves costs on long-term patient care and social services [61].

Patients with ischemic stroke eligible for thrombectomy are selected based on multiple variables: baseline mRS, severity of symptoms (NIHSS scale), extension of early signs in CT or DWI, and time of onset. Collateral assessment and perfusion analysis are added in extended time window cases. Selection is heavily dependent on imaging.

Guidelines were stablished to mentor clinicians regarding thrombectomy [62–64].

In 2015 Guidelines of the American Heart Association, thrombectomy in the presence of LVO of anterior circulation (either ICA or M1) should be considered in selected patients independently of having done tPA; if age ≥ 18 and <80 years, previous mRS score 0–1, ASPECTS ≥ 6, and NIHSS ≥ 6, treatment has to be initiated within 6 h from onset to femoral puncture.

However, despite the great results obtained in trials there is still room for improvement, better rates of complete recanalization, and better mRS in outcome (Table 6.4).

Some patients do not fit all the recommended features but they still may have some benefit from treatment, such as elderly patients (>80 years) and when the time

Table 6.4 Summary of mRS (0–2), mRS 3, and TICI 2b-3 results of the "big" five RCTs as a percentage

	mRS (0–2)	mRS (3)	TICI 2b-3
MR CLEAN	33	18	59
REVASCAT	43.7	18.4	65.6
ESCAPE	54	16	72.4
SWIFT PRIME	60.2	12.2	88
EXTEND-IA	72	17	86

window exceeds 6 h [65]. Advanced age is no longer an exclusion criteria. After the
DAWN and DEFUSE 3 trial's results, the time window of treatment was extended
in some patients to between 6 and 24 h.

6.3.1.1 Criteria Selection for Thrombectomy

Patients that are eligible for tPA should receive IV tPA even if thrombectomy is
considered and if thrombectomy is subsequently indicated, there should be no delay
to access clinical response from tPA.

In time window from 0 to 6 h thrombectomy should be done if pre-stroke mRS
score is 0–1; occlusion vessel is in ICA or M1 segment of MCA; age is ≥18 years;
NIHSS score is ≥6; and ASPECTS is ≥6 and treatment can be initiated (arterial
puncture) within 6 h of symptom onset (Fig. 6.41).

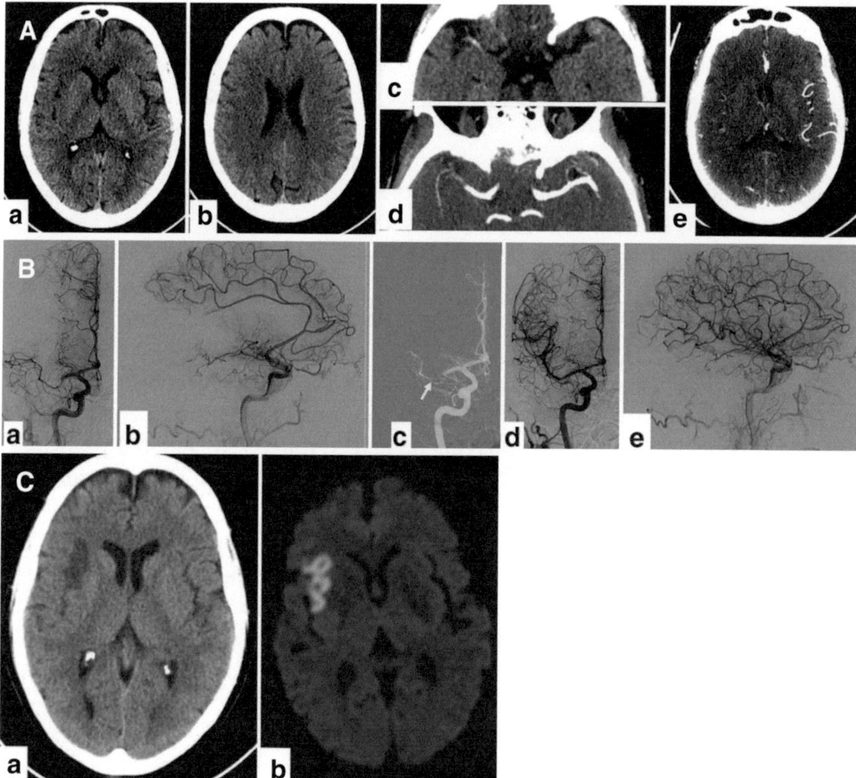

Fig. 6.41 (**A**) 72-Year-old man with sudden onset of left hemiparesis at 14:00 h. Did not do tPA
due to unknown medication for arrhythmia. NIHSS is 12. CT/CTA at 15:30 h shows ASPECTS-9
(**a, b**) and middle third M1 occlusion (**c, d**). Fair collateral circulation (**e**). (**B**) Angiogram at
17:16 h confirms occlusion of right M1 (**a, b**). Thrombectomy with one catheter aspiration (**c**) with
complete recanalization at 17:39 h (**d, e**). (**C**) Twenty-four-hour follow-up. NCCT (**a**) and DWI
(**b**)—infarct in insular ribbon

In time window from 6 to 24 h, thrombectomy should be done in selected patients within 6–16 h of last known well that meet DEFUSE 3 criteria and in selected patients within 16–24 h of last known well that meet DAWN criteria.

In both DAWN and DEFUSE only patients with small to moderate size of core are included.

Benefits are uncertain but thrombectomy may be reasonable in occlusion of M2 or M3 segments of MCA; occlusion of ACA, BA, or PCA; pre-stroke mRS score >1; ASPECTS <6; and NIHSS score <6.

Regarding imaging criteria ASPECTS ≥6 means infarcts with small/moderate core, less than 70 mL, and less than 1/3 of middle cerebral artery territory.

Time window is a major predictor of outcome especially in those patients that have poor collaterals. Since collateral circulation can only be evaluated when imaging is performed, all patients that may have an ischemic stroke with LVO are emergent. Between extremes of good and bad collaterals there are all the intermediate scenarios as each patient has his/her own individual genetic and biomarker patrimony.

DAWN criteria (DWI or CTP assessment with clinical mismatch in the triage of wake-up and late-presenting strokes undergoing neurointervention with trevo) (Table 6.5).

Assessment time window from 6 to 24 h.

Occlusion of ICA and/or MCA (M1), ≥18 years, pre-stroke mRS (0–1), infarct volume less than 1/3 of MCA territory.

DEFUSE criteria (endovascular therapy following imaging evaluation for ischemic stroke) (Table 6.6).

Assessment time window from 6 to 16 h.

Occlusion of ICA and/or MCA (M1); NIHSS ≥6.

The technical goal of the intervention procedure is to achieve the opening of the vessels that are occluded as soon as possible and at first pass. The result is measured by the **mTICI** (thrombolysis in cerebral infarction) score tool [66] (Table 6.7).

Table 6.5 NIHSS and infarct volume values in DAWN criteria

Mismatch between clinical deficit (NIHSS) and infarct volume		
<80 years		≥80 years
NIHSS >10	NIHSS >20	NIHSS ≥10
Vol <31 mL	Vol >31 to <51 mL	Vol <21 mL

Table 6.6 Volume of penumbra tissue and infarct in DEFUSE 3 criteria

Volume of ischemic tissue in perfusion/infarct volume
Core. Infarct volume <70 mL
"Target" mismatch ratio ≥1.8 (MTT/core)
"Mismatch volume" = perfusion lesion volume = penumbra ≥15 mL with a Tmax 6 s (MTT-core)

Table 6.7 mTICI score

Grade 0—no recanalization
Grade 1—anterograde recanalization past the initial occlusion, but limited distal branch filling with little or slow distal flow (Fig. 6.42)
Grade 2
2A—anterograde recanalization <50% of the previously occluded target (Fig. 6.43)
2B—anterograde recanalization >50% of the previously occluded target (Fig. 6.44)
Grade 3—complete recanalization (Fig. 6.45)

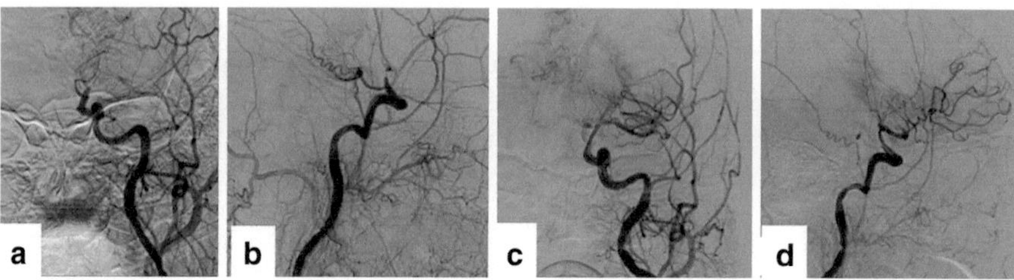

Fig. 6.42 TICI 1. Angiogram of left ICA before (**a**, **b**) and after (**c**, **d**) thrombectomy

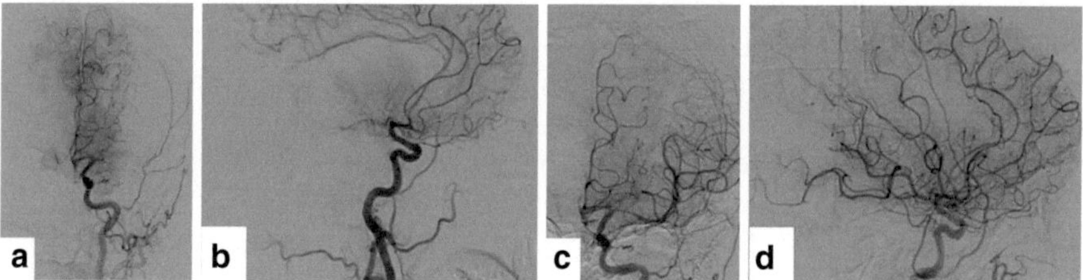

Fig. 6.43 TICI 2a. Angiogram of left ICA before (**a**, **b**) and after (**c**, **d**) thrombectomy

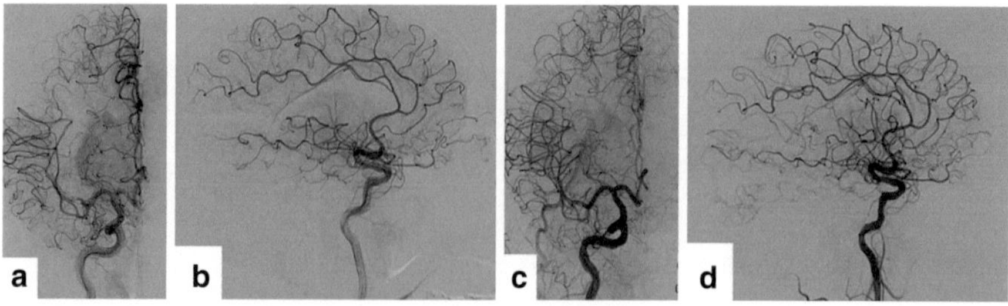

Fig. 6.44 TICI 2b. Angiogram of right ICA (**a**, **b**) and after (**c**, **d**) thrombectomy

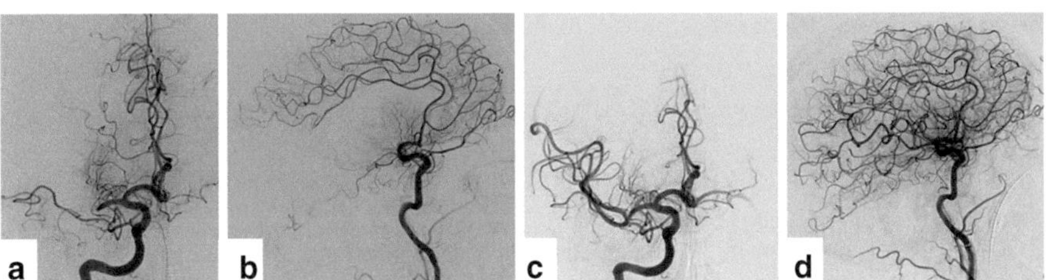

Fig. 6.45 TICI 3. Angiogram of right ICA (**a**, **b**) and after (**c**, **d**) thrombectomy

It is considered adequate if recanalization of TICI 2b/3 is achieved. A NCCT 24-h follow-up is performed to evaluate parenchyma and exclude complications such as mass effect or hemorrhage. An echo Doppler of cervical vessels and transcranial is routinely performed at 24 h in our institution.

The procedure is performed under conscious sedation or general anesthesia depending on the patient's baseline condition and reperfusion should not be delayed. Arterial pressure should not drop during the procedure. Thrombectomy, particularly in distal vessels, should be performed with the patient lying as still as possible so a standard safe condition to rescue the thrombus can be guaranteed. The decision should always be a balance between cost and benefit [67].

A stent retriever technique and aspiration devices with large catheters that are capable of navigating far enough to reach the thrombus safely and aspirate the clot were also developed. No differences in results exist between stent retrievers and aspiration techniques. The choice depends on the intervention team's experience [68, 69]. In some situations a combined technique is performed.

In around 8–18% of patients, recanalization cannot be achieved [4–8]. Multiple factors are implied such as tortuous anatomy with difficult anatomical access and resistant thrombus by either composition, size, or location. As thrombectomy is a surgical technique, results are also dependent on operator experience and a learning curve is needed.

From RCT the overall complication rate is around 15% which can be at the access site of puncture or intracranial such as vessel perforation, vessel dissection, vasospasm, and fragmentation of clot with embolization to new territories.

Symptomatic hemorrhage after thrombectomy is around 4.3%. In late time window trials, Dawn is 6% and in Defuse 3 is 7%.

Classification of hemorrhage in NCCT according to ECASS III definition of symptomatic intracranial hemorrhage is any hemorrhage with neurologic deterioration, as indicated by an NIHSS score that is higher by four or more points than the value at baseline or the lowest value in the first 7 days, or that led to death or was identified as the predominant cause of the neurologic deterioration (Table 6.8). PH2 hemorrhage is the only hemorrhage pattern with the risk of early neurological deterioration and 3-month mortality.

Good collaterals and early recanalization of blood flow in the occluded vessel dictate clinical outcome.

Table 6.8 Hemorrhagic transformation classification

Hemorrhagic infarction (HI)
HI 1—Small petechial hemorrhage at the infarct margins. Tiny punctate regions of hyperattenuation in CT.
HI 2—Confluent petechial hemorrhage through the infarct. No mass effect due to hemorrhage
Parenchymatous hematoma (PH)
PH 1—Clot less than 30% of the infarct area. Minor mass effect due to hemorrhage. Patchy hyperattenuation surrounded by the hypoattenuated parenchyma on CT. Some mass effect due to hemorrhage
PH 2—Dense blood clot more than 30% of the infarct area with mass effect due to hemorrhage

Infarct volume is only a part of treatment effect of EVT. Follow-up infarct volume is a strong independent predictor of outcome; nevertheless combined image and clinical values have more predictive value than imaging alone since the size of final infarct does not always correlate with the outcome [70].

It is important to streamline patient management to avoid any delay in treatment and monitor several target times. Time from symptom onset to hospital admission reflects the quality of transportation. Time from admission to needle or time from admission to artery puncture reflects the hospital organization. Time from artery puncture to recanalization reflects endovascular team performance.

Guidelines are helpful in decision-making and in preservation of quality standards and safe care of patients ensuring that the more adequate treatment option is taken based on scientific evidence. They should rather be used to include patients and not overselect patients to not be submitted to treatment. The questions are: Which are the patients that for sure will no longer benefit from treatment independently of time window? Does the treatment bring any benefit for the patient?

If these patients are identified it will avoid futile recanalization with the consequences of potential harm, costs, false hopes, and expectations.

Three case examples (Figs. 6.46, 6.47, and 6.48):

However, we still have concerns about patients that do not fit into the standard parameters of the guidelines, yet may benefit from treatment. The inclusion criteria that clinical trials used to guide treatment should not function as a limitation but as a guide to promote a treatment with a proven efficacy. When the high morbimortality of ischemic strokes is considered against a therapy with substantial benefit and low complication rate, the goal should be to include as many patients as possible while analyzing which patients to exclude.

In the guidelines, baseline functional status mRS should be less than or equal to 1 to meet the criteria to receive thrombectomy. Within 6 h of symptom onset, benefits are considered uncertain but treatment may be reasonable if mRS >1. There is a long-standing debate as to whether patients with preexisting disabilities should be included or not for invasive therapies [71]. They are excluded from RCTs because of the enhancing likelihood of detecting a treatment effect. No evidence of increased mortality was demonstrated in higher mRS and intravenous thrombolysis or thrombectomy may be effective [72].

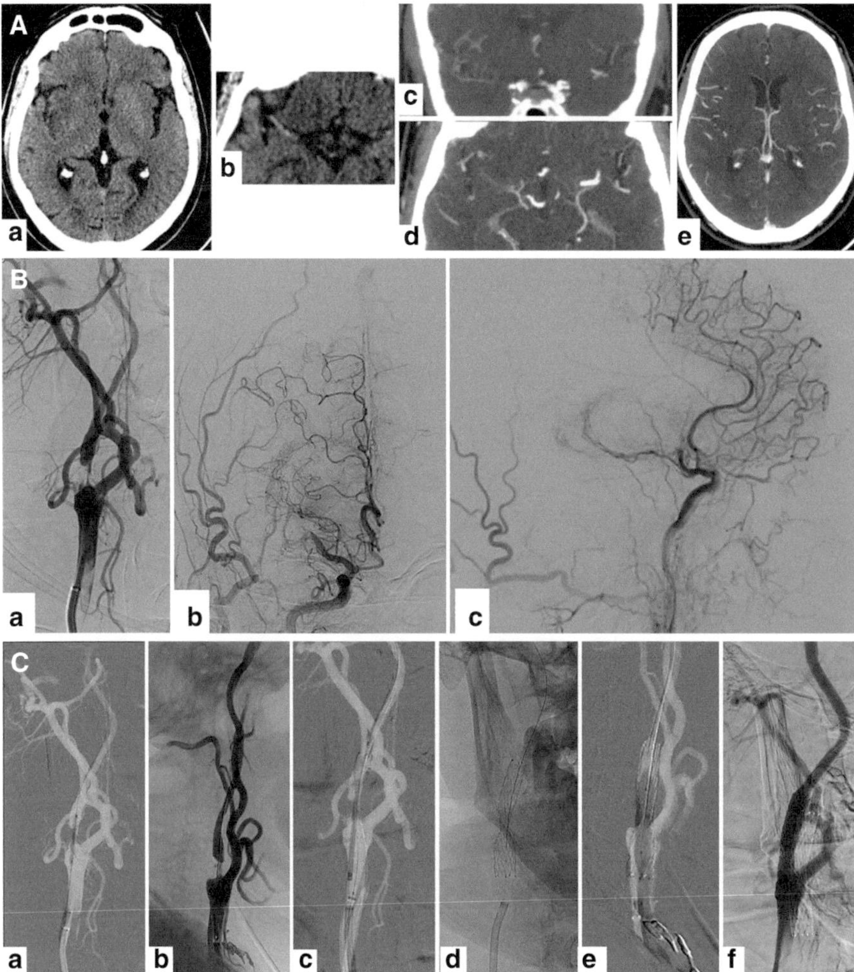

Fig. 6.46 (A) 72-Year-old male, sudden right hemisphere symptoms with NIHSS 13 at 20:00 h, mothership transportation, NCCT/CTA at 23:40 h, tPA at 0:15 h. ASPECTS 7–8 (**a**). Hyperdense thrombus in R MCA (**b**). Filling defect in R M1 confirms occlusion (**c, d**). Good collateral circulation (**e**). (**B**) Thrombectomy at 1:00 h. Tandem occlusion. Preocclusive stenosis in carotid bulb (**a**) and M1 occlusion (**b**) and distal A2 occlusion (**c**). (**C**) Before thrombectomy, stent implantation in ICA stenosis. Predilatation with 2 × 20 angioplasty ballon (**a**). Placement of stent 7 × 40 (**b, c**). Opening of stent (**d**). Postdilatation with 5 × 20 angioplasty ballon (**e**). Final result (**f**). (**D**) Thrombectomy of M1 (**c, d**) and A2 (**a, b**). (**E**) TICI 2b for MCA (**a**) and total recanalization in A2 (**b**). (**F**) NCCT 12 h later to exclude hemorrhage or large infarct so DAPT may be initiated (**a, b**). Twenty-four-hour control (**c, d**). Contrast retention in infarcted zone (**a**). Small petechial hemorrhagic transformation (**c**). (**G**) Echo Doppler follow-up—permeability of ICA

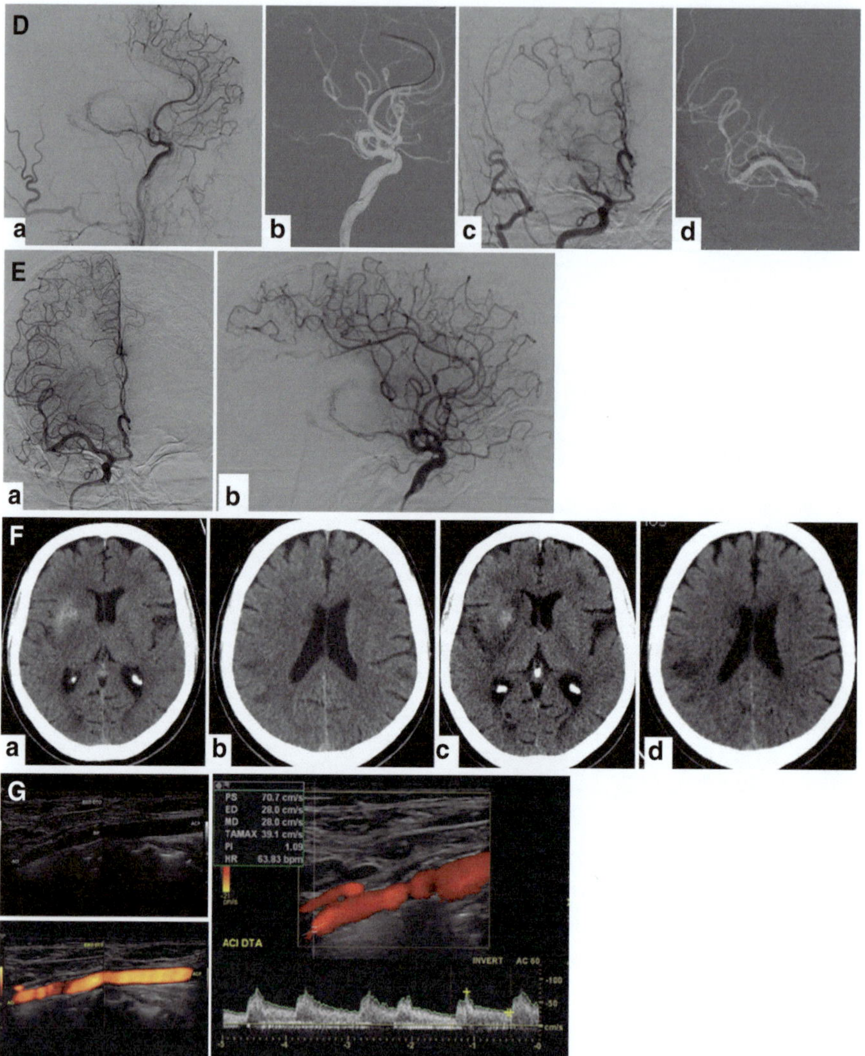

Fig. 6.46 (continued)

Should a patient that is paraplegic (previous vehicle accident) not be treated because their mRS is not less than or equal to 1?

Each case should be evaluated individually and the decision strengthened with other parameters like cognitive performance, other comorbidities, and age to risk/benefit.

Evaluation of treatment is based on mRS between 0 and 2, but results that cover all the mRS need to be considered and not all good results are from those in between 0 and 2. A patient recovering from a 4 to 3 is a significant success; it means that the patient will require some help but is able to walk unassisted, well-being increases, and socioeconomic costs could be lowered.

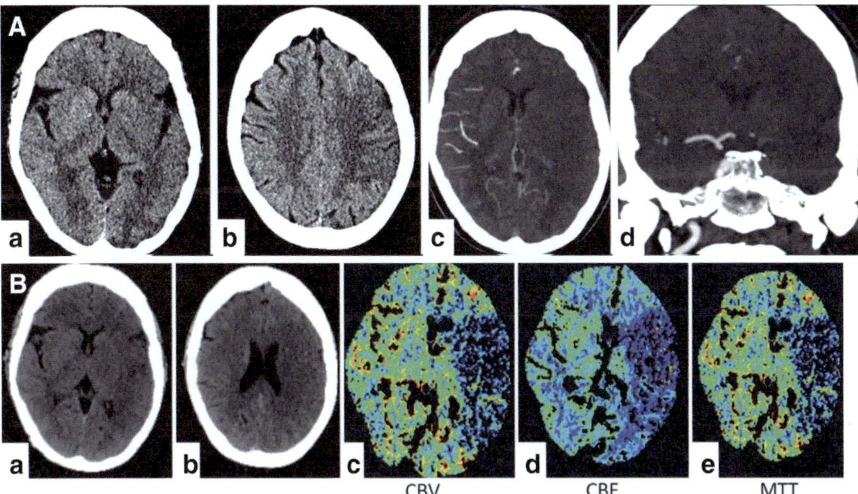

Fig. 6.47 (**A**) 64-Year-old woman with sudden onset of left hemisphere symptoms is fast transported to primary hospital. CT/CTA at 13:30 h. ASPECTS 5 (**a, b**). Poor collateral circulation (**c**). Left "T" ICA occlusion (**d**). (**B**) At comprehensive stroke center repeat NCCT and CTP at 16:29 h. "Fast progressor." ASPECTS 2 (**a, b**). No mismatch (**c–e**). Decided for no thrombectomy

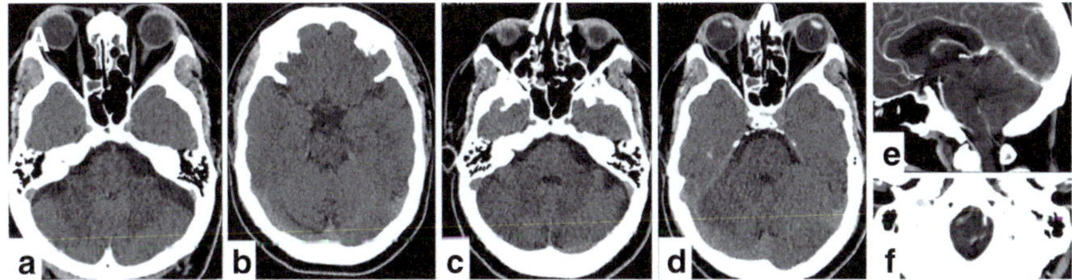

Fig. 6.48 (**A**) 53-Year-old man. Heavy smoker. Three days before with vertigo and headache. First attendee in primary hospital NCCT normal (**a, b**). Second attendee next day to same hospital with vertigo, headache, and ataxia. NCCT/CTA. Hypoattenuation of right cerebellum hemisphere (**c, d**). No intracranial vessel occlusion (**e, f**). (**B**) Three days later clinical deterioration with consciousness impairment (NIHSS 30), intubation needed. Repeat NCCT/CTA. No new hypoattenuation; more mass effect (**a, b**). Filling defect in basilar artery (**c, d**). (**C**) Patient transported to comprehensive stroke center. MR performed. ADC (**a, b**), DWI (**c**), and FLAIR (**d, e**) show no mismatch in cerebellum lesion but brain stem is spared. Mass effect in midline structures. (**D**) Right vertebral dissection was the cause of stroke that happened two times. Stenosis and irregularity of vertebral lumen artery (**a**). Normal filling of basilar tip and PCAs from collateral circulation through PComs (**b, c**). Basilar artery occlusion (**d**). Thrombectomy with two aspirations and complete recanalization (**e, f**). Two days later the patient was extubated with NIHSS 7

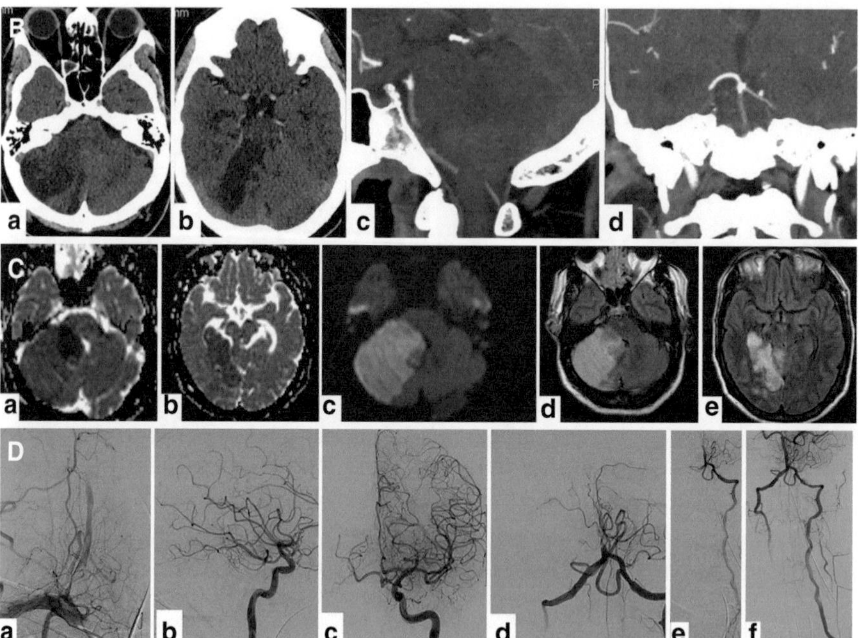

Fig. 6.48 (continued)

6.4 Still in Debate …

6.4.1 Previous mRS

As the global population is ageing stroke incidence will increase in people with preexisting disability. The risk/benefit balance for good outcome in treatment is multifactorial and previous disability should be less and less an excluding criterion.

6.4.2 Low ASPECTS

The ASPECTS scale has some limitations; it does not take into account the more or less eloquent locations of points. It assigns the same value to the head of the caudate nucleus as the rolandic area for example. It only analyzes the middle cerebral media territory, and it is difficult to punctuate in very early scans or patients with leukoaraiosis or a previous stroke. Regarding the cutoff of more or less than ASPECTS 6, it is rather difficult to not treat a patient based on such a weak tool when they could benefit from thrombectomy.

In current guidelines it is considered of uncertain benefit (class IIb) to treat patients with ASPECTS <6 even if symptom onset was within 6 h from the anterior circulation being impaired. In the RCT in which these guidelines are based, most of the patients included had small cores so there is a lack of evidence of thrombectomy efficacy in such patients. Nevertheless, large core infarcts may still benefit from endovascular treatment and were excluded from trials.

RCTs such as TENSION, IN EXTREMIS, Select-2, and TESLA are still waiting for results.

In a recent meta-analysis [73], including 1400 patients with ASPECTS lower than 6, it was demonstrated that thrombectomy with a result (TICI 2b/3) was associated with better outcome than conservative/medical treatment alone. The subgroup 5–6 had comparable and better outcome and in subgroup 0–4 good outcomes were markedly reduced but without increased rate of ICH. One in four patients may regain independency at 3 months in ASPECTS 4 and only 14% of patients with aspects 0–3 will benefit from thrombectomy. The effect of treatment was higher in younger patients (age continues to be a strong predictor of final outcome). These findings were confirmed in other studies [74, 75]. In Hermes meta-analysis there was no benefit of thrombectomy in ASPECTS 0–2 and there was higher rate of symptomatic ICH in patients with ASPECTS 0–4 but with ASPECTS 3–5 a significant benefit from thrombectomy exists.

The larger the core the less the tissue at risk exists, it is less likely to benefit from reperfusion, and there is less chance to good outcome, but in those patients with large core that still may benefit from treatment it is a "race against time" since they are likely more time dependent probably because they are "fast progressors."

Three groups of ASPECTS may be considered regarding outcome: good (8–10), moderate (5–7), and bad (0–4) according to results: good outcome (mRS 0–2) 46%, 38.6%, and 5% and mortality of 19%, 28.9%, and 55%, respectively [21].

When considering treatment in low ASPECTS (large core) patients that accounts for 20–25% of all anterior circulation with LVO strokes, other factors like previous comorbidities, previous stroke, leukoaraiosis, and age have a higher strength in outcome and should be carefully evaluated in an attempt to lower risks of treatment (increased ICH) and avoid futile recanalization. The expectations of treatment have to take into account the already infarcted tissue and deficit baseline. In such patients a mRS 3 at 90 days may still be considered a good outcome. Discussion with relatives is encouraged.

6.4.3   Low NIHSS

NIHSS is the most frequent clinical LVO prediction instrument.

Ischemic strokes with mild neurological symptoms but with LVO are still debatable regarding treatment options, current data is limited, and no RCTs are available [76].

About one-third of ischemic stroke is associated with LVO and 10–20% with mild neurological symptoms are associated with LVO.

It may be considered to perform vessel imaging even in low-NIHSS patients to exclude LVO as the low NIHSS may represent a stroke that will aggravate if an LVO subsists to an undesirable outcome.

Nevertheless, some studies have shown better results in patients with LVO and low NIHSS submitted to thrombectomy without increase of hemorrhagic complications, but others did not demonstrate a statistical difference in results and showed an even higher rate of intracranial hemorrhage. Variability may be related to the definition of low NIHSS and the location of LVO.

In ischemic stroke with LVO and low NIHSS there is a need to correlate the location of thrombus with the clinical symptoms and determine if there is still tissue to rescue and benefit from thrombectomy. They are patients in which cost/benefit has to be carefully balanced. More data is needed.

Another group with LVO is patients that have fluctuating symptoms which begin with a moderate NIHSS and then, with or without IV tPA, improve their clinical status, lowering their NIHSS (<6). In such cases a new vessel imaging evaluation should be done. Two situations may present: vessel recanalization or maintenance of the occlusion with tissue perfusion being supported by collaterals. In the latter, the risk of collaterals failing leading to worsening of clinical status may be high and thrombectomy may be the best option.

Trials to evaluate the efficacy and safety of EVT in low NIHSS are ongoing such as ENDOLOW and IN-EXTREMIS.

6.5 Tandem Occlusions

Tandem occlusion is an ischemic stroke that occurs simultaneously with LVO and extracranial carotid steno-occlusive disease. Frequency of tandem occlusion is variable around 10–15% in ischemic stroke due to LVO. It occurs in about 10% and is associated with poor outcome.

There is still no data available from RCTs about which is the best treatment, if medical, angioplasty, or stenting, in the acute phase but there is increased evidence that carotid artery stenting in thrombectomy leads to a better outcome. This data strengthens the need for acquisition imaging to be performed from aortic arch to the convexity, so disease in the carotid bifurcation like atherosclerotic stenosis, dissection, or even "pseudo-occlusion" due to a "T" thrombus in the distal extremity of the ICA may be seen.

In an analysis of a nonrandomized study of LVO with stenosis of bifurcation superior to 90% stented (TITAN study) there was no increase in hemorrhagic events (according to ECASS II classification of hemorrhage) in those patients that were stented compared to the control group [77] and there were similar ICH and good outcome in patients that received tPA compared with patients that did not receive (STRATIS study).

6.6 Intracranial Stenosis

Intracranial large vessel stenosis is an important cause of stroke and is often the cause of unsuccessful thrombectomy by stent retriever or aspiration. Therefore it is important to identify this entity in acute procedures. Intracranial atheroma stenosis represents almost half of the cases of unsuccessful reperfusion procedures in thrombectomy, which accounts for 10–30% of thrombectomy cases of RCT with a high morbimortality (only 21% of mRS 0–2 at 3 months and around 30% mortality) [78]. Contrary to elective cases where vessel wall imaging by MR can be scheduled, in emergency situations it is not feasible. Some indirect signs like mural calcification in vessel walls may raise the suspicion. In digital angiography it is almost impossible to detect and differentiate from a regular thrombus. Some of them have a tiny tail rather than a simple cutoff image. In a thrombectomy when several stent retriever passes or aspiration is unfruitful a stenosis may be the cause. Intracranial stent delivery may be the only option to recanalize the vessel knowing that it requires antithrombotic therapy and the decision should be made on an individualized basis regarding extension of infarct and clinical status.

6.7   Thrombolysis Before Thrombectomy or Not?

When the patient arrives outside the time window for tPA there is a consensus that the only treatment option in ischemic stroke with LVO is thrombectomy.

In guidelines it is considered that patients with LVO within the therapeutic time window for thrombolysis should do tPA followed by thrombectomy.

There is no total agreement how these patients should be treated if they arrive directly to a comprehensive stroke center that can do thrombectomy straightaway without tPA and if tPA will provide additional benefit over thrombectomy. Those that are pro doing tPA defend that tPA may work as a co-adjuvant in the treatment and have some benefit if fragmentation of the clot occurs. Others that are against defend that tPA can work in a negative way making the clot more fragile and prone to migrate and fragmentate.

Recent results from RCT DIRECT-MT showed that going directly to thrombectomy had similar results concerning functional outcome to doing tPA prior to thrombectomy [79]. However, the rate of recanalization was higher in the group that received tPA plus thrombectomy. Disparity between high rate of recanalization and not so high good clinical outcome may be due to individualized factors like being "fast progressors" or lack of fast transportation.

New thrombolytic agents (tenecteplase) are being used in trials (EXTEND-IA TNK) [80] and may be more effective than alteplase. This showed that IV tenecteplase before thrombectomy led to "spontaneous" recanalization in around 22% at the time of angiography and was associated with better outcomes.

6.8   Stroke in COVID-19 Era

Incidence of ischemic stroke in COVID-19 patients remains unknown.

COVID-19 pandemic affected the way diseases have been treated all over the world either by the influence of the infection itself or by the delay of diagnosis due to overburdened health systems or some fear of patients going to hospital. These had severe consequences in outcomes of diseases and institutions had to adapt to a new reality [81].

Patients infected with COVID-19 have a possible increase in incidence of stroke due to a procoagulant effect of the virus or the immune response to it. They have an increase in-hospital mortality rate and high rate of thrombotic complications [82].

Treatment of patients infected by COVID-19 imposes additional measures of personal protection measures that can delay procedures, so strict organization should implement special workflow and training of staff for these patients. Most of the patients attending for thrombectomy are of undocumented COVID-19 status; they are tested at the admission to hospital but the procedure is performed before results are known, so all patients are treated as potentially COVID-19 positive and extra measures have to be taken regarding protection.

6.9   Conclusions

In the last 5 years a global revolution in the treatment of acute ischemic stroke has been achieved with thrombectomy and imaging has been in the epicenter of selecting tools.

Imaging parameters are of paramount importance to guide decision-making, allowing adequate treatment tailored to a specific patient as precision medicine requires. Crucially, we still need to settle the equilibrium between selecting more or treating more patients by development of new imaging tools so better selection can be achieved and futile recanalization avoided.

Advancements in investigating clot composition and imaging tools that could influence the retrieval of clot and successful recanalization are needed.

Faster transportation of patients with acute ischemic stroke to hospitals where diagnosis can be done by either CT or MR will strengthen the battle against the passivity that results in approximately 40–50% of patients with ischemic stroke failing to reach a stroke center. Furthermore, despite recent progress, only 10–15% receive specific, precise treatment.

References

1. Garraway WM, Akhtar AJ, Prescott RJ, Hockey L. Management of acute stroke in the elderly: preliminary results of a controlled trial. Br Med J. 1980;280:1040–3.
2. The National Institute of Neurological Disorders and Stroke Rt-Pa Stroke Study Group. Tissue plasminogen activator for acute ischemic stroke. N Engl J Med. 1995;333:1581–7.
3. Wolpert SM, Bruckmann H, Greenlee R, Wechsler L, Pessin MS, Zoppo GJ, the rt-PA Acute Stroke Study Group. Neuroradiologic evaluation of patients with acute stroke treated with recombinant tissue plasminogen activator. AJNR. 1993;14:3–13.
4. Berkhemer OA, Fransen PS, Beumer D, et al., for the MR CLEAN Investigators. A randomized trial of intraarterial treatment for acute ischemic stroke. N Engl J Med. 2015;372:11–20.
5. Campbell BC, Mitchell PJ, Kleinig TJ, for the EXTEND-IA Investigators. Endovascular therapy for ischemic stroke with perfusion-imaging selection. N Engl J Med. 2015;372:1009–18.

6. Goyal M, Demchuk AM, Menon BK, et al., for the ESCAPE Trial Investigators. Randomized assessment of rapid endovascular treatment of ischemic stroke. N Engl J Med. 2015;372:1019–30.

7. Saver JL, Goyal M, Bonafe A, et al., for the SWIFT PRIME Investigators. Stent-retriever thrombectomy after intravenous t-PA vs. t-PA alone in stroke. N Engl J Med. 2015;372:2285–95.

8. Jovin TG, Chamorro A, Cobo E, et al., for the REVASCAT Trial Investigators. Thrombectomy within 8 hours after symptom onset in ischemic stroke. N Engl J Med. 2015;372:2296–2306.

9. Kidwell CS, Villablanca JP, Saver JL. Advances in neuroimaging of acute stroke. Curr Atheroscler Rep. 2000;2:126–35.

10. Hinman JD, Rost NS, Leung TW, Montaner J, Muir KW, Brown S, Arenillas JF, Feldmann E, Liebeskind DS. Principles of precision medicine in stroke. J Neurol Neurosurg Psychiatry. 2017;88:54–61.

11. Hansen K, Christensen A, Ovesen C, Havsteen I, Christensen H. Stroke severity and incidence of acute large vessel occlusions in patients with hyper-acute cerebral ischemia: results from a prospective cohort study based on CT-angiography (CTA). Int J Stroke. 2015;10(3):336–42.

12. Duffy S, McCarthy R, Farrell M, Thomas S, Brennan P, Power S, O'Hare A, Morris L, Rainsford E, MacCarthy E, Thornton J, Gilvarry M. Per-pass analysis of thrombus composition in patients with acute ischemic stroke undergoing mechanical thrombectomy. Stroke. 2019;50:1156–63.

13. Luthman AS, Bouchez L, Botta D, Vargas MI, Machi P, Lövblad KO. Imaging clot characteristics in stroke and its possible implication on treatment. Clin Neuroradiol. 2019; https://doi.org/10.1007/s00062-019-00841-w.

14. Jones TH, Morawetz RB, Crowell RM, Marcoux FW, Fitzgirbon SJ, Degirolami U, OEmann RG. Thresholds of focal cerebral ischemia in awake monkeys. J Neurosurg. 1981;54:773–82.

15. Jovin TG, Yonas H, Gebel JM, Kanal E, Chang YF, Grahovac SZ, Goldstein S, Wechsler LR. The cortical ischemic core and not the consistently present penumbra is a determinant of clinical outcome in acute middle cerebral artery occlusion. Stroke. 2003;34:2426–35.

16. Astrup J, Siesjo BK, Symon L. Thresholds in cerebral ischemia—the ischemic penumbra. Stroke. 1981;12(6):723.

17. Saver JL. Time is brain—quantified. Stroke. 2006;37:263–6.

18. von Kummer R, Dzialowski I. Imaging of cerebral ischemic edema and neuronal death. Neuroradiology. 2017;59:545–53.

19. Lev MH, Farkas J, Gemmete JJ. Acute stroke: improved nonenhanced CT detection—benefits of soft-copy interpretation by using variable window width and center level settings. Radiology. 1999;213:150–5.

20. Barber PA, Demchuk AM, Zhang J, Buchan AM, for the ASPECTS Study Group. Validity and reliability of a quantitative computed tomography score in predicting outcome of hyperacute stroke before thrombolytic therapy. Lancet. 2000;355:1670–4.

21. Yoo AJ, Zaidat OO, Chaudhry ZA, Berkhemer OA, González RG, Goyal M, Demchuk AM, Menon BK, Mualem E, Ueda D, Buell H, Sit SP, Bose A, on behalf of the Penumbra Pivotal and Penumbra Imaging Collaborative Study (PICS) Investigators. Impact of pretreatment non-contrast CT Alberta stroke program early CT score on clinical outcome after intra-arterial stroke therapy. Stroke. 2014;45:746–51.

22. Kim AC, Kiruluta A, Gonzalez RG, Schaefer P. Diffusion MR of acute stroke. In: Gonzalez RG, et al., editors. Acute ischemic stroke. 2nd ed. Berlin: Springer; 2011.

23. Fiehler J, von Bezold M, Kucinski T, Knab R, Eckert B, Wittkugel O, Zeumer H, Röther J. Cerebral blood flow predicts lesion growth in acute stroke patients. Stroke. 2002;33:2421–5.

24. Purushotham A, Campbell BCV, Straka M, Mlynash M, Olivot J-M, Bammer R, Kemp SM, Albers GW, Lansberg MG. Apparent diffusion coefficient threshold for delineation of ischemic core. Int J Stroke. 2015;10(3):348–53.

25. Goyal M, Ospel JM, Menon B, Almekhlafi M, Jayaraman M, Fiehler J, Psychogios M, Chapot R, Lugt A, Liu J, Yang P, Agid R, Hacke W, Walker M, Fischer U, Asdaghi N, McTaggart R, Srivastava P, Nogueira RG, Moret J, Saver JL, Hill MD, Dippel D, Fisher M. Challenging the ischemic core concept in acute ischemic stroke imaging. Stroke. 2020;51:3147–55.

26. Bhatia R, Hill MD, Shobha N, Menon B, Bal S, Kochar P, Watson T, Goyal M, Demchuk AM. Low rates of acute recanalization with intravenous recombinant tissue plasminogen activator in ischemic stroke real-world experience and a call for action. Stroke. 2010;41:2254–8.

27. Puetz V, Dzialowski I, Hill MD, Subramaniam S, Sylaja PN, Krol A, O'Reilly C, Hudon ME, Hu WY, Coutts SB, Barber PA, Watson T, Roy J, Demchuk AM, for the Calgary CTA Study Group. Intracranial thrombus extent predicts clinical outcome, final infarct size and hemorrhagic transformation in ischemic stroke: the clot burden score. Int J Stroke. 2008;3:230–6.

28. Dutra BG, Tolhuisen ML, Alves HCBR, Treurniet KM, Kappelhof M, Yoo AJ, Jansen IGH, Dippel DWJ, van Zwam WH, van Oostenbrugge RJ, Rocha AJ, Lingsma HF, van der Lugt A, Roos YBWEM, Marquering HA, Majoie CBLM, the MR CLEAN Registry Investigators. Thrombus imaging characteristics and outcomes in acute ischemic stroke patients undergoing endovascular treatment. Stroke. 2019;50:2057–64.

29. Maekawaa K, Shibataa M, Nakajimab H, Mizutanic A, Kitanob Y, Seguchia M, Yamasakic M, Kobayashia K, Sanob T, Morib G, Yabanad T, Naitoc Y, Shimizub S, Miyab F. Erythrocyte-rich thrombus is associated with reduced number of maneuvers and procedure time in patients with acute ischemic stroke undergoing mechanical thrombectomy. Cerebrovasc Dis Extra. 2018;8:39–49.

30. Riedel CH, Zimmermann P, Jensen-Kondering U, Stingele R, Deuschl G, Jansen O. The importance of size: successful recanalization by intravenous thrombolysis in acute anterior stroke depends on thrombus length. Stroke. 2011;42:1775–7.

31. Tomsick TA, Brott TG, Chambers AA, Fox AJ, Gaskill MF, Lukin RR, Pleatman CW, Wiot JG, Bourekas E. Hyperdense middle cerebral artery sign on CT: efficacy in detecting middle cerebral artery thrombosis. AJNR. 1990;11:473–7.

32. Jagani M, Kallmes DF, Brinjikji W. Correlation between clot density and recanalization success or stroke etiology in acute ischemic stroke patients. Interv Neuroradiol. 2017;23(3):274–8.

33. Luthman AS, Bouchez L, Botta D, Vargas MI, Machi P, Lövblad KO. Imaging clot characteristics in stroke and its possible implication on treatment. Clin Neuroradiol. 2020;30:27–35.

34. Schramm P, Schellinger PD, Klotz E, Kallenberg K, Fiebach JB, Kulkens S, Heiland S, Knauth M, Sartor K. Comparison of perfusion computed tomography and computed tomography angiography source images with perfusion-weighted imaging and diffusion-weighted imaging in patients with acute stroke of less than 6 hours' duration. Stroke. 2004;35:1652–8.

35. Lev MH, Farkas J, Rodriguez VR, Schwamm LH, Hunter GJ, Putman CM, Rordorf GA, Buonanno FS, Budzik R, Koroshetz WJ, Gonzalez GR. CT angiography in the rapid triage of patients with hyperacute stroke to intraarterial thrombolysis: accuracy in the detection of large vessel thrombus. J Comput Assist Tomogr. 2001;25(4):520–8.

36. Mayer SA, Viarasilpa T, Panyavachiraporn N, Brady M, Scozzari D, Van Harn M, Miller D, Katramados A, Hefzy H, Malik S, Marin H, Kole M, Chebl A, Lewandowski C, Mitsias PD. CTA-for-all impact of emergency computed tomographic angiography for all patients with stroke presenting within 24 hours of onset. Stroke. 2020;51:331–4.

37. Nael K, Khan R, Choudhary G, Meshksar A, Villablanca P, Tay J, Drake K, Coull BM, Kidwell CS. Six-minute magnetic resonance imaging protocol for evaluation of acute ischemic stroke pushing the boundaries. Stroke. 2014;45:1985–91.

38. Menon B, Smith EE, Coutts SB, Welsh DG, Faber JE, Goyal M, Hill MD, Demchuk AM, Damani Z, Cho K-H, Chang H, Hong J-H, Sohn SI. Leptomeningeal collaterals are associated with modifiable metabolic risk factors. Ann Neurol. 2013;74(2):241–8.

39. Zhang H, Prabhakar P, Sealock R, Faber JE. Wide genetic variation in the native pial collateral circulation is a major determinant of variation in severity of stroke. J Cereb Blood Flow Metab. 2010;30:923–34.

40. Liebeskind DS. Collateral circulation. Stroke. 2003;34:2279–84.

41. Lippert H, Pabst R. Arterial variations in man. Munich: JF Bergmann Verlag; 1985. p. 92–3.

42. Rocha M, Jovin TG. Fast versus slow progressors of infarct growth in large vessel occlusion stroke clinical and research implications. Stroke. 2017;48:2621–7.

43. Liebeskind DS, Tomsick TA, Foster LD, Yeatts SD, Carrozzella J, Demchuk AM, Jovin TG, Khatri P, von Kummer R, Sugg RM, Zaidat OO, Hussain SI, Goyal M, Menon BK, Al Ali F,

Yan B, Palesch YY, Broderick JP, for the IMS III Investigators. Collaterals at angiography and outcomes in the interventional management of stroke III trial. Stroke. 2014;45(3):759–64.

44. Mlynash M, Lansberg MG, De Silva DA, Lee J, Christensen S, Straka M, Campbell BCV, Bammer R, Olivot JM, Desmond P, Donnan GA, Davis SM, Albers GW, on behalf of the DEFUSE-EPITHET Investigators. Refining the definition of the malignant profile: insights from the DEFUSE-EPITHET pooled dataset. Stroke. 2011;42(5):1270–5.

45. Azizyan A, Sanossian N, Mogensen MA, Liebeskind DS. Fluid-attenuated inversion recovery vascular hyperintensities: an important imaging marker for cerebrovascular disease. Am J Neuroradiol. 2011;32:1771–5.

46. Tan JC, Dillon WP, Liu S, Adler F, Smith WS, Wintermark M. Systematic comparison of perfusion-CT and CT-angiography in acute stroke patients. Ann Neurol. 2007;61:533–43.

47. Parthasarathy R, Kate M, Rempel JL, Liebeskind DS, Jeerakathil T, Butcher KS, Shuaib A. Prognostic evaluation based on cortical vein score difference in stroke. Stroke. 2013;44:2748–54.

48. Menon BK, Bai HD, Modi J, Demchuk AM, Hudon M, Goyal M, TWJ W. The ICV sign as a marker of increased cerebral blood transit time. Can J Neurol Sci. 2013;40:187–91.

49. Johanna Mucke J, Möhlenbruch M, Kickingereder P, Kieslich PJ, Bäumer P, Gumbinger C, Purrucker J, Mundiyanapurath S, Schlemmer HP, Bendszus M, Radbruch A. Asymmetry of deep medullary veins on susceptibility weighted MRI in patients with acute MCA stroke is associated with poor outcome. PLoS One. 2015;10(4):e0120801.

50. Koopman MS, Berkhemer OA, Geuskens RR, Emmer BJ, van Walderveen MA, Jenniskens SF, van Zwam WH, van Oostenbrugge RJ, van der Lugt A, Dippel DW, Beenen LF, Roos YB, Marquering HA, Majoie CB, on behalf of the MR CLEAN Trial Investigators. Comparison of three commonly used CT perfusion software packages in patients with acute ischemic stroke. J NeuroIntervent Surg. 2019;11:1–8.

51. Dávalos A, Blanco M, Pedraza S, Leira R, Castellanos M, Pumar JM, Silva Y, Serena J, Castillo J. The clinical–DWI mismatch. A new diagnostic approach to the brain tissue at risk of infarction. Neurology. 2004;62:2187–92.

52. Eastwood JD, Lev MH, Azhari T, Lee TY, Barboriak DP, Delong DM, Fitzek C, Herzau M, Wintermark M, Meuli R, Brazier D, Provenzale JM. Perfusion scanning with deconvolution analysis: pilot study in patients with acute middle cerebral artery stroke. Radiology. 2002;222:227–36.

53. Sorensen AG, Copen WA, Østergaard L, Buonanno FS, Gonzalez RG, Rordorf G, Rosen BR, Schwamm LH, Weisskoff RM, Koroshetz WJ. Hyperacute stroke: simultaneous measurement of relative cerebral blood volume, relative cerebral blood flow, and mean tissue transit time. Radiology. 1999;210:519–27.

54. Heit JJ, Wintermark M. Perfusion computed tomography for the evaluation of acute ischemic stroke strengths and pitfalls. Stroke. 2016;47:1153–8.

55. Hacke W, Kaste M, Bluhmki E, Brozman M, Dávalos A, Guidetti D, Larrue V, Lees KR, Medeghri Z, Machnig T, Schneider D, von Kummer R, Wahlgren N, Toni D, for the ECASS Investigators. Thrombolysis with Alteplase 3 to 4.5 hours after acute ischemic stroke. N Engl J Med. 2008;359(13):1317–29.

56. Albers GW, Marks MP, Kemp S, Christensen S, Tsai JP, Ortega-Gutierrez S, McTaggart RA, Torbey MT, Kim-Tenser M, Leslie-Mazwi T, Sarraj A, Kasner SE, Ansari SA, Yeatts SD, Hamilton S, Mlynash M, Heit JJ, Zaharchuk G, Kim S, Carrozzella J, Palesch YY, Demchuk AM, Bammer R, Lavori PW, Broderick JP, Lansberg MG, for the DEFUSE 3 Investigators. Thrombectomy for stroke at 6 to 16 hours with selection by perfusion imaging. N Engl J Med. 2018;378(8):708–18.

57. Nogueira RG, Jadhav AP, Haussen DC, Bonafe A, Budzik RF, Bhuva P, Yavagal DR, Ribo M, Cognard C, Hanel RA, Sila CA, Hassan AE, Millan M, Levy EI, Mitchell P, Chen M, English JD, Shah QA, Silver FL, Pereira VM, Mehta BP, Baxter BW, Abraham MG, Cardona P, Veznedaroglu E, Hellinger FR, Feng L, Kirmani JF, Lopes DK, Jankowitz BT, Frankel MR, Costalat V, Vora NA, Yoo AJ, Malik AM, Furlan AJ, Rubiera M, Aghaebrahim A, Olivot JM, Tekle WG, Shields R, Graves T, Lewis RJ, Smith WS, Liebeskind DS, Saver JL, Jovin TG,

for the DAWN Trial Investigators. Thrombectomy 6 to 24 hours after stroke with a mismatch between deficit and infarct. N Engl J Med. 2018;378(1):11–21.

58. Goyal M, Menon BK, van Zwam WH, DWJ D, Mitchell PJ, Demchuk AM, Dávalos A, Majoie CB, van der Lugt A, de Miquel MA, Donnan GA, Roos YB, Bonafe A, Jahan R, Diener HC, van den Berg LA, Levy EI, Berkhemer OA, Pereira VM, Rempel J, Millán M, Davis SM, Roy D, Thornton J, Román LS, Ribó M, Beumer D, Stouch B, Brown S, Campbell BC, van Oostenbrugge RJ, Saver JL, Hill MD, Jovin TG, for the HERMES Collaborators. Endovascular thrombectomy after large-vessel ischaemic stroke: a meta-analysis of individual patient data from five randomised trials. Lancet. 2016;387:1723–31.

59. Pierot L, Jayaraman MV, Szikora I, et al. Standards of practice in acute ischemic stroke intervention: international recommendations. J NeuroIntervent Surg. 2018;10:1121–6.

60. Smith EE, Schwamm LH. Endovascular clot retrieval therapy implications for the Organization of Stroke Systems of Care in North America. Stroke. 2015;46:1462–7.

61. Carlsson KS, Andsberg G, Petersson J, Norrving B. Long-term cost-effectiveness of thrombectomy for acute ischaemic stroke in real life: an analysis based on data from the Swedish stroke register (Riksstroke). Int J Stroke. 2017;12:1–13.

62. Powers W, Derdeyn CP, Biller J, Coffey CS, Hoh BL, Jauch EC, Johnston KC, Johnston SC, Khalessi AA, Kidwell CS, Meschia JF, Ovbiagele B, Yavagal DR, on behalf of the American Heart Association Stroke Council. 2015 American Heart Association/American Stroke Association focused update of the 2013 guidelines for the early management of patients with acute ischemic stroke regarding endovascular treatment. Stroke. 2015;46:3024–39.

63. Turc G, Bhogal P, Fischer U, et al. European Stroke Organisation (ESO)—European Society for Minimally Invasive Neurological Therapy (ESMINT) guidelines on mechanical thrombectomy in acute ischemic stroke. J NeuroIntervent Surg. 2019:1–30. https://doi.org/10.1136/neurintsurg-2018-014569.

64. Powers WJ, Rabinstein AA, Ackerson T, Adeoye OM, Bambakidis NC, Becker K, Biller J, Brown M, Demaerschalk BM, Hoh B, Jauch EC, Kidwell CS, Leslie-Mazwi TM, Ovbiagele B, Scott PA, Sheth KN, Southerland AM, Summers DV, Tirschwell DL, on behalf of the American Heart Association Stroke Council. Guidelines for the early management of patients with acute ischemic stroke: 2019 update to the 2018 guidelines for the early management of acute ischemic stroke a guideline for healthcare professionals from the American Heart Association/American Stroke Association endorsed by the Society for Academic Emergency Medicine and the Neurocritical Care Society. Stroke. 2019;50:e344. https://doi.org/10.1161/STR.0000000000000211.

65. Goyal N, Tsivgoulis G, Frei D, et al. A multicenter study of the safety and effectiveness of mechanical thrombectomy for patients with acute ischemic stroke not meeting top-tier evidence criteria. J NeuroIntervent Surg. 2018;10:10–6.

66. Higashida RT, Furlan AJ, for the Technology Assessment Committees of the American Society of Interventional and Therapeutic Neuroradiology and the Society of Interventional Radiology. Trial design and reporting standards for intra-arterial cerebral thrombolysis for acute ischemic stroke. Stroke. 2003;34:e109–37.

67. Sørensen LH, Speiser L, Karabegovic S, et al. A safety and quality of endovascular therapy under general anesthesia and conscious sedation are comparable: results from the GOLIATH trial. J NeuroIntervent Surg. 2019;11:1070–2.

68. Turk AS, Siddiqui A, Fifi JT, De Leacy RA, Fiorella DJ, Gu E, Levy EI, Snyder KV, Hanel RA, Aghaebrahim A, Woodward BK, Hixson HR, Chaudry MI, Spiotta AM, Rai AT, Frei D, Almandoz JED, Kelly M, Arthur A, Baxter B, English J, Linfante I, Fargen KM, Mocco J. Aspiration thrombectomy versus stent retriever thrombectomy as first-line approach for large vessel occlusion (COMPASS): a multicentre, randomised, open label, blinded outcome, non-inferiority trial. Lancet. 2019;393:998–1008.

69. Ducroux C, Piotin M, Gory B, Labreuche J, Blanc R, Maacha MB, Lapergue B, Fahed R, for the ASTER Trial Investigators. First pass effect with contact aspiration and stent retrievers in the aspiration versus stent retriever (ASTER) trial. J NeuroIntervent Surg. 2020;12:386–91.

70. Boers AMM, Jansen IGH, Beenen LFM, et al. Association of follow-up infarct volume with functional outcome in acute ischemic stroke: a pooled analysis of seven randomized trials. J NeuroIntervent Surg. 2018;10:1–6.
71. Bahouth MN, Leys D. Baseline functional status as a variable in personalized acute stroke care. Neurology. 2019;93:869–70.
72. Gumbinger C, Ringleb P, Ippen F, Ungerer M, Reuter B, Bruder I, Daffertshofer M, Stock C, for the Stroke Working Group of Baden-Wurttemberg. Outcomes of patients with stroke treated with thrombolysis according to prestroke Rankin Scale scores. Neurology. 2019;93:e1–e10.
73. Cagnazzo F, Derraz I, Dargazanli C, Lefevre P-H, Gascou G, Riquelme C, Bonafe A, Vincent CV. Mechanical thrombectomy in patients with acute ischemic stroke and ASPECTS ≤6: a meta-analysis. J NeuroIntervent Surg. 2020;12:350–5.
74. Kaesmacher J, Chaloulos-Iakovidis P, Panos L, Mordasini P, Michel P, Hajdu S, Ribo M, Requena M, Maegerlein C, Friedrich B, Costalat V, Benali A, Pierot L, Gawlitza M, Schaafsma J, Pereira VM, Gralla J, Fischer U. Mechanical thrombectomy in ischemic stroke patients with Alberta stroke program early computed tomography score 0–5. Stroke. 2019;50:880–8.
75. Mourand I, Abergel E, Mantilla D, et al. Favorable revascularization therapy in patients with ASPECTS ≤5 on DWI in anterior circulation stroke. J NeuroIntervent Surg. 2018;10:5–9.
76. Ospel J, Kim B, Heo J-H, Yoshimura S, Kashani N, Menon B, Almekhlafi M, Demchuk A, Hill M, Saposnik G, Goyal M. Endovascular treatment decision-making in acute ischemic stroke patients with large vessel occlusion and low National Institutes of Health Stroke Scale: insights from UNMASK EVT, an international multidisciplinary survey. Neuroradiology. 2020;62:715–21.
77. Anadani M, Spiotta AM, Alawieh A, Turjman F, Piotin M, Haussen DC, Nogueira RG, Papanagiotou P, Siddiqui AH, Lapergue B, Dorn F, Cognard C, Ribo M, Psychogios MN, Labeyrie MA, Mazighi M, Biondi A, Anxionnat R, Bracard S, Richard S, Gory B, on behalf of the TITAN (Thrombectomy in TANdem lesions) Investigators. Emergent carotid stenting plus thrombectomy after thrombolysis in tandem strokes analysis of the TITAN Registry. Stroke. 2019;50:2250–2.
78. Premat K, Dechartres A, Lenck S, Shotar E, Le Bouc R, Degos V, Sourour N, Alamowitch S, Samson Y, Clarençon F. Rescue stenting versus medical care alone in refractory large vessel occlusions: a systematic review and meta-analysis. Neuroradiology. 2020;62:629–37.
79. Yang P, Zhang Y, Zhang L, et al. Endovascular thrombectomy with or without intravenous alteplase in acute stroke. N Engl J Med. 2020; https://doi.org/10.1056/NEJMoa2001123.
80. Campbell BCV, Mitchell PJ, Churilov L, et al. Tenecteplase versus alteplase before thrombectomy for ischemic stroke. N Engl J Med. 2018;378:1573–82.
81. Nguyen TN, Abdalkader M, Jovin TG, Nogueira RG, Jadhav AP, Haussen DC, Hassan AE, Novakovic R, Sheth SA, Ortega-Gutierrez S, Panagos PD, Cordina SM, Linfante I, Mansour OY, Malik AM, Narayanan S, Masoud HE, Chou SH-Y, Khatri R, Janardhan V, Yavagal DR, Zaidat OO, Greer DM, Liebeskind DS. Mechanical thrombectomy in the era of the COVID-19 pandemic: emergency preparedness for neuroscience teams a guidance statement from the Society of Vascular and Interventional Neurology. Stroke. 2020;51:1896–901.
82. Pop R, Hasiu A, Bolognini F, Mihoc D, Quenardelle V, Gheoca R, Schluck E, Courtois S, Delaitre M, Musacchio M, Pottecher J, Chamaraux-Tran TN, Sellal F, Wolff V, Lebedinsky PA, Beaujeux R. Stroke thrombectomy in patients with COVID-19: initial experience in 13 cases. AJNR. 2020; https://doi.org/10.3174/ajnr.A6750.

Current Applications of Precision Medicine in Haemorrhagic Stroke

Jonathan G. Best and David J. Werring

7.1   Introduction

Of the various forms of intracranial haemorrhage, which also encompasses sub-arachnoid, subdural, intraventricular, traumatic, and venous haemorrhages, as well as haemorrhagic transformation of infarcted brain tissue, spontaneous intracerebral haemorrhage (ICH)—non-traumatic haemorrhage originating within brain paren-chyma—is the most likely to present to stroke physicians or neurologists with a clinical stroke syndrome. It accounts for 10–20% of strokes worldwide, with a higher incidence in low- and middle-income countries [1, 2] and East Asian popula-tions [3]. Despite advances in cardiovascular risk factor management, the age-standardised incidence of ICH remains static, in part due to the increasing use of oral anticoagulants [4], while the absolute incidence continues to increase in ageing populations. Unlike ischaemic stroke, there are no proven disease-modifying treat-ments for ICH, and its morbidity and mortality are considerably higher, with 30-day mortality of around 40% and a risk of long-term dependency of at least 60% [5]. Despite its lower incidence, the burden of disability associated with ICH is similar to that of ischaemic stroke, with 18 million people estimated to be living with the consequences of ICH [6], and 5% of all deaths are attributed to ICH worldwide [7]. The effective treatment and prevention of ICH is therefore a major unmet global health need.

The concept of precision medicine has its origins in the selection of treatment based on individual pathophysiology, with a focus on pharmacogenomics and oncogenomics [8]. ICH, a largely sporadic condition with no established treatments, may seem a difficult target for such an approach. However, in the broader sense of clinical care tailored to the characteristics of individuals or groups with shared char acteristics [9], opportunities for precision medicine exist in the care of patients with

J. G. Best · D. J. Werring (✉)
Stroke Research Centre, UCL Queen Square Institute of Neurology, London, UK
e-mail: jonathan.best@ucl.ac.uk; d.werring@ucl.ac.uk

© Springer Nature Switzerland AG 2021   127
A. C. Fonseca, J. M. Ferro (eds.), *Precision Medicine in Stroke*,
https://doi.org/10.1007/978-3-030-70761-3_7

ICH. These include the rational investigation of ICH aetiology, selection of secondary prevention strategies, and individualised prognostication. The recent successes of imaging-based patient selection in extending hyperacute treatment in ischaemic stroke to previously untreatable groups [10–13] raise the possibility that detailed phenotyping based on pathophysiology might also have a role in developing new treatments in ICH. In this chapter, we review the current practice of precision medicine in ICH, and discuss the outlook for progress in this field in the near future.

7.2 Aetiology

The diagnosis of acute ICH is usually straightforward, at least in healthcare systems with widespread access to computed tomography (CT). Establishing the cause of the ICH is often more challenging, but is an essential first step towards precision medical care, with major implications for recurrence risk and secondary prevention. Indeed, the concept of a 'new taxonomy' of disease based on pathophysiology was a major focus of the influential report by the US National Research Council which proposed the term 'precision medicine'. In this respect, the historic classification of ICH into 'primary' and 'secondary' haemorrhages is inadequate: 'primary' haemorrhage is not without cause, but is usually caused by a cerebral small arteriopathy, while 'secondary' haemorrhage includes a wide range of conditions and risk factors with very different underlying pathology [14]. This classification is therefore of little clinical or prognostic value. The term 'primary' provides a spurious diagnostic certainty, and discourages adequate investigation and appropriate classification. Classification systems based on aetiology do exist, notably the 'SMASH-U' classification [15], which groups ICH into groups caused by structural vascular lesions, antithrombotic medication, cerebral amyloid angiopathy, systemic disease, hypertension, and undetermined causes, and the H-ATOMIC classification [16], which includes additional categories for tumours and combined causes, and replaces 'systemic disease' with 'infrequent causes'. Both systems show excellent interrater reliability, and SMASH-U classification is associated with mortality risk [15]. In clinical practice, our approach to investigation is first to exclude a structural vascular cause (preferring the term 'macrovascular', as small vessel diseases are also associated with abnormal vascular structure), and to consider whether an unusual cause, such as a genetic small vessel disease, might be present requiring additional targeted investigations. Most remaining cases can be attributed to sporadic small vessel disease, which we aim to classify in as much detail as possible. We regard antithrombotic medication as an exacerbating factor with particular implications for treatment, rather than an independent cause, as antithrombotic medication does not in itself cause arterial wall rupture, the prerequisite for ICH.

7.2.1 Macrovascular Lesions

The overall prevalence of an underlying macrovascular lesion in ICH patients is around 20% [17, 18]. Of these, around half are arteriovenous malformations, with dural arteriovenous fistulae, aneurysms, and cavernomas making up the remainder. Apart from cavernomas, which are angiographically occult low-flow capillary lesions best diagnosed using blood-sensitive MRI sequences, digital subtraction angiography is the gold standard for the diagnosis of these lesions and should be considered in all ICH patients in whom non-invasive imaging has not yielded a definitive aetiology. However, invasive angiography is associated with a small but appreciable risk of ischaemic stroke, vessel wall perforation, and death (up to 1%, 1%, and 0.1%, respectively) [19], risks which must be balanced against the anticipated yield of the procedure, and the fitness of the patient to undergo treatment of any lesion identified.

Many risk factors for the presence of a macrovascular lesion have been described. Most obviously, a younger age and the absence of conventional cardiovascular risk factors, such as hypertension, diabetes, and smoking, reduce the probability a patient will have significant cerebral small vessel disease, and therefore increase the probability that an alternative cause is present. The absence of radiological signs of small vessel disease on CT and MRI, such as leukoaraiosis/white matter hyperintensities, lacunes, cerebral microbleeds, and enlarged perivascular spaces, provides evidence against the presence of cerebral small vessel disease, and is associated with a very low risk of intracranial haemorrhage overall [20]. ICH in such patients is therefore unusual and should be thoroughly investigated. Other predictors of macrovascular lesion presence include posterior fossa and lobar haemorrhage locations [18] and the presence of suggestive abnormalities on CT angiography [21]. The interaction between haemorrhage location and risk factor profile should be considered: the absence of signs of cerebral amyloid angiopathy may be more important in a patient with a lobar haemorrhage than a deep haemorrhage, while diabetes, male sex, alcohol abuse, and black or Hispanic ethnicity may be risk factors for non-lobar haemorrhage only [22].

A clinical prediction model summarising these risk factors, the DIAGRAM score, has been proposed for selecting ICH patients for catheter angiography [23]. Developed in a multicentre prospective cohort of 298 patients undergoing investigation after non-traumatic ICH, the score incorporates age >50 years, lobar and posterior ICH locations, absence of leukoaraiosis and lacunes on CT, and, where available, suggestive findings on CT angiography as independent predictors of a macrovascular lesion (Fig. 7.1). In external validation in a cohort of 173 consecutive ICH patients undergoing catheter angiography at an independent centre, the model incorporating CTA findings showed excellent discrimination ($c = 0.88$). Using DIAGRAM, patients with small vessel disease and deep ICH, and patients >50 years with small vessel disease and a negative CTA, had a 1–2% risk of a macrovascular lesion, a level at which a DSA might not be justified. However, the model

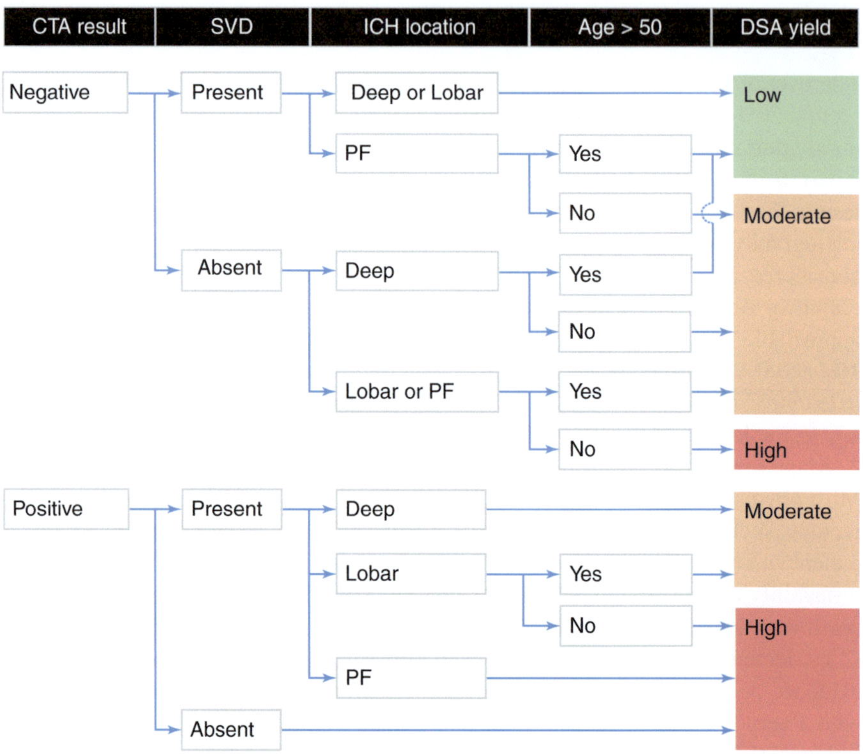

Fig. 7.1 Algorithm for predicted probability of macrovascular lesion presence, based on the DIAGRAM CTA-based risk model (DIAGRAM+; Ref. [23]). 'Low' DSA yield corresponds to predicted probability of macrovascular lesion presence $\leq$5%, 'moderate' 6–25%, and 'high' >25%. *PF* posterior fossa, *SVD* small vessel disease

without CTA showed more modest discrimination ($c = 0.66$), both models systematically underestimated risk prior to recalibration, and the confidence intervals for observed risks across all levels of the score were relatively wide, reflecting a relatively small sample size. Patients >70 years were excluded, reducing widespread applicability. Although macrovascular lesion prevalence might be expected to be low in this group, a predictive tool to identify older patients who should undergo DSA despite negative non-invasive vascular imaging would be of value.

The use of more detailed imaging might allow more accurate prediction of macrovascular lesion risk. Although the DIAGRAM score pragmatically uses CT to assess small vessel disease, MRI is often performed before deciding if catheter angiography is needed, and is sensitive to small vessel disease markers such as perivascular spaces and cerebral microbleeds that CT cannot detect. This allows more accurate identification of patients without small vessel disease, and better assessment of its severity when present, by individual markers or using validated composite small vessel disease burden scores [24]. The characteristics of the haematoma itself might also be informative, with the hypothesis that the type of bleeding source affects haematoma shape or texture. A study using radiomics features from manually segmented ICH cases to train a range of classification algorithms found excellent discrimination ($c = 0.96$) and negative predictive value (0.97) for the highest-performing algorithm, an adaptive boosted decision tree classifier [25]. Positive predictive value was good (0.80), comparable to an experienced radiologist. However, the use of such highly flexible algorithms and many input variables in small study populations is prone to overfitting, and rigorous external validation was not performed. The requirement for lesion segmentation is another barrier to the implementation of similar approaches in routine clinical practice.

7.2.2 Genetic Causes of ICH

Although ICH risk shows substantial heritability—up to 44%, based on data from the International Stroke Genetics Consortium [26]—monogenic causes of ICH, in the sense of a penetrant disorder showing Mendelian inheritance, are rare. Their recognition is nevertheless important, with important prognostic implications for affected patients and their families. These patients, in whom dysfunction of a specific molecular pathway leads with high probability to ICH, may also be candidates for the development of targeted therapies in the future—a core aim of precision medicine—and their study may offer insights into the pathogenesis of ICH in general.

Many monogenic disorders causing ICH are small vessel diseases, including COL4A1/2-related disorders, CARASAL, CADASIL, Fabry disease, and familial cerebral amyloid angiopathy. While these disorders may show distinctive neurological and systemic features (Table 7.1, Fig. 7.2), these may not be apparent unless specifically sought, and may show variable expression. The clinical spectrum associated with these disorders may expand with the increased use of genetic testing [27], and a family history may be absent due to unrecognised mild disease, incomplete penetrance, or censoring. Deciding when to perform genetic testing in patients presenting with ICH and radiological evidence of cerebral small vessel disease can be challenging. The European Academy of Neurology has recently published consensus guidelines in this area [28]. Proposed 'red flags' for genetic small vessel diseases include young age at onset, family history or consanguinity, and characteristic clinical or neuroimaging phenotypes. The absence of traditional vascular risk factors may prompt consideration of genetic small vessel disease, but their presence should not prevent testing if otherwise indicated, and testing does not need to be reserved only for cases in which sporadic causes have been exhaustively excluded. Gene panels, where available, can allow more efficient investigation than sequential tests for individual genetic variants or genes.

Genetic disorders may also be considered in patients with macrovascular lesions, particularly in the presence of multiple lesions or a family history of similar lesions or ICH. Mutations in three genes, KRIT1, CCM2/malcavernin, and PCD10, are associated with CCM1, 2, and 3, respectively, disorders characterised by multiple cerebral cavernous malformations (Fig. 7.3), with autosomal dominant inheritance

Table 7.1 Summary of sporadic and monogenic cerebral small vessel diseases associated with ICH

	DPA (arteriolosclerosis)	CAA	COL4A1/2	CADASIL	CARASAL	Fabry disease
Hereditability	Sporadic	Sporadic; rare familial forms exist	AD	AD	AR	X-linked; female heterozygotes may be symptomatic
Aetiology	Conventional vascular risk factors, especially hypertension	Age related; APOε2 and APOε4 alleles; iatrogenic cases described (neurosurgery, HGH)	Missense/null mutations in COL4A1 or COL4A2, encoding type 4 collagen	NOTCH3 mutation leading to abnormal aggregation and sequestration of ECM proteins	CTSA mutation; encodes cathepsin-A, involved in lysosomal function and degradation of endothelin-1	GLA gene variants (~900 reported); lysosomal storage disease with accumulation of GL-3/lyso-GL-3
Age at symptom onset	Usually >65 years; also younger patients with additional risk factors, e.g. secondary hypertension	Usually >65 years; Boston criteria exclude patients <55 years	Stroke onset in 30s; congenital brain malformations and paediatric ICH may occur	Stroke onset between 40 and 60 years; migraine with aura onset between 20 and 40 years	20–40s	Stroke onset usually 20–50 years
Neurological features	ICH, especially deep Small vessel IS Cognitive impairment (slowed processing, executive dysfunction) Gait disorder Urinary incontinence	Lobar ICH Convexity SAH and TFNE High recurrence risk Lobar lacunar infarcts Cortical microinfarcts Cognitive impairment (including amnestic features if associated with AD)	Stroke (ICH twice as common as IS) Intracranial aneurysms Porencephaly Schizencephaly	Small vessel IS ICH (rare) Migraine with aura Acute encephalopathy Cognitive impairment Gait disorder	IS and ICH Late cognitive decline Headache, migraine Vertigo Dystonia Gait disorder	IS (large and small vessel) ICH Posterior circulation involvement CVST Tinnitus, deafness Acroparesthesias

	DPA (arteriolosclerosis)	CAA	COL4A1/2	CADASIL	CARASAL	Fabry disease
Systemic features	Cardiovascular comorbidities common	–	Retinal vasculopathy Premature cataracts Renal and hepatic cysts CKD and proteinuria	–	Refractory hypertension Dry eyes and mouth Muscle cramps	Angiokeratomas Hypohidrosis Corneal opacity Ischaemic heart disease Cardiomyopathy Arrhythmias CKD
Radiological signs	WMH, deep lacunes, BGPVS, deep CMBs	WMH, lobar lacunes, CSOPVS, lobar CMBs, cSS	Evidence of previous ICH (e.g. haemosiderin-lined cavities), CMBs, WMH, lacunes	WMH, lacunes, PVS, CMBs; anterior temporal lobe involvement characteristic but may be absent	Leukoencephalopathy with brainstem involvement; may be disproportionate to clinical features	WMH Lacunes and CMBs Basilar dolichoectasia Pulvinar sign (T1 hyperintensity of lateral pulvinar)
Management	Vascular risk factor control (esp. BP)	sBP <130 mmHg Avoid antithrombotics	Avoid antithrombotics, prolonged exercise, and activities with risk of head injury	Vascular risk factor control; antiplatelets not indicated unless previous IS	No specific treatment recommended; very limited data (19 cases as of early 2020)	Control of vascular risk factors; antiplatelets if previous IS; enzyme replacement therapy reduces systemic complications and may reduce stroke risk (limited data)

DPA deep perforator arteriopathy, *CAA* cerebral amyloid angiopathy, *HGH* human growth hormone, *TFNE* transient focal neurological episodes, *CADASIL* cerebral autosomal dominant arteriopathy with subcortical infarcts and leukoencephalopathy, *ECM* extracellular matrix, *CARASAL* cathepsin-A-related arteriopathy with strokes and leukoencephalopathy, *CVST* cerebral venous sinus thrombosis, *CKD* chronic kidney disease, *BP* blood pressure

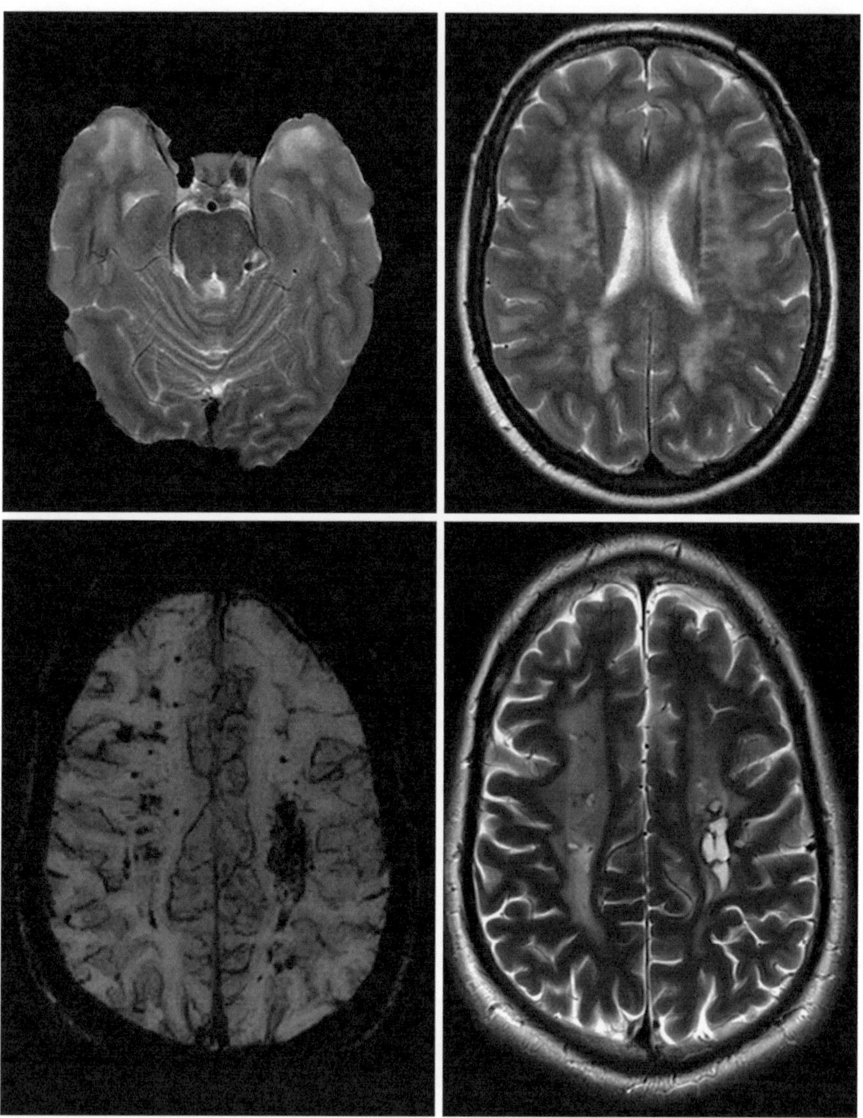

Fig. 7.2 Monogenic small vessel diseases. Top: CADASIL—extensive white matter hyperintensity with distinctive involvement of anterior temporal lobes, only rarely associated with ICH. Bottom: COL4A1-related small vessel disease, with extensive microhaemorrhages and cystic lesions, frequently associated with ICH

[29]. The diagnostic yield of genetic testing may be more than 75% in patients with a positive family history of cavernomas, or multiple cavernomas without previous brain radiotherapy (which can cause cavernoma development within the radiation field) [30]. Although somatic KRAS and BRAF mutations are common within endothelial cells from cerebral arteriovenous malformations [31, 32], nearly all

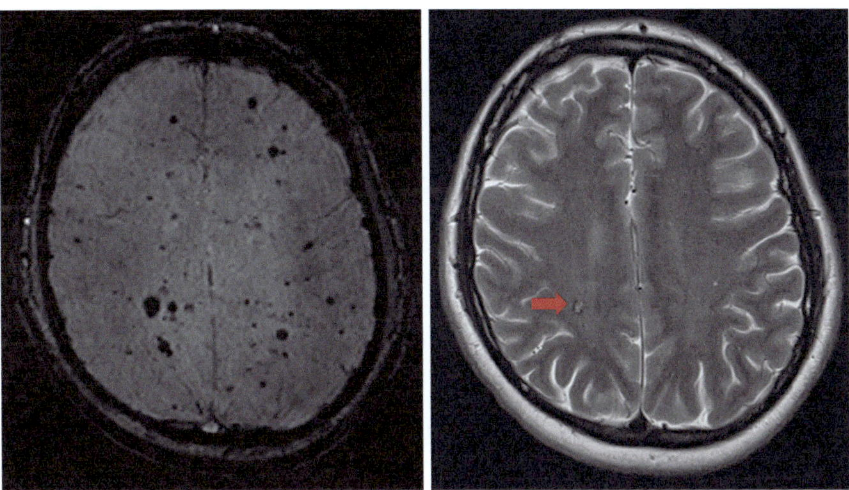

Fig. 7.3 Left: Multiple foci of hypointensity on susceptibility-weighted MR imaging corresponding to cerebral cavernomas in a patient with KRIT-1 mutation. Right: T2-weighted MRI shows small hyperintense lesion with hypointense rim (arrowed), typical of a cavernoma and corresponding to a larger focus of susceptibility on SWI

arteriovenous malformations are sporadic. A suggestive family history, recurrent epistaxis, mucocutaneous telangiectasia, gastrointestinal bleeding, or known arteriovenous malformations at other sites raise the possibility of hereditary haemorrhagic telangiectasia (HHT), caused by mutations in the TGF-β signalling pathway leading to abnormal VEGF expression and dysfunctional angiogenesis. The use of bevacizumab, a monoclonal antibody targeting VEGF-A, to reduce transfusion requirements and epistaxis in HHT is a rare example of a targeted molecular treatment for a disorder associated with ICH [33], although whether bevacizumab reduces ICH risk is unknown.

7.2.3 Sporadic Cerebral Small Vessel Disease

After excluding macrovascular lesions and genetic disorders, the vast majority of ICH is caused by sporadic cerebral small vessel disease. Two main forms exist. Firstly, arteriolosclerosis, in which the walls of small arteries and arterioles become thickened and inelastic, probably due to the extravasation of plasma components across damaged vascular endothelium. This form of small vessel disease is strongly, but not exclusively, associated with hypertension [34], and is contributed to by other cardiovascular risk factors such as diabetes and smoking. It particularly affects small perforating vessels supplying the basal regions of the brain. These arise directly from large cerebral arteries, without the protection of preceding long, branching arteries afforded to cortical arterioles, so are exposed directly to high pulse pressures [35]. Cerebral arteriolosclerosis is therefore also termed 'deep perforator arteriopathy' (DPA). The other main cerebral small vessel disease, sporadic cerebral amyloid angiopathy (CAA), is an age-related disorder which occurs independently of other conventional vascular risk factors, in which amyloid-β accumulates within the walls of cortical and leptomeningeal small arteries and arterioles (as well as venules and, less commonly, capillaries) leading to smooth muscle loss, vascular fragility, and a risk of ICH exceeding 15% per year in certain forms of the disease [36]. The pathophysiology of CAA is incompletely understood, but may be contributed by impaired perivascular clearance of amyloid-β [37] and presence of APOε2 and APOε4 alleles of the apolipoprotein E gene, which influence amyloid-β clearance from brain parenchyma and transport across the blood-brain barrier [38].

Neuroimaging, especially MRI with blood-sensitive T2*GRE or SWI sequences, is the most helpful tool for distinguishing these two small vessel diseases in vivo (Fig. 7.4). The Boston criteria for CAA were proposed in 1995, and modified to include cortical superficial siderosis in 2010 [39]. Under these criteria, a definite diagnosis of CAA can only be made through a full post-mortem examination showing evidence of severe CAA; however, a diagnosis of 'probable' CAA can be made in patients over 55 years old in whom MRI shows evidence of multiple macro- or micro-haemorrhages within cortex or subcortical white matter only, or a single such haemorrhage and cortical superficial siderosis, indicating previous convexity subarachnoid haemorrhage. In patients with ICH, a rating of probable CAA by modified Boston criteria shows 94.7% sensitivity and 81.2% specificity for a pathological diagnosis of CAA [40]. These criteria do have several limitations. Firstly, the performance of the modified Boston criteria in patients without previous symptomatic ICH is uncertain, while the sensitivity of the original criteria appears low in these patients [41]. Secondly, the requirement for a strictly lobar pattern of haemorrhage excludes the diagnosis of CAA in patients with any evidence of deep haemorrhage. This is problematic, as DPA and CAA probably coexist in many older patients [42]. Criteria acknowledging patients with a 'mixed' small arteriopathy would be helpful in clinical practice and prognostic research. Thirdly, non-haemorrhagic markers of CAA are emerging, including enlarged perivascular spaces within the centrum semiovale [43], posterior-predominant white matter hyperintensities [44], and cortical microinfarcts [45]. These may be early markers of CAA, and their incorporation into diagnostic criteria, if validated, might facilitate study of the early natural history of CAA and trials of disease-modifying treatment [39]. An international effort to update the Boston criteria is currently underway, and aims to address many of these issues [46].

Beyond the Boston criteria, the Edinburgh criteria aim to provide a means to diagnose CAA using CT, supplemented by genetic data on APOE genotype where available [47]. In its derivation cohort of 62 consecutive participants with lobar ICH who subsequently underwent autopsy, the combination of subarachnoid haemorrhage and either fingerlike projections (Fig. 7.5) or APOε4 possession showed 96% specificity for the diagnosis at post-mortem of moderate or severe CAA, while the absence of these markers showed 100% rule-out sensitivity. A simplified neuroimaging-only model without APOE genotype showed similar performance, suggesting that these criteria might have particular applications in lower resource

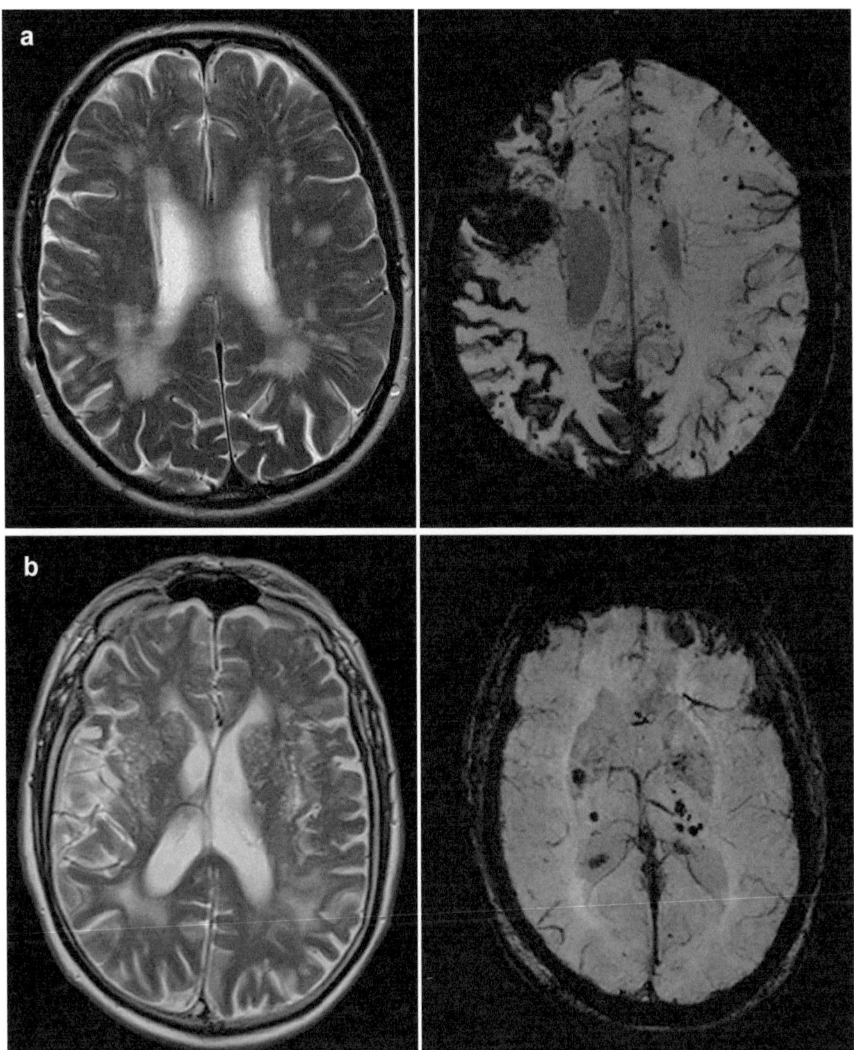

Fig. 7.4 (**a**) Cerebral amyloid angiopathy. Left: T2 MRI shows white matter hyperintensity with posterior predominance and enlarged perivascular spaces within deep white matter. Right: SWI demonstrates multiple lobar microhaemorrhages, disseminated cortical siderosis, and evidence of previous lobar macrohaemorrhage. (**b**) Deep perforator arteriopathy. Left: White matter hyperintensity and enlarged basal ganglia perivascular spaces on T2 MRI. Right: Deep microhaemorrhages on SWI

settings without access to MRI. However, the criteria have not yet been externally validated, and their generalisability to younger patients and those with smaller volume non-fatal haemorrhage is uncertain. The role of other non-imaging data in the diagnosis of CAA is also under investigation: a recent small study identified a global reduction in CSF amyloid species compared to healthy controls, while elevated tau,

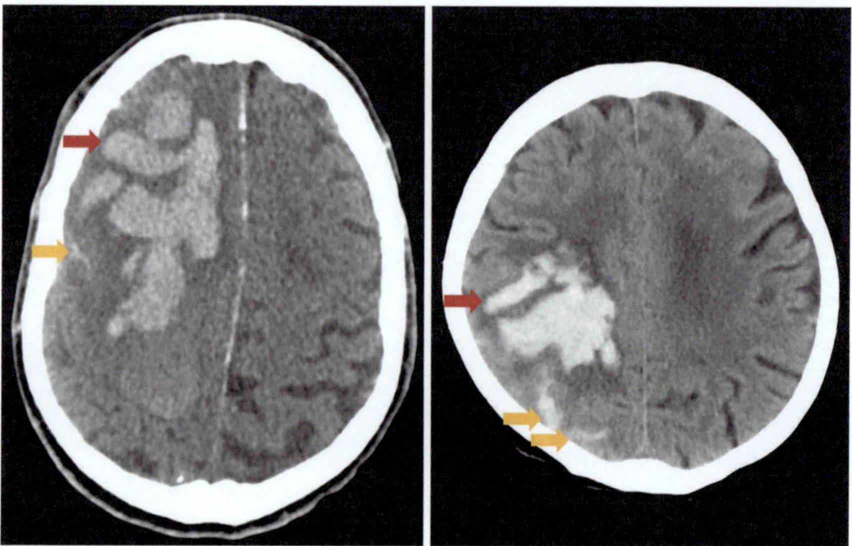

Fig. 7.5 Two examples of lobar haemorrhages demonstrating fingerlike projections (red arrows) and subarachnoid extension (yellow arrows), consistent with Edinburgh CT diagnostic criteria for CAA

phospho-tau, and neurogranin distinguished Alzheimer's disease from CAA [48]. A meta-analysis of previous data also found lower CSF tau and phospho-tau in CAA compared to AD, but also significantly lower amyloid-β40 [49].

Unlike CAA, formal diagnostic criteria for DPA do not exist. However, the presence of deep ICH or deep cerebral microbleeds suggests previous deep perforator rupture, while deep lacunes suggest previous perforator occlusion, both providing direct evidence that DPA may be present. Indirectly, enlarged perivascular spaces within the basal ganglia and a peri-basal ganglia pattern of white matter hyperintensity are associated with deep ICH and microhaemorrhages [43, 50]. A diagnosis of DPA based on these markers may be of greater prognostic significance than one simply based on the presence of hypertension and absence of CAA, but ideally pathological validation of imaging findings is needed.

7.3 Recurrence Risk and Secondary Prevention

The modifiable risk factors for ICH in general include hypertension, excessive alcohol intake [51] and the use of recreational drugs (particularly sympathomimetic vasoactive drugs including cocaine or amphetamines). Diabetes, especially if poorly controlled, and smoking may also increase ICH risk [52–55]. These factors should be managed as fully as possible in all ICH survivors. Around one-quarter of ICH patients are taking antithrombotic medication at onset, an important potentially modifiable risk factor [56], but the decision as to whether to stop or continue this medication requires careful consideration of the increased risk of ICH recurrence with continuation, against the increased risk of thrombotic events related to the original indication for treatment if it is stopped. An individualised approach to this dilemma is an excellent example of precision medicine, and benefits from an increasing body of evidence. More generally, accurately estimating recurrence risk and selecting the optimal secondary prevention strategy in ICH survivors require consideration of both risk factors and the actual cause of the ICH.

7.3.1 Macrovascular Lesions

The management of macrovascular lesions is a major neurosurgical subspecialty in its own right, and an important part of interventional neuroradiological practice. However, stroke physicians and neurologists should be aware of which lesions are likely to be of high bleeding risk and require urgent intervention, and which are unlikely to be good candidates for interventional treatment. Importantly, many macrovascular lesions, particularly cavernomas, are identified as incidental findings on neuroimaging for another indication, or present with seizures. The role of interventional treatment for these lesions is uncertain. The ARUBA randomised controlled trial (RCT) of symptomatic medical versus interventional management of unruptured cerebral arteriovenous malformations found worse outcomes in the intervention group [57], although its generalisability, follow-up duration, and definition of outcome events have been criticised, and subsequent observational studies have challenged the high rate of adverse outcomes observed in its interventional arm [58]. Similar RCT evidence does not exist for cavernomas, but guidelines recommend observation of unruptured lesions [30].

Macrovascular lesions encountered in ICH patients have generally already bled, and therefore present a much higher risk of future haemorrhage [59]. The exact risk is further influenced by lesion type and anatomy. In patients with arteriovenous malformations, the annual risk of haemorrhage is around 4.8% in those with haemorrhagic presentations, against 1.3% in those without. Age, and possibly female sex and exclusively deep venous drainage on angiography, also predicts ICH, but not lesion size [60]. In patients with untreated cavernomas, an individual patient data meta-analysis of 1620 patients from seven centres found an annual risk of haemorrhage in those presenting with ICH or focal neurological deficit (which might indicate previous ICH) of 6.2% in those with a brainstem lesion, and 3% in those with a supratentorial or cerebellar lesion. Without previous ICH or focal deficit, the annual risk for a brainstem cavernoma was 1.6%, and 0.8% for non-brainstem lesions. The risk in patients with multiple cavernomas was similar to that in those with a single lesion. Dural arteriovenous fistulae are rare lesions, so many studies of predictors of haemorrhage from these lesions are small and cross-sectional [61]. They are usually graded by Borden or Cognard classifications, in which cortical venous drainage is an important factor, as these small vessels are less able to withstand increased flow than large venous sinuses. The Cognard classification additionally considers the direction of flow at the drainage site, and the presence of venous ectasia. Both classifications show association with haemorrhagic presentation in cross-sectional analysis [62]. Heterogeneity between prospective studies limits the accuracy with which ICH rates in patients with untreated dural arteriovenous fistulae can be estimated [61], but may be around 1.5% in patients with lesions showing cortical venous drainage which have not bled, and 7.4–19% in those which have [63, 64].

Based on these data, macrovascular lesions which have bled are usually considered for interventional treatment, which can include embolisation, open microsurgery, or stereotactic radiotherapy. In patients with arteriovenous malformations, the Spetzler-Martin grading system predicts adverse surgical outcomes based on increasing lesion size, eloquent adjacent brain tissue, and deep venous drainage [65]. A revised system has been proposed which improves predictive performance by considering increasing age, absence of prior bleeding, and noncompact morphology as additional adverse features [66]. Patients with lower grade lesions are likely to be treated surgically, whereas high-grade lesions may require embolisation (either alone or to reduce lesion grade prior to surgery) or radiosurgery. Although non-invasive, lesion obliteration and reduction of ICH risk after radiosurgery may take months or years, a key disadvantage of this technique [58]. In patients with cavernomas that have bled, the risk of recurrence is similar to that in patients with arteriovenous malformations, but haemorrhage from these low-pressure lesions is often less severe. Guidelines therefore reserve surgery for ICH patients with supratentorial lesions (which are more accessible) and those with recurrent ICH [30]. The role of radiosurgery is unclear: although the rate of recurrence declines from around 2 years after treatment in ICH patients, the same phenomenon has been reported in untreated patients, and may reflect the natural history of the lesion [59]. A recent systematic review found similar outcomes in treated and untreated patients [67].

7.3.2 Cerebral Small Vessel Disease

Classification of the underlying arteriopathy allows more accurate estimation of the risk of recurrence in survivors of ICH attributed to small vessel disease. The most important distinction is that between CAA and DPA. In survivors of lobar ICH, who are likely to meet Boston criteria for possible or probable CAA, the risk of recurrence is around four times that of those with deep or infratentorial ICH [68, 69], while in a meta-analysis of the prognostic significance of the Boston criteria in ICH survivors, the annual risk of recurrence in those with possible or probable CAA was 7.4%, compared to 1.1% in those without [70]. Although these studies did not report recurrence risks for possible and probable CAA separately, the risk is likely to be even higher in patients meeting probable CAA criteria, as the specificity of a 'possible CAA' diagnosis for pathologically confirmed CAA might be less than 50% [71]. Based on a secondary analysis of the PROGRESS trial, patients with probable

CAA may benefit from tighter blood pressure control (<130/80 mmHg) than patients with ICH due to other mechanisms [72].

Individual neuroimaging markers of small vessel disease can also improve prediction of future ICH, through more detailed assessment of the nature or severity of a patient's small vessel disease. In patients with CAA, cortical superficial siderosis (cSS) is an important diagnostic marker, but also an indicator of particularly high ICH risk, with an annual rate of 9.1% in patients with focal siderosis (siderosis limited to three or fewer sulci) and 12.5% in those with disseminated siderosis [73]. Siderosis progression over time further increases ICH risk [74]. The mechanism of these associations is unclear. Pathologically, cSS corresponds to haemosiderin deposition following convexity subarachnoid haemorrhage. It therefore implies clinically significant involvement of leptomeningeal arteries, and affected patients might also have more severely diseased intraparenchymal vessels. An additional factor might be APOε2 presence, which is associated with both disseminated cSS and increased ICH risk, and increases the severity of pathologically-defined vasculopathic changes in patients with CAA [75].

Other markers are relevant to patients with and without CAA. Cerebral microbleeds (CMB), small ovoid hypointense lesions observed on blood-sensitive MRI sequences and thought to correspond to haemosiderin-containing macrophages accumulating at the site of extravasation of blood from a small artery or arteriole, are thought to be markers of vascular fragility and therefore of future ICH risk. The largest relevant study to date, an individual patient data meta-analysis of over 20,000 patients from 38 studies, identified a clear exposure-response relationship, with an adjusted hazard ratio for ICH in antithrombotic-treated patients of 1.89 for those with a single microbleed, 4.55 for those with five or more, and 8.61 for those with >20 [76]. Unexpectedly, a lobar distribution of CMBs was not associated with additional risk, possibly reflecting the limited diagnostic accuracy of the Boston criteria in patients without previous ICH, who made up the vast majority of the study sample. Non-haemorrhagic markers may also show prognostic value: an association between extensive white matter hyperintensity burden and ICH risk (HR 3.82) has been confirmed by a recent meta-analysis [77], while recent prospective studies suggest that enlarged basal ganglia perivascular spaces might be markers of ICH risk [20, 78, 79]. Further investigation is required into whether clinical prediction models incorporating any of these markers, or composite small vessel disease scores [24], can improve on the performance of existing bleeding risk scores, such as HASBLED, ATRIA, and ORBIT, which show limited performance for predicting ICH, rather than all-cause major bleeding [80, 81].

7.3.3 Antithrombotic-Associated ICH

Cardiovascular comorbidities are common in patients with ICH, including atrial fibrillation and ischaemic stroke. Antithrombotic use prior to ICH is therefore also common. This is almost always suspended in the hyperacute phase after ICH, due to the risk of haemorrhage expansion. Deciding whether to restart antithrombotic medication after this is a challenging decision, which requires weighing the increased risk of recurrent ischaemic events if antithrombotics are withheld against the additional risk of major bleeding if they are reinstated. The risk of ICH is the most difficult to quantify, given the limitations of current prognostic models, but also the risk most relevant to stroke patients. Even after a decision to restart antithrombotic therapy, a decision as to *when* to restart it is also required.

In patients taking antiplatelets, the RESTART trial offers important new evidence [82]. In this multicentre open-label trial, 537 patients with previous antithrombotic-associated ICH were randomised to start or avoid antiplatelet therapy, with a median time from ICH to randomisation of 80 days (IQR 30—149 days). Over a median follow-up of 2 years, the rate of recurrent ICH was 4% in the antiplatelet arm, compared to 9% in the comparator arm, with an adjusted HR of 0.51 (95% CI 0.25–1.03). These results suggest that, for most patients, resuming antiplatelet therapy several weeks after ICH is unlikely to increase the risk of recurrence sufficiently to outweigh its benefits, which include a roughly 20% reduction in recurrent ischaemic stroke and coronary events [83]. Reassuringly, in subgroup analyses, lobar ICH, which accounted for just under two-thirds of the study population, was not associated with increased risk of harm from resuming antiplatelets. No evidence was obtained for harm in patients with probable CAA by Boston or Edinburgh criteria, patients with more than five CMBs, and patients with siderosis; however, the incomplete use of baseline MR imaging and size of the study limit the strength with which conclusions can be drawn for these high-risk groups [84].

The management of patients taking anticoagulants is less certain. These patients often have a very high risk of thrombotic events if untreated—for example, non-valvular atrial fibrillation (AF) increases the risk of ischaemic stroke fivefold [85]—but anticoagulants pose a higher risk of ICH than antiplatelets. While observational studies suggest that resuming anticoagulation 4–8 weeks after ICH in patients with AF may be of net benefit [86, 87], these might have been influenced by selection bias, and lacked information on ICH location and aetiology. The risk-benefit balance may also differ between vitamin K antagonists (VKAs) and direct oral anticoagulants (DOACs), with much existing evidence concerning VKAs only. Several current randomised controlled trials (RCTs) (including SoSTART, PRESTIGE-AF, APACHE-AF, ENRICH-AF, and ASPIRE) will compare resuming anticoagulation, in most cases with a DOAC, to antiplatelet or no antithrombotic treatment after ICH. The A_3ICH trial will be important for patients with AF, as it includes an arm for left atrial appendage occlusion, which avoids long-term anticoagulation and is of similar net benefit to anticoagulation with warfarin [88], and possibly DOACs [89], for stroke prevention in AF overall. Well-powered subgroup analyses based on markers of future ICH risk will be vital to enable an evidence-based, personalised approach to this issue in future, noting that some markers of haemorrhagic risk may also be associated with increased ischaemic stroke risk [76]. An individual patient data meta-analysis of trials in this area is planned through the COCROACH collaboration [90].

7.4   Prognostication

Formulating an individualised prognosis is an example of precision medicine in itself, and provides context with which to make and communicate decisions about medical care. Potentially burdensome interventions such as intensive care and neurosurgery should be targeted at patients who are likely to benefit from them, but should also not be withheld inappropriately on the basis of an unduly pessimistic outlook. Clinical prediction models are intended to allow objective, evidence-based prognostication, and may be particularly useful for non-specialist or less experienced clinicians. This is particularly important in ICH patients, in whom a wide spectrum of outcomes is possible, from complete recovery to permanent severe disability or death, and who may be at risk of a self-fulfilling prophecy of care limitation and poor outcomes if prognostication is inaccurate [91]. Beyond clinical care, accurate prognostication may have applications in research studies, for instance, in stratification in clinical trials of new treatments, and in clinical governance.

7.4.1   Clinical Prediction Models for Functional Outcome

Over 20 published clinical prediction models exist for early mortality or functional outcome after ICH [92, 93]. These models include combinations of demographic variables, medical history, bedside observations and scales, and simple radiological variables such as gross haematoma location, haematoma volume by ABC/2 method [94], and intraventricular or subarachnoid extension. For ease of use, most models categorise continuous variables and dichotomise ordinal outcome scales such as the modified Rankin scale (mRS), though at differing thresholds. In head-to-head comparative studies in independent cohorts, most scores perform reasonably well but similarly, reflecting considerable overlap between their components [92, 95]. The extent of external validation varies widely between scores, and this may be a better criterion for selecting a prognostic model to use, as well as simplicity. The four most extensively validated prognostic scores are summarised in Table 7.2, and perform similarly in meta-analysis, with c-statistics around 0.8 for death and poor functional outcome [93]. However, several limitations apply to all these scores. Importantly, it is unclear whether they perform better than informal clinical predictions by experienced clinicians in neuroscience or comprehensive stroke centres, the locations in which ICH patients should ideally be cared for [96]. Additionally, without recalibration, their performance in contemporary practice may not correspond to their performance at original derivation or validation, due to secular trends in healthcare. For example, the original ICH score, described in 2001, now appears overly pessimistic [97], raising the possibility that overreliance on it could lead to withdrawal of care from patients who might otherwise survive. The optimal time point at which a score should be calculated is unclear [98], and a one-off assessment of prognosis may be less accurate than one incorporating clinical change over time [99, 100]. Finally, whether a policy of using a prognostic model to inform ICH care actually improves outcomes or other care metrics is largely unstudied.

Table 7.2 Components of original ICH (oICH), modified ICH (mICH), FUNC, and ICH Grading Scale (ICH-GS) scores—adapted from Ref. [93]

	oICH	mICH	ICH-GS	FUNC
Age	80+: 1	80+: 1	65+: 2	80+: 2
	<80: 0	<80: 0	45–64: 1	70–79: 1
			<45: 0	<70: 0
GCS	3–4: 2		3–8: 2	3–8: 2
	5–12: 1		9–12: 1	9–15: 0
	13–15: 0		13–15: 0	
NIHSS		21–40: 2		
		11–20: 1		
		0–10: 0		
ICH location	Infratentorial: 1	Infratentorial: 1	Infratentorial: 1	Infratentorial: 2
	Supratentorial: 0	Supratentorial: 0	Supratentorial: 0	Lobar: 1
				Supratentorial: 0
ICH volume	30 mL+: 1	30 mL+: 1	*IT:* 20 mL+: 2	>60 mL: 4
	<30 mL: 0	<30 mL: 0	10–20 mL: 1	30–60 mL: 2
			<10 mL: 0	<30 mL: 0
			ST: 70 mL+: 2	
			40–70 mL: 1	
			<40 mL: 0	
IV extension	Present: 1	Present: 1	Present: 1	
	Absent: 0	Absent: 0	Absent: 0	
Cognitive impairment				Present: 1
				Absent: 0
Score range	0–6	0–6	0–8	0–11

For comparison, the FUNC scoring has been inverted (in the unmodified version, a higher score predicts better outcome) and the ICH-GS recentred (unmodified, the lowest score for each item is 1, giving a range of 5–13)

7.4.2 Imaging Biomarkers: The Haematoma

As imaging is a routine part of stroke care, the use of imaging variables is an attractive strategy for improving ICH prognostication. CT and CT angiography are the key initial diagnostic investigations for ICH patients, and most studies focus on these. The CTA spot sign, visible contrast within an intracerebral haematoma, is thought to indicate active bleeding, and has been linked to an increased risk of haemorrhage expansion—with a positive likelihood ratio approaching 5 in a meta-analysis of 26 studies [101]. The clinical significance of this is that haematoma expansion is an important risk factor for poor outcome [102, 103], and might be modifiable through haemostatic or other therapies. The CTA spot sign is in turn associated with poor functional outcome and mortality [101, 104, 105]. However, although a fairly specific marker of expansion risk, the CTA spot sign shows more limited sensitivity, and is absent in a substantial proportion of haematomas which do subsequently expand [106]. It is uncertain whether incorporating this marker into existing prognostic models would improve their performance. In a secondary analysis of the PREDICT cohort, the CTA spot sign was independently associated with poor outcome after adjusting for the components of the original ICH score, but adding the spot sign failed to improve the discrimination of the ICH score [107]. Discrimination is only one aspect of model performance, and reporting of the effect of biomarkers on other indices, such as calibration and classification accuracy, should also be considered [108].

As not all ICH patients undergo hyperacute CT angiography, due to resource limitations or contraindications such as severe renal impairment, a number of non-contrast counterparts to the spot sign have been described (Fig. 7.6). These are also associated with haematoma expansion [109]. The 'black hole' and 'swirl' signs correspond to variation in density within the haematoma caused by hypodense plasma-rich regions of fresh bleeding, while the 'blend' sign refers to adjacent hypodense and hyperdense regions. These markers have a similar pathophysiological basis, and considering the presence of any hypodensity within the haemorrhage may be as informative as considering individual markers [110]. Other non-contrast CT markers linked to expansion or poor outcomes include irregular shape or margins (also termed the 'island' sign) [111, 112], and fluid levels within the haematoma, which is strongly associated with anticoagulant use [113]. As with the CTA spot sign, while associations independent of major ICH prognostic score components have been reported, limited evidence exists on how including these radiological signs might affect the predictive accuracy of existing clinical risk scores.

More detailed parameterisation of haematoma properties is becoming possible with advances in medical image analysis. Rather than subjective visual rating of haematoma morphology or heterogeneity, more complex representations can be extracted algorithmically. For instance, a relatively simple objective measure of variation in haematoma texture might be the variance in Hounsfield density across the voxels it contains. A more complex 'second-order' measure might take into account the relative spatial distribution of voxels of similar intensity. These features can then be assessed as candidate predictors in prognostic models. A few relatively

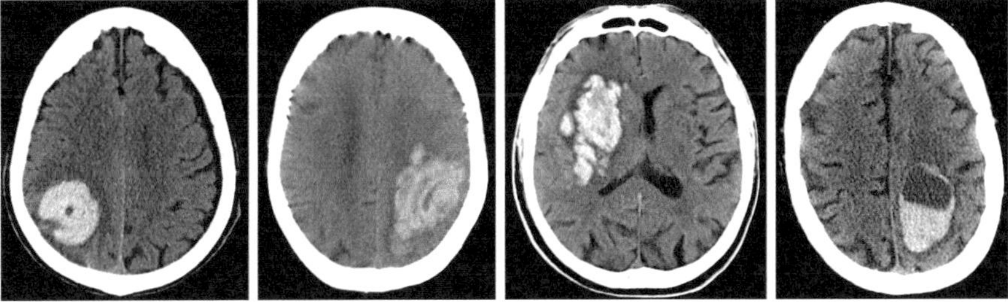

Fig. 7.6 Prognostic markers on non-contrast CT. Left to right: Black hole sign, swirl sign, island sign (note small discrete foci of haemorrhage around main haematoma), fluid level (in patient taking warfarin)

small studies suggest that this radiomics approach might improve the prediction of haematoma expansion [114]. Another approach entails detailed consideration of haematoma location, which can be considered in varying levels of complexity, from the involvement of large brain regions analogous to the ASPECTS used in ischaemic stroke [115], or ICH-specific anatomical classifications such as CHARTS [116], to overlap with maps of influential voxels derived from lesion-deficit mapping approaches [117]. As relationships between voxel injury and outcomes may be complex and influenced by underlying vascular anatomy, maps generated through high-dimensional approaches are more likely to be reliable than those derived through mass-univariate techniques [118]. For either of these approaches to be used in clinical practice, rapid automated lesion segmentation is required. This is well established for segmenting lesions from diffusion-weighted imaging in ischaemic stroke, but has limited progress in ICH. New algorithms using convolutional neural networks show promise for segmenting haemorrhage from non-contrast CTs and may address this [119, 120].

7.4.3 Imaging Biomarkers: Cerebral Small Vessel Disease and 'Brain Frailty'

Prognosis after ICH is influenced by both the severity of the injury and the physiological capacity of the patient to recover. Existing prognostic models often include age and comorbidities, but imaging allows a more direct insight into the resilience of the injured brain. Patients with significant small vessel disease or brain atrophy may have not only a higher risk of recurrent stroke and more cardiovascular comorbidities, but also reduced cerebral functional reserve and structural connectivity between brain regions, and therefore less ability to reorganise brain networks and recover. Supporting this, in analyses adjusted for age and ICH severity, MRI-detected periventricular white matter hyperintensities, CT-detected leukoaraiosis, and quantitative measures of brain atrophy all correlate with worse functional outcomes [121–123]. The prognostic importance of cerebral microbleeds and MR-visible perivascular spaces, which less directly indicate focal brain injury, is uncertain. For use in clinical practice, a simple CT-based 'brain frailty' score which summarises the presence of leukoaraiosis, chronic lacunar infarcts, and atrophy has potential, having been shown to predict adverse functional and cognitive outcomes in a large clinical trial population of acute stroke patients, including around 600 patients with ICH [124]. More detailed MRI measures of brain health, such as diffusion tensor imaging (DTI), which can measure microstructural changes in connectivity which cannot be assessed on clinical MRI scans, show promise for more precise prediction of functional recovery [125], including more specific aspects of function such as upper limb recovery, but may be difficult to acquire in the acute phase in clinically unstable patients.

7.4.4 Non-imaging Biomarkers

Although imaging provides the most direct insight into ICH severity and brain health, biomarkers from other modalities are under investigation. APOε2 genotype is associated with poor outcome after ICH, but as this association is mediated by increased haematoma volume [126], this may not add to existing prognostic scores that include haematoma volume directly. Similarly, a non-coding region at 17p12 is associated with ICH volume and outcome in non-lobar ICH [127]. Larger genome-wide association studies in ischaemic stroke patients have identified genetic variants which may influence recovery independent of initial stroke severity, including an intronic variant (rs1842681) which influences the expression of PPP1R21, a protein implicated in neuroplasticity, and variants in PATJ, involved in ion channel transport and signalling [127, 128]. Such large studies are more difficult to perform in ICH, but the identification of genetic variants influencing outcome independent of ICH volume could improve prognostication and provide new pathophysiological insights. In the rehabilitation setting, neurophysiological measures such as transcranial magnetic stimulation (TMS) can provide information on nervous system function to complement structural information from imaging. The validation of the TMS- and DTI-based PREP algorithm for predicting upper limb motor recovery in patients with ischaemic stroke or ICH provides an example of this in current practice [129].

7.5 Acute Treatment and Future Directions

The acute management of ICH remains almost entirely supportive, with prompt admission to a stroke unit being the most important intervention for reducing death and dependency [130]. Although supportive care within a stroke unit (or critical care unit) is personalised, this is difficult to quantify as a 'precision medicine' treatment. Control of blood pressure is a routine practice, with a reduction to 130–140 mmHg over around an hour probably the most beneficial [131, 132]. There is little evidence on whether the blood pressure target should be individualised, though very recent evidence suggests that BP reduction below 140 mmHg may be harmful in patients with very severe (>220 mmHg) hypertension at presentation [133]. The main current example of precision medicine in ICH in treatment is therefore in patients taking anticoagulants, as specific reversal agents are available: vitamin K and four-factor prothrombin complex concentrate for vitamin K antagonists [134], the neutralising monoclonal antibody idarucizumab for dabigatran [135], and the decoy protein andexanet alfa for factor Xa inhibitors [136], though the clinical benefit of the latter two drugs has not been established in clinical trials. However, the recognition of pathophysiological factors associated with poor outcome, such as haematoma expansion and perihaematomal oedema, has created new targets for treatment, and the role of surgery continues to be studied. Although platelet transfusion is not beneficial in ICH patients taking antiplatelets [137], the role of desmopressin as a potential reversal agent is under active investigation [138]. More broadly, selecting patients for clinical trials based on pathophysiology and accounting as fully as possible for confounding factors might lead to more successful translation of candidate treatments into practice.

7.5.1 Haematoma Expansion

Patients at high risk of clinical deterioration from haematoma expansion can be identified through the CTA spot sign and related non-contrast CT markers. In theory, these patients might benefit particularly from treatments designed to limit haematoma expansion—broadly, intensive blood pressure control and haemostatic agents. Unfortunately, these have not yet been shown to be beneficial. In the TICH-2 trial, tranexamic acid did not improve functional outcome at 90 days after ICH, but was associated with reduced risk of early death and haematoma expansion [139]. A subsequent analysis therefore investigated whether tranexamic acid might be of greater benefit in patients with blend, black hole, island, or hypodensity signs, but failed to find an interaction between these signs and treatment [140]. A similar analysis of the CTA spot sign in TICH-2 is in progress, but the STOP-AUST trial of tranexamic acid in spot sign-positive patients did not find evidence of benefit [141, 142]. Similarly, secondary analyses of the ATACH-II trial, which did not support intensive blood pressure control after ICH overall, found no greater benefit in patients with the CTA spot sign or non-contrast CT signs [143, 144]. Both parent trials had limitations which may have reduced their ability to detect an effect of treatment and its interaction with markers of expansion risk: in TICH-2, most patients received tranexamic acid more than 3 h after ICH, a time point beyond which its benefit is lost in other forms of major bleeding [145], while the difference in achieved blood pressures between intensive and control arms in ATACH-II was relatively small. The investigation of these markers in future trials may therefore still be merited.

7.5.2 Perihaematomal Oedema

After ICH, oedema frequently develops around the haematoma through osmotic and cytotoxic mechanisms, and can continue to grow for up to 3 weeks [146]. This perihaematomal oedema (PHO) is thought to be an important marker of secondary brain injury and can contribute to clinical deterioration through local mass effect and increased intracranial pressure. The relationship between PHO and clinical outcomes is complex, as studies have used a range of measurement methods (including absolute volume, relative volume to haematoma size, and mean extension distance beyond the haematoma) and time points (including serial measurements to assess for oedema growth). However, overall, PHO is likely to be associated with adverse outcomes, and it has therefore been investigated as a therapeutic target and a surrogate outcome measure for early-phase clinical trials [147]. A number of putative neuroprotective agents have been shown to reduce PHO in clinical trials, including deferoxamine [148], fingolimod [149], and celecoxib [150]; however, these have not yet been shown to be of clinical benefit in phase three studies (and the more recent iDEF phase two study suggested that such a trial of deferoxamine would likely be futile) [151]. Kinaret, an interleukin 1 receptor antagonist with potential to reduce perihaematomal inflammation, and therefore PHO, is currently under phase two investigation in the BLOC-ICH trial [152].

7.5.3 The Role of Surgery

Surgical evacuation of the haematoma is an alternative approach to limiting secondary brain injury after ICH, reducing mass effect and production of toxic blood breakdown products. This is accepted practice in infratentorial haemorrhage, as the anatomy of the posterior fossa means ICH here presents a high risk of brainstem compression and hydrocephalus [153]. The role of craniotomy in supratentorial haemorrhage is more controversial, with limited evidence from the STICH-II trial for increased survival in patients with superficial lobar ICH without intraventricular haemorrhage [154]. However, it should be noted that trials are less likely to include patients for whom surgery is perceived as immediately life-saving, due to lack of equipoise, and a high crossover rate to the surgical treatment arm occurred. More recently, minimally invasive clot evacuation via an indwelling thrombolysis and drainage catheter has been evaluated in the MISTIE III trial in patients with supratentorial ICH >30 mL (a threshold associated with poor outcomes). Although there was no overall difference in functional outcomes, a secondary analysis suggested benefit in patients with a residual haematoma volume <15 mL [155]. Identifying baseline or operative factors able to predict successful evacuation might allow the development of a truly precise neurosurgical intervention in the future.

7.5.4 Precision Clinical Trials?

ICH is uncommon compared to ischaemic stroke and is more frequently disabling. As a result, recruitment to clinical trials of ICH can be difficult, reducing feasible sample sizes and power to detect small treatment effects. Adjustment for covariates of known prognostic significance can increase statistical power, and is recommended practice in clinical trials [156]. As the predictors of ICH outcome become better understood, the number of variables which could be corrected for will increase. With advances in ICH lesion segmentation, even adjusting for the pattern of brain injury may become possible. A recent simulation study using segmented DWI lesions from over 1000 ischaemic stroke patients found that correcting for a covariate representing an outcome prediction made from the distribution of injured voxels significantly improved the power to detect a simulated intervention [157]. In this way, accounting for individual variability, a key component of precision medicine, might improve the development of new treatments, not just the selection of which existing treatments to use. Adjusting for imaging biomarkers may also be useful in designing trials of stroke prevention strategies: a secondary analysis of the PICASSO trial, which compared aspirin and cilostazol in ischaemic stroke patients at high risk of intracerebral haemorrhage, suggests that cilostazol might be preferable specifically in patients with cerebral microbleeds [158].

7.6   Conclusion

ICH remains a major cause of morbidity and mortality, and advances in the care of affected patients are sorely needed. Although the precision treatment of ICH is yet to be realised, its causes and prognostic factors are increasingly understood. As comprehensive electronic healthcare records become commonplace, the integration of multimodal data from clinical, imaging, and paraclinical data sources may enable personalised prediction of ICH aetiology and outcome in routine clinical practice. Advances in predicting recurrent ICH should enable more effective secondary prevention, including in patients with indications for antithrombotic therapy. Disease-modifying treatments remain elusive, but trials targeting specific aspects of ICH pathophysiology in carefully selected patients are more likely to be fruitful than trials in heterogenous populations with 'primary' ICH, and embedding mechanistic and biomarker substudies into future RCTs should be strongly considered. It is therefore likely that precision medicine will play an important role in improving outcomes for ICH patients in the future.

References

1. Feigin VL, Lawes CM, Bennett DA, Barker-Collo SL, Parag V. Worldwide stroke incidence and early case fatality reported in 56 population-based studies: a systematic review. Lancet Neurol. 2009;8(4):355–69.
2. Krishnamurthi RV, Ikeda T, Feigin VL. Global, regional and country-specific burden of ischaemic stroke, intracerebral haemorrhage and subarachnoid haemorrhage: a systematic analysis of the Global Burden of Disease Study 2017. Neuroepidemiology. 2020;54(Suppl. 2):171–9.
3. Mehndiratta MM, Khan M, Mehndiratta P, Wasay M. Stroke in Asia: geographical variations and temporal trends. J Neurol Neurosurg Psychiatry. 2014;85(12):1308–12.
4. Lioutas V-A, Beiser AS, Aparicio HJ, Himali JJ, Selim MH, Romero JR, et al. Assessment of incidence and risk factors of intracerebral hemorrhage among participants in the Framingham Heart Study between 1948 and 2016. JAMA Neurol. 2020 [cited 2020 Aug 17]. Available from: https://jamanetwork.com/journals/jamaneurology/fullarticle/2766800.
5. van Asch CJ, Luitse MJ, Rinkel GJ, van der Tweel I, Algra A, Klijn CJ. Incidence, case fatality, and functional outcome of intracerebral haemorrhage over time, according to age, sex, and ethnic origin: a systematic review and meta-analysis. Lancet Neurol. 2010;9(2):167–76.
6. James SL, Abate D, Abate KH, Abay SM, Abbafati C, Abbasi N, et al. Global, regional, and national incidence, prevalence, and years lived with disability for 354 diseases and injuries for 195 countries and territories, 1990–2017: a systematic analysis for the Global Burden of Disease Study 2017. Lancet. 2018;392(10159):1789–858.

7. Roth GA, Abate D, Abate KH, Abay SM, Abbafati C, Abbasi N, et al. Global, regional, and national age-sex-specific mortality for 282 causes of death in 195 countries and territories, 1980–2017: a systematic analysis for the Global Burden of Disease Study 2017. Lancet. 2018;392(10159):1736–88.

8. Ashley EA. Towards precision medicine. Nat Rev Genet. 2016;17(9):507–22.

9. Collins FS, Varmus H. A new initiative on precision medicine. N Engl J Med. 2015;372(9):793–5.

10. Albers GW, Marks MP, Kemp S, Christensen S, Tsai JP, Ortega-Gutierrez S, et al. Thrombectomy for stroke at 6 to 16 hours with selection by perfusion imaging. N Engl J Med. 2018;378(8):708–18.

11. Nogueira RG, Jadhav AP, Haussen DC, Bonafe A, Budzik RF, Bhuva P, et al. Thrombectomy 6 to 24 hours after stroke with a mismatch between deficit and infarct. N Engl J Med. 2018;378(1):11–21.

12. Thomalla G, Simonsen CZ, Boutitie F, Andersen G, Berthezene Y, Cheng B, et al. MRI-guided thrombolysis for stroke with unknown time of onset. N Engl J Med. 2018;379(7):611–22.

13. Ma H, Campbell BCV, Parsons MW, Churilov L, Levi CR, Hsu C, et al. Thrombolysis guided by perfusion imaging up to 9 hours after onset of stroke. N Engl J Med. 2019;380(19):1795–803.

14. Cordonnier C, Demchuk A, Ziai W, Anderson CS. Intracerebral haemorrhage: current approaches to acute management. Lancet. 2018;392(10154):1257–68.

15. Meretoja A, Strbian D, Putaala J, Curtze S, Haapaniemi E, Mustanoja S, et al. SMASH-U: a proposal for etiologic classification of intracerebral hemorrhage. Stroke. 2012;43(10):2592–7.

16. Martí-Fàbregas J, Prats-Sánchez L, Guisado-Alonso D, Martínez-Domeño A, Delgado-Mederos R, Camps-Renom P. SMASH-U versus H-ATOMIC: a head-to-head comparison for the etiologic classification of intracerebral hemorrhage. J Stroke Cerebrovasc Dis. 2018;27(9):2375–80.

17. Almandoz JED, Schaefer PW, Forero NP, Falla JR, Gonzalez RG, Romero JM. Diagnostic accuracy and yield of multidetector CT angiography in the evaluation of spontaneous intra-parenchymal cerebral hemorrhage. Am J Neuroradiol. 2009;30(6):1213–21.

18. van Asch CJJ, Velthuis BK, Rinkel GJE, Algra A, de Kort GAP, Witkamp TD, et al. Diagnostic yield and accuracy of CT angiography, MR angiography, and digital subtraction angiography for detection of macrovascular causes of intracerebral haemorrhage: prospective, multicentre cohort study. BMJ. 2015;351:h5762.

19. Alakbarzade V, Pereira AC. Cerebral catheter angiography and its complications. Pract Neurol. 2018;18(5):393–8.

20. Lau KK, Li L, Schulz U, Simoni M, Chan KH, Ho SL, et al. Total small vessel disease score and risk of recurrent stroke. Neurology. 2017;88(24):2260–7.

21. Wilson D, Ogungbemi A, Ambler G, Jones I, Werring DJ, Jäger HR. Developing an algorithm to identify patients with intracerebral haemorrhage secondary to a macrovascular cause. Eur Stroke J. 2017 [cited 2020 Aug 17]. Available from: https://journals.sagepub.com/doi/10.1177/2396987317732874.

22. Jolink WMT, Wiegertjes K, Rinkel GJE, Algra A, de Leeuw F-E, Klijn CJM. Location specific risk factors for intracerebral hemorrhage: systematic review and meta-analysis. Neurology. 2020; https://doi.org/10.1212/WNL.0000000000010418.

23. Hilkens NA, van Asch CJJ, Werring DJ, Wilson D, Rinkel GJE, Algra A, et al. Predicting the presence of macrovascular causes in non-traumatic intracerebral haemorrhage: the DIAGRAM prediction score. J Neurol Neurosurg Psychiatry. 2018;89(7):674–9.

24. Staals J, Makin SDJ, Doubal FN, Dennis MS, Wardlaw JM. Stroke subtype, vascular risk factors, and total MRI brain small-vessel disease burden. Neurology. 2014;83(14):1228–34.

25. Zhang Y, Zhang B, Liang F, Liang S, Zhang Y, Yan P, et al. Radiomics features on non-contrast-enhanced CT scan can precisely classify AVM-related hematomas from other spontaneous intraparenchymal hematoma types. Eur Radiol. 2019;29(4):2157–65.

26. Devan WJ, Falcone GJ, Anderson CD, Jagiella JM, Schmidt H, Hansen BM, et al. Heritability estimates identify a substantial genetic contribution to risk and outcome of intracerebral hemorrhage. Stroke. 2013;44(6):1578–83.

27. Werring DJ, Lynch DS. Monogenic small vessel diseases—rare but still important. Nat Rev Neurol. 2020;16(8):407–8.

28. Mancuso M, Arnold M, Bersano A, Burlina A, Chabriat H, Debette S, et al. Monogenic cerebral small-vessel diseases: diagnosis and therapy. Consensus recommendations of the European Academy of Neurology. Eur J Neurol. 2020;27(6):909–27.

29. Zafar A, Quadri Syed A, Farooqui M, Ikram A, Robinson M, Hart Blaine L, et al. Familial cerebral cavernous malformations. Stroke. 2019;50(5):1294–301.

30. Akers A, Al-Shahi Salman R, Awad I, Dahlem K, Flemming K, Hart B, et al. Synopsis of guidelines for the clinical management of cerebral cavernous malformations: consensus recommendations based on systematic literature review by the Angioma Alliance Scientific Advisory Board Clinical Experts Panel. Neurosurgery. 2017;80(5):665–80.

31. Nikolaev SI, Vetiska S, Bonilla X, Boudreau E, Jauhiainen S, Jahromi BR, et al. Somatic activating KRAS mutations in arteriovenous malformations of the brain. N Engl J Med. 2018 [cited 2020 Aug 18]. Available from: https://www.nejm.org/doi/10.1056/NEJMoa1709449?url_ver=Z39.88-2003&rfr_id=ori%3Arid%3Acrossref.org&rfr_dat=cr_pub++0pubmed.

32. Hong T, Yan Y, Li J, Radovanovic I, Ma X, Shao YW, et al. High prevalence of KRAS/BRAF somatic mutations in brain and spinal cord arteriovenous malformations. Brain J Neurol. 2019;142(1):23–34.

33. Iyer VN, Apala DR, Pannu BS, Kotecha A, Brinjikji W, Leise MD, et al. Intravenous bevacizumab for refractory hereditary hemorrhagic telangiectasia–related epistaxis and gastrointestinal bleeding. Mayo Clin Proc. 2018;93(2):155–66.

34. Wardlaw JM, Smith C, Dichgans M. Small vessel disease: mechanisms and clinical implications. Lancet Neurol. 2019;18(7):684–96.

35. Blanco PJ, Müller LO, Spence JD. Blood pressure gradients in cerebral arteries: a clue to pathogenesis of cerebral small vessel disease. Stroke Vasc Neurol. 2017;2(3):108–17.

36. Charidimou A, Boulouis G, Roongpiboonsopit D, Auriel E, Pasi M, Haley K, et al. Cortical superficial siderosis multifocality in cerebral amyloid angiopathy. Neurology. 2017;89(21):2128–35.

37. Hawkes CA, Härtig W, Kacza J, Schliebs R, Weller RO, Nicoll JA, et al. Perivascular drainage of solutes is impaired in the ageing mouse brain and in the presence of cerebral amyloid angiopathy. Acta Neuropathol (Berl). 2011;121(4):431–43.

38. Yamazaki Y, Zhao N, Caulfield TR, Liu C-C, Bu G. Apolipoprotein E and Alzheimer disease: pathobiology and targeting strategies. Nat Rev Neurol. 2019;15(9):501–18.

39. Greenberg SM, Charidimou A. Diagnosis of cerebral amyloid angiopathy: evolution of the Boston criteria. Stroke. 2018;49(2):491–7.

40. Linn J, Halpin A, Demaerel P, Ruhland J, Giese AD, Dichgans M, et al. Prevalence of superficial siderosis in patients with cerebral amyloid angiopathy. Neurology. 2010;74(17):1346–50.

41. Martinez-Ramirez S, Romero J-R, Shoamanesh A, McKee AC, Van Etten E, Pontes-Neto O, et al. Diagnostic value of lobar microbleeds in individuals without intracerebral hemorrhage. Alzheimers Dement J Alzheimers Assoc. 2015;11(12):1480–8.

42. Schreiber S, Wilisch-Neumann A, Schreiber F, Assmann A, Scheumann V, Perosa V, et al. Invited review: the spectrum of age-related small vessel diseases: potential overlap and interactions of amyloid and nonamyloid vasculopathies. Neuropathol Appl Neurobiol. 2020;46(3):219–39.

43. Charidimou A, Boulouis G, Pasi M, Auriel E, van Etten ES, Haley K, et al. MRI-visible perivascular spaces in cerebral amyloid angiopathy and hypertensive arteriopathy. Neurology. 2017;88(12):1157–64.

44. Thanprasertsuk S, Martinez-Ramirez S, Pontes-Neto OM, Ni J, Ayres A, Reed A, et al. Posterior white matter disease distribution as a predictor of amyloid angiopathy. Neurology. 2014;83(9):794–800.

45. Xiong L, van Veluw Susanne J, Bounemia N, Charidimou A, Pasi M, Boulouis G, et al. Cerebral cortical microinfarcts on magnetic resonance imaging and their association with cognition in cerebral amyloid angiopathy. Stroke. 2018;49(10):2330–6.

46. Charidimou A, Frosch MP, Salman RA-S, Baron J-C, Cordonnier C, Hernandez-Guillamon M, et al. Advancing diagnostic criteria for sporadic cerebral amyloid angiopathy: study protocol for a multicenter MRI-pathology validation of Boston criteria v2.0. Int J Stroke. 2019;14(9):956–71.
47. Rodrigues MA, Samarasekera N, Lerpiniere C, Humphreys C, McCarron MO, White PM, et al. The Edinburgh CT and genetic diagnostic criteria for lobar intracerebral haemorrhage associated with cerebral amyloid angiopathy: model development and diagnostic test accuracy study. Lancet Neurol. 2018;17(3):232–40.
48. Banerjee G, Ambler G, Keshavan A, Paterson RW, Foiani MS, Toombs J, et al. Cerebrospinal fluid biomarkers in cerebral amyloid angiopathy. J Alzheimers Dis. 2020;74(4):1189–201.
49. Charidimou A, Friedrich JO, Greenberg SM, Viswanathan A. Core cerebrospinal fluid biomarker profile in cerebral amyloid angiopathy: a meta-analysis. Neurology. 2018;90(9):e754–62.
50. Charidimou A, Boulouis G, Haley K, Auriel E, van Etten ES, Fotiadis P, et al. White matter hyperintensity patterns in cerebral amyloid angiopathy and hypertensive arteriopathy. Neurology. 2016;86(6):505–11.
51. O'Donnell MJ, Chin SL, Rangarajan S, Xavier D, Liu L, Zhang H, et al. Global and regional effects of potentially modifiable risk factors associated with acute stroke in 32 countries (INTERSTROKE): a case-control study. Lancet. 2016;388(10046):761–75.
52. Boulanger M, Poon MTC, Wild SH, Al-Shahi Salman R. Association between diabetes mellitus and the occurrence and outcome of intracerebral hemorrhage. Neurology. 2016;87(9):870–8.
53. Saliba W, Barnett-Griness O, Gronich N, Molad J, Naftali J, Rennert G, et al. Association of diabetes and glycated hemoglobin with the risk of intracerebral hemorrhage: a population-based cohort study. Diabetes Care. 2019 [cited 2020 Aug 19]. Available from: https://care.diabetesjournals.org/content/early/2019/01/31/dc18-2472.
54. Kurth T, Kase CS, Berger K, Schaeffner ES, Buring JE, Gaziano JM. Smoking and the risk of hemorrhagic stroke in men. Stroke. 2003;34(5):1151–5.
55. Kurth T, Kase CS, Berger K, Gaziano JM, Cook NR, Buring JE. Smoking and risk of hemorrhagic stroke in women. Stroke. 2003;34(12):2792–5.
56. Béjot Y, Cordonnier C, Durier J, Aboa-Eboulé C, Rouaud O, Giroud M. Intracerebral haemorrhage profiles are changing: results from the Dijon population-based study. Brain. 2013;136(2):658–64.
57. Mohr JP, Overbey JR, Hartmann A, von Kummer R, Al-Shahi Salman R, Kim H, et al. Medical management with interventional therapy versus medical management alone for unruptured brain arteriovenous malformations (ARUBA): final follow-up of a multicentre, non-blinded, randomised controlled trial. Lancet Neurol. 2020;19(7):573–81.
58. Feghali J, Huang J. Updates in arteriovenous malformation management: the post-ARUBA era. Stroke Vasc Neurol. 2020 [cited 2020 Aug 28];5(1). Available from: https://svn.bmj.com/content/5/1/34.
59. Horne MA, Flemming KD, Su I-C, Stapf C, Jeon JP, Li D, et al. Clinical course of untreated cerebral cavernous malformations: a meta-analysis of individual patient data. Lancet Neurol. 2016;15(2):166–73.
60. Kim H, Al-Shahi Salman R, McCulloch CE, Stapf C, Young WL, for the MARS Coinvestigators. Untreated brain arteriovenous malformation: patient-level meta-analysis of hemorrhage predictors. Neurology. 2014;83(7):590–7.
61. Kobayashi A, Salman RA-S. Prognosis and treatment of intracranial dural arteriovenous fistulae: a systematic review and meta-analysis. Int J Stroke. 2014;9(6):670–7.
62. Davies MA, TerBrugge K, Willinsky R, Coyne T, Saleh J, Wallace MC. The validity of classification for the clinical presentation of intracranial dural arteriovenous fistulas. J Neurosurg. 1996;85(5):830–7.
63. Strom RG, Botros JA, Refai D, Moran CJ, Cross DT, Chicoine MR, et al. Cranial dural arteriovenous fistulae asymptomatic cortical venous drainage portends less aggressive clinical course. Neurosurgery. 2009;64(2):241–8.

64. Söderman M, Pavic L, Edner G, Holmin S, Andersson T. Natural history of dural arteriovenous shunts. Stroke. 2008;39(6):1735–9.

65. Spetzler RF, Martin NA. A proposed grading system for arteriovenous malformations. J Neurosurg. 1986;65(4):476–83.

66. Kim H, Abla AA, Nelson J, McCulloch CE, Bervini D, Morgan MK, et al. Validation of the supplemented Spetzler-Martin grading system for brain arteriovenous malformations in a multicenter cohort of 1009 surgical patients. Neurosurgery. 2015;76(1):25–33.

67. Poorthuis MHF, Rinkel LA, Lammy S, Al-Shahi Salman R. Stereotactic radiosurgery for cerebral cavernous malformations: a systematic review. Neurology. 2019;93(21):e1971–9.

68. Poon MTC, Fonville AF, Al-Shahi Salman R. Long-term prognosis after intracerebral haemorrhage: systematic review and meta-analysis. J Neurol Neurosurg Psychiatry. 2014;85(6):660–7.

69. Li L, Luengo-Fernandez R, Zuurbier SM, Beddows NC, Lavallee P, Silver LE, et al. Ten-year risks of recurrent stroke, disability, dementia and cost in relation to site of primary intracerebral haemorrhage: population-based study. J Neurol Neurosurg Psychiatry. 2020;91(6):580–5.

70. Charidimou A, Imaizumi T, Moulin S, Biffi A, Samarasekera N, Yakushiji Y, et al. Brain hemorrhage recurrence, small vessel disease type, and cerebral microbleeds. Neurology. 2017;89(8):820–9.

71. Knudsen KA, Rosand J, Karluk D, Greenberg SM. Clinical diagnosis of cerebral amyloid angiopathy: validation of the Boston criteria. Neurology. 2001;56(4):537–9.

72. Arima H, Tzourio C, Anderson C, Woodward M, Bousser M-G, MacMahon S, et al. Effects of perindopril-based lowering of blood pressure on intracerebral hemorrhage related to amyloid angiopathy. Stroke. 2010;41(2):394–6.

73. Charidimou A, Boulouis G, Greenberg SM, Viswanathan A. Cortical superficial siderosis and bleeding risk in cerebral amyloid angiopathy: a meta-analysis. Neurology. 2019;93(24):e2192–202.

74. Pongpitakmetha T, Fotiadis P, Pasi M, Boulouis G, Xiong L, Warren AD, et al. Cortical superficial siderosis progression in cerebral amyloid angiopathy. Neurology. 2020;94(17):e1853–65.

75. Charidimou A, Martinez-Ramirez S, Shoamanesh A, Oliveira-Filho J, Frosch M, Vashkevich A, et al. Cerebral amyloid angiopathy with and without hemorrhage. Neurology. 2015;84(12):1206–12.

76. Wilson D, Ambler G, Lee K-J, Lim J-S, Shiozawa M, Koga M, et al. Cerebral microbleeds and stroke risk after ischaemic stroke or transient ischaemic attack: a pooled analysis of individual patient data from cohort studies. Lancet Neurol. 2019;18(7):653–65.

77. Debette S, Schilling S, Duperron M-G, Larsson SC, Markus HS. Clinical significance of magnetic resonance imaging markers of vascular brain injury: a systematic review and meta-analysis. JAMA Neurol. 2019;76(1):81–94.

78. Duperron M-G, Tzourio C, Schilling S, Zhu Y-C, Soumaré A, Mazoyer B, et al. High dilated perivascular space burden: a new MRI marker for risk of intracerebral hemorrhage. Neurobiol Aging. 2019;84:158–65.

79. Best JG, Barbato C, Ambler G, Du H, Banerjee G, Wilson D, et al. Association of enlarged perivascular spaces and anticoagulant-related intracranial hemorrhage. Neurology. 2020;95:e2192–9.

80. Chao T-F, Lip GYH, Lin Y-J, Chang S-L, Lo L-W, Hu Y-F, et al. Major bleeding and intracranial hemorrhage risk prediction in patients with atrial fibrillation: attention to modifiable bleeding risk factors or use of a bleeding risk stratification score? A nationwide cohort study. Int J Cardiol. 2018;254:157–61.

81. Friberg L, Rosenqvist M, Lip GYH. Evaluation of risk stratification schemes for ischaemic stroke and bleeding in 182 678 patients with atrial fibrillation: the Swedish Atrial Fibrillation cohort study. Eur Heart J. 2012;33(12):1500–10.

82. Salman RA-S, Dennis MS, Sandercock PAG, Sudlow CLM, Wardlaw JM, Whiteley WN, et al. Effects of antiplatelet therapy after stroke due to intracerebral haemorrhage (RESTART): a randomised, open-label trial. Lancet. 2019;393(10191):2613–23.

83. Antithrombotic Trialists' (ATT) Collaboration. Aspirin in the primary and secondary prevention of vascular disease: collaborative meta-analysis of individual participant data from randomised trials. Lancet. 2009;373(9678):1849–60.

84. Salman RA-S, Minks DP, Mitra D, Rodrigues MA, Bhatnagar P, du Plessis JC, et al. Effects of antiplatelet therapy on stroke risk by brain imaging features of intracerebral haemorrhage and cerebral small vessel diseases: subgroup analyses of the RESTART randomised, open-label trial. Lancet Neurol. 2019;18(7):643–52.

85. Wolf PA, Dawber TR, Thomas HE, Kannel WB. Epidemiologic assessment of chronic atrial fibrillation and risk of stroke: the Framingham study. Neurology. 1978;28(10):973–7.

86. Murthy SB, Gupta A, Merkler AE, Navi BB, Mandava P, Iadecola C, et al. Restarting anticoagulant therapy after intracranial hemorrhage. Stroke. 2017;48(6):1594–600.

87. Pennlert J, Overholser R, Asplund K, Carlberg B, Van Rompaye B, Wiklund P-G, et al. Optimal timing of anticoagulant treatment after intracerebral hemorrhage in patients with atrial fibrillation. Stroke. 2017;48(2):314–20.

88. Reddy VY, Doshi SK, Kar S, Gibson DN, Price MJ, Huber K, et al. 5-Year outcomes after left atrial appendage closure: from the prevail and protect AF trials. J Am Coll Cardiol. 2017;70(24):2964–75.

89. Osmancik P, Herman D, Neuzil P, Hala P, Taborsky M, Kala P, et al. Left atrial appendage closure versus direct oral anticoagulants in high-risk patients with atrial fibrillation. J Am Coll Cardiol. 2020;75(25):3122–35.

90. COCROACH. The University of Edinburgh [cited 2020 Sept 6]. Available from: https://www.ed.ac.uk/clinical-brain-sciences/research/so-start/for-collaborators.

91. Hemphill JC, White DB. Clinical nihilism in neuro-emergencies. Emerg Med Clin North Am. 2009;27(1):27–37, viii.

92. Satopää J, Mustanoja S, Meretoja A, Putaala J, Kaste M, Niemelä M, et al. Comparison of all 19 published prognostic scores for intracerebral hemorrhage. J Neurol Sci. 2017;379:103–8.

93. Gregório T, Pipa S, Cavaleiro P, Atanásio G, Albuquerque I, Chaves PC, et al. Assessment and comparison of the four most extensively validated prognostic scales for intracerebral hemorrhage: systematic review with meta-analysis. Neurocrit Care. 2019;30(2):449–66.

94. Kothari RU, Brott T, Broderick JP, Barsan WG, Sauerbeck LR, Zuccarello M, et al. The ABCs of measuring intracerebral hemorrhage volumes. Stroke. 1996;27(8):1304–5.

95. Parry-Jones AR, Abid KA, Di Napoli M, Smith CJ, Vail A, Patel HC, et al. Accuracy and clinical usefulness of intracerebral hemorrhage grading scores. Stroke. 2013;44(7):1840–5.

96. Hwang DY, Dell CA, Sparks MJ, Watson TD, Langefeld CD, Comeau ME, et al. Clinician judgment vs. formal scales for predicting intracerebral hemorrhage outcomes. Neurology. 2016;86(2):126–33.

97. McCracken DJ, Lovasik BP, McCracken CE, Frerich JM, McDougal ME, Ratcliff JJ, et al. The intracerebral hemorrhage score: a self-fulfilling prophecy? Neurosurgery. 2019;84(3):741–8.

98. Lun R, Yogendrakumar V, Demchuk AM, Aviv RI, Rodriguez-Luna D, Molina CA, et al. Calculation of prognostic scores, using delayed imaging, outperforms baseline assessments in acute intracerebral hemorrhage. Stroke. 2020;51(4):1107–10.

99. Maas MB, Francis BA, Sangha RS, Lizza BD, Liotta EM, Naidech AM. Refining prognosis for intracerebral hemorrhage by early reassessment. Cerebrovasc Dis. 2017;43(3–4):110–6.

100. Yogendrakumar V, Smith EE, Demchuk AM, Aviv RI, Rodriguez Luna D, Molina CA, et al. Lack of early improvement predicts poor outcome following acute intracerebral hemorrhage. Crit Care Med. 2018;46(4):e310–7.

101. Phan TG, Krishnadas N, Lai VWY, Batt M, Slater L-A, Chandra RV, et al. Meta-analysis of accuracy of the spot sign for predicting hematoma growth and clinical outcomes. Stroke. 2019;50(8):2030–6.

102. Delcourt C, Huang Y, Arima H, Chalmers J, Davis SM, Heeley EL, et al. Hematoma growth and outcomes in intracerebral hemorrhage: the INTERACT1 study. Neurology. 2012;79(4):314–9.

103. Davis SM, Broderick J, Hennerici M, Brun NC, Diringer MN, Mayer SA, et al. Hematoma growth is a determinant of mortality and poor outcome after intracerebral hemorrhage. Neurology. 2006;66(8):1175–81.

104. Demchuk AM, Dowlatshahi D, Rodriguez-Luna D, Molina CA, Blas YS, Dzialowski I, et al. Prediction of haematoma growth and outcome in patients with intracerebral haemorrhage using the CT-angiography spot sign (PREDICT): a prospective observational study. Lancet Neurol. 2012;11(4):307–14.

105. Delgado Almandoz Josser E, Yoo AJ, Stone MJ, Schaefer PW, Oleinik A, Brouwers HB, et al. The spot sign score in primary intracerebral hemorrhage identifies patients at highest risk of in-hospital mortality and poor outcome among survivors. Stroke. 2010;41(1):54–60.

106. Xu X, Zhang J, Yang K, Wang Q, Xu B, Chen X. Accuracy of spot sign in predicting hematoma expansion and clinical outcome. Medicine (Baltimore). 2018 [cited 2020 Sept 20];97(34). Available from: https://www.ncbi.nlm.nih.gov/pmc/articles/PMC6113011/.

107. Schneider H, Huynh TJ, Demchuk AM, Dowlatshahi D, Rodriguez-Luna D, Silva Y, et al. Combining spot sign and intracerebral hemorrhage score to estimate functional outcome. Stroke. 2018;49(6):1511–4.

108. Cook NR. Quantifying the added value of new biomarkers: how and how not. Diagn Progn Res. 2018;2(1):14.

109. Boulouis G, Morotti A, Charidimou A, Dowlatshahi D, Goldstein JN. Noncontrast computed tomography markers of intracerebral hemorrhage expansion. Stroke. 2017;48(4):1120–5.

110. Boulouis G, Morotti A, Brouwers HB, Charidimou A, Jessel MJ, Auriel E, et al. Association between hypodensities detected by computed tomography and hematoma expansion in patients with intracerebral hemorrhage. JAMA Neurol. 2016;73(8):961–8.

111. Delcourt C, Zhang S, Arima H, Sato S, Al-Shahi Salman R, Wang X, et al. Significance of hematoma shape and density in intracerebral hemorrhage: the intensive blood pressure reduction in acute intracerebral hemorrhage trial study. Stroke. 2016;47(5):1227–32.

112. Li Q, Liu Q-J, Yang W-S, Wang X-C, Zhao L-B, Xiong X, et al. Island sign. Stroke. 2017;48(11):3019–25.

113. Sato S, Delcourt C, Zhang S, Arima H, Heeley E, Zheng D, et al. Determinants and prognostic significance of hematoma sedimentation levels in acute intracerebral hemorrhage. Cerebrovasc Dis Basel Switz. 2016;41(1–2):80–6.

114. Chen Q, Xia T. Radiomics in stroke neuroimaging: techniques, applications, and challenges. Aging Dis. 2021;12:143–54.

115. Rangaraju S, Streib C, Aghaebrahim A, Jadhav A, Frankel M, Jovin TG. Relationship between lesion topology and clinical outcome in anterior circulation large vessel occlusions. Stroke J Cereb Circ. 2015;46(7):1787–92.

116. Charidimou A, Schmitt A, Wilson D, Yakushiji Y, Gregoire SM, Fox Z, et al. The Cerebral Haemorrhage Anatomical RaTing inStrument (CHARTS): development and assessment of reliability. J Neurol Sci. 2017;372:178–83.

117. Wu O, Cloonan L, Mocking Steven JT, Bouts Mark JRJ, Copen WA, Cougo-Pinto PT, et al. Role of acute lesion topography in initial ischemic stroke severity and long-term functional outcomes. Stroke. 2015;46(9):2438–44.

118. Xu T, Jha A, Nachev P. The dimensionalities of lesion-deficit mapping. Neuropsychologia. 2018;115:134–41.

119. Ironside N, Chen C-J, Mutasa S, Sim JL, Marfatia S, Roh D, et al. Fully automated segmentation algorithm for hematoma volumetric analysis in spontaneous intracerebral hemorrhage. Stroke. 2019;50(12):3416–23.

120. Dhar R, Falcone GJ, Chen Y, Hamzehloo A, Kirsch EP, Noche RB, et al. Deep learning for automated measurement of hemorrhage and perihematomal edema in supratentorial intracerebral hemorrhage. Stroke. 2020;51(2):648–51.

121. Uniken Venema SM, Marini S, Lena UK, Morotti A, Jessel M, Moomaw CJ, et al. Impact of cerebral small vessel disease on functional recovery after intracerebral hemorrhage. Stroke. 2019;50(10):2722–8.

122. Sato S, Delcourt C, Heeley E, Arima H, Zhang S, Al-Shahi Salman R, et al. Significance of cerebral small-vessel disease in acute intracerebral hemorrhage. Stroke. 2016;47(3):701–7.
123. Caprio FZ, Maas MB, Rosenberg NF, Kosteva AR, Bernstein RA, Alberts MJ, et al. Leukoaraiosis on magnetic resonance imaging correlates with worse outcomes after spontaneous intracerebral hemorrhage. Stroke. 2013;44(3):642–6.
124. Appleton JP, Woodhouse LJ, Adami A, Becker JL, Berge E, Cala LA, et al. Imaging markers of small vessel disease and brain frailty, and outcomes in acute stroke. Neurology. 2020;94(5):e439–52.
125. Moura LM, Luccas R, de Paiva JPQ, Amaro E, Leemans A, Leite CDC, et al. Diffusion tensor imaging biomarkers to predict motor outcomes in stroke: a narrative review. Front Neurol. 2019 [cited 2020 Sept 7];10. Available from: https://www.ncbi.nlm.nih.gov/pmc/articles/PMC6530391/.
126. Biffi A, Anderson CD, Jagiella JM, Schmidt H, Kissela B, Hansen BM, et al. APOE genotype and extent of bleeding and outcome in lobar intracerebral haemorrhage: a genetic association study. Lancet Neurol. 2011;10(8):702–9.
127. Marini S, Devan WJ, Radmanesh F, Miyares L, Poterba T, Hansen BM, et al. 17p12 Influences hematoma volume and outcome in spontaneous intracerebral hemorrhage. Stroke. 2018;49(7):1618–25.
128. Mola-Caminal M, Carrera C, Soriano-Tárraga C, Giralt-Steinhauer E, Díaz-Navarro RM, Tur S, et al. PATJ low frequency variants are associated with worse ischemic stroke functional outcome. Circ Res. 2019;124(1):114–20.
129. Stinear CM, Byblow WD, Ackerley SJ, Barber PA, Smith M-C. Predicting recovery potential for individual stroke patients increases rehabilitation efficiency. Stroke. 2017;48(4):1011–9.
130. Langhorne P, Fearon P, Ronning OM, Kaste M, Palomaki H, Vemmos K, et al. Stroke unit care benefits patients with intracerebral hemorrhage. Stroke. 2013;44(11):3044–9.
131. Moullaali TJ, Wang X, Martin RH, Shipes VB, Robinson TG, Chalmers J, et al. Blood pressure control and clinical outcomes in acute intracerebral haemorrhage: a preplanned pooled analysis of individual participant data. Lancet Neurol. 2019;18(9):857–64.
132. Overview | Stroke and transient ischaemic attack in over 16s: diagnosis and initial management | Guidance | NICE. NICE [cited 2020 Sept 20]. Available from: https://www.nice.org.uk/guidance/ng128.
133. Qureshi AI, Huang W, Lobanova I, Barsan WG, Hanley DF, Hsu CY, et al. Outcomes of intensive systolic blood pressure reduction in patients with intracerebral hemorrhage and excessively high initial systolic blood pressure: post hoc analysis of a randomized clinical trial. JAMA Neurol. 2020 [cited 2020 Sept 9]. Available from: https://jamanetwork.com/journals/jamaneurology/fullarticle/2769857.
134. Steiner T, Poli S, Griebe M, Hüsing J, Hajda J, Freiberger A, et al. Fresh frozen plasma versus prothrombin complex concentrate in patients with intracranial haemorrhage related to vitamin K antagonists (INCH): a randomised trial. Lancet Neurol. 2016;15(6):566–73.
135. Pollack CVJ, Reilly PA, van Ryn J, Eikelboom JW, Glund S, Bernstein RA, et al. Idarucizumab for dabigatran reversal—full cohort analysis. Massachusetts Medical Society; 2017 [cited 2020 Sept 4]. https://doi.org/10.1056/NEJMoa1707278. Available from: https://www.nejm.org/doi/10.1056/NEJMoa1707278.
136. Connolly SJ, Crowther M, Eikelboom JW, Gibson CM, Curnutte JT, Lawrence JH, et al. Full study report of andexanet alfa for bleeding associated with factor Xa inhibitors. N Engl J Med. 2019;380(14):1326–35.
137. Baharoglu MI, Cordonnier C, Salman RA-S, de Gans K, Koopman MM, Brand A, et al. Platelet transfusion versus standard care after acute stroke due to spontaneous cerebral haemorrhage associated with antiplatelet therapy (PATCH): a randomised, open-label, phase 3 trial. Lancet. 2016;387(10038):2605–13.
138. Desmopressin for reversal of antiplatelet drugs in stroke due to haemorrhage—full text view—ClinicalTrials.gov [cited 2020 Sept 20]. Available from: https://clinicaltrials.gov/ct2/show/NCT03696121.

139. Sprigg N, Flaherty K, Appleton JP, Salman RA-S, Bereczki D, Beridze M, et al. Tranexamic acid for hyperacute primary IntraCerebral Haemorrhage (TICH-2): an international randomised, placebo-controlled, phase 3 superiority trial. Lancet. 2018 [cited 2020 Sept 8]. Available from: https://www.thelancet.com/journals/lancet/article/PIIS0140-6736(18)31033-X/abstract.

140. Law ZK, Ali A, Krishnan K, Bischoff A, Appleton JP, Scutt P, et al. Noncontrast computed tomography signs as predictors of hematoma expansion, clinical outcome, and response to tranexamic acid in acute intracerebral hemorrhage. Stroke. 2020;51(1):121–8.

141. Ovesen C, Jakobsen JC, Gluud C, Steiner T, Law Z, Flaherty K, et al. Prevention of haematoma progression by tranexamic acid in intracerebral haemorrhage patients with and without spot sign on admission scan: a statistical analysis plan of a pre-specified sub-study of the TICH-2 trial. BMC Res Notes. 2018;11(1):379.

142. Meretoja A, Churilov L, Campbell BCV, Aviv RI, Yassi N, Barras C, et al. The spot sign and tranexamic acid on preventing ICH growth—AUStralasia Trial (STOP-AUST): protocol of a phase II randomized, placebo-controlled, double-blind, multicenter trial. Int J Stroke. 2014;9(4):519–24.

143. Morotti A, Brouwers HB, Romero JM, Jessel MJ, Vashkevich A, Schwab K, et al. Intensive blood pressure reduction and spot sign in intracerebral hemorrhage. JAMA Neurol. 2017;74(8):950–60.

144. Morotti A, Boulouis G, Romero JM, Brouwers HB, Jessel MJ, Vashkevich A, et al. Blood pressure reduction and noncontrast CT markers of intracerebral hemorrhage expansion. Neurology. 2017;89(6):548–54.

145. Gayet-Ageron A, Prieto-Merino D, Ker K, Shakur H, Ageron F-X, Roberts I, et al. Effect of treatment delay on the effectiveness and safety of antifibrinolytics in acute severe haemorrhage: a meta-analysis of individual patient-level data from 40 138 bleeding patients. Lancet. 2018;391(10116):125–32.

146. Ironside N, Chen C-J, Ding D, Mayer SA, Connolly ES. Perihematomal edema after spontaneous intracerebral hemorrhage. Stroke. 2019;50(6):1626–33.

147. Parry-Jones AR, Wang X, Sato S, Mould WA, Vail A, Anderson CS, et al. Edema extension distance. Stroke. 2015;46(6):e137–40.

148. Zeng L, Tan L, Li H, Zhang Q, Li Y, Guo J. Deferoxamine therapy for intracerebral hemorrhage: a systematic review. PLoS One. 2018 [cited 2020 Sept 8];13(3). Available from: https://www.ncbi.nlm.nih.gov/pmc/articles/PMC5863956/.

149. Fu Y, Hao J, Zhang N, Ren L, Sun N, Li Y-J, et al. Fingolimod for the treatment of intracerebral hemorrhage: a 2-arm proof-of-concept study. JAMA Neurol. 2014;71(9):1092–101.

150. Lee S-H, Park H-K, Ryu W-S, Lee J-S, Bae H-J, Han M-K, et al. Effects of celecoxib on hematoma and edema volumes in primary intracerebral hemorrhage: a multicenter randomized controlled trial. Eur J Neurol. 2013;20(8):1161–9.

151. Selim M, Foster LD, Moy CS, Xi G, Hill MD, Morgenstern LB, et al. Deferoxamine mesylate in patients with intracerebral haemorrhage (i-DEF): a multicentre, randomised, placebo-controlled, double-blind phase 2 trial. Lancet Neurol. 2019;18(5):428–38.

152. BLOC-ICH: interleukin-1 receptor antagonist in intracerebral haemorrhage—full text view—ClinicalTrials.gov [cited 2020 Sept 20]. Available from: https://clinicaltrials.gov/ct2/show/NCT03737344.

153. Hostettler IC, Seiffge DJ, Werring DJ. Intracerebral hemorrhage: an update on diagnosis and treatment. Expert Rev Neurother. 2019;19(7):679–94.

154. Mendelow AD, Gregson BA, Rowan EN, Murray GD, Gholkar A, Mitchell PM, et al. Early surgery versus initial conservative treatment in patients with spontaneous supratentorial lobar intracerebral haematomas (STICH II): a randomised trial. Lancet Lond Engl. 2013;382(9890):397–408.

155. Hanley DF, Thompson RE, Rosenblum M, Yenokyan G, Lane K, McBee N, et al. Efficacy and safety of minimally invasive surgery with thrombolysis in intracerebral haemorrhage evacuation (MISTIE III): a randomised, controlled, open-label, blinded endpoint phase 3 trial. Lancet. 2019;393(10175):1021–32.

156. Kahan BC, Jairath V, Doré CJ, Morris TP. The risks and rewards of covariate adjustment in randomized trials: an assessment of 12 outcomes from 8 studies. Trials. 2014;15(1):139.
157. Xu T, Rolf Jäger H, Husain M, Rees G, Nachev P. High-dimensional therapeutic inference in the focally damaged human brain. Brain. 2018;141(1):48–54.
158. Kim BJ, Kwon SU, Park J-H, Kim Y-J, Hong K-S, Wong LKS, et al. Cilostazol versus aspirin in ischemic stroke patients with high-risk cerebral hemorrhage: subgroup analysis of the PICASSO trial. Stroke. 2020;51(3):931–7.

Blood Biomarkers in the Diagnosis of Acute Stroke

8

Gian Marco De Marchis and Tolga D. Dittrich

8.1 Introduction

Acute stroke represents a leading cause of death in industrialized countries and has a considerable socioeconomic impact due to its attached high morbidity leaving up to 50% of the survivors chronically disabled [1].

Two pathophysiological types of stroke can be distinguished: the ischemic stroke due to an occlusion of an arterial blood vessel leading to local oxygen undersupply of the brain tissue and the hemorrhagic stroke, which is caused by a disruption of the integrity of a vascular wall within the brain with subsequent extravasation of blood into the surrounding tissue or subarachnoid space, potentially leading to neuronal demise [2].

Despite the intuitiveness of these underlying pathophysiological mechanisms, the diagnostic and therapeutic workup in cases of suspected stroke holds several difficulties: Acute stroke represents a heterogeneous syndrome with a variety of clinical manifestations encompassing evident deficits, such as acute facial or limb weakness, but also more subtle, unspecific symptoms such as dizziness, gait disturbance, or severe headache. As the absence of the mentioned symptoms above does not safely preclude a severe cerebrovascular event, every patient with newly developed focal neurological deficits requires prompt radiological evaluation [3, 4].

The distinction between ischemic and hemorrhagic stroke is crucial as their therapeutic approaches are diametrical: systemic thrombolysis with recombinant tissue plasminogen activator (rt-PA) represents a therapeutic core element in cases of acute occlusions of intracranial arteries due to its ability to restore cerebral blood supply by the dissolution of a blood clot. In contrast, hemodilution in cases of

G. M. De Marchis (✉) · T. D. Dittrich
Department of Neurology & Stroke Center, University Hospital Basel, Basel, Switzerland
e-mail: gian.demarchis@usb.ch; tolga.dittrich@usb.ch

© Springer Nature Switzerland AG 2021
A. C. Fonseca, J. M. Ferro (eds.), *Precision Medicine in Stroke*,
https://doi.org/10.1007/978-3-030-70761-3_8

intracranial hemorrhage may fuel its growth and is therefore strictly contraindicated. In this context, time is the most critical factor especially in cases of large vessel occlusion, as the potentially salvageable brain tissue gradually diminishes over time leading to a narrow therapeutic window with an increased risk for neurologic sequelae and worse outcome in cases of treatment delay [5, 6].

Current diagnostic algorithms recommend computed tomography (CT) or magnetic resonance imaging (MRI) of the head to rule out intracranial hemorrhage and to determine whether there is an underlying vascular occlusion.

Nevertheless, unremarkable initial brain imaging findings do not rule out a transient insufficient blood supply or lacunar ischemic event as the underlying cause for observed neurologic deficits. Against this background, the differentiation between a causative vascular problem and a stroke mimic (such as migraine, hypertensive crisis, or epileptic seizures) can be difficult [7].

In recent years, interest in the field of novel biomarker research has steadily increased. Biomarkers are generally referred to as objective indicators of an individual's (patho-) biological state, which can be measured reproducibly and accurately [8]. Studied areas of application within stroke biomarker research involve the rapid biomarker-based differentiation between stroke subtypes and stroke mimics to further streamline the prehospital management in patients with suspected stroke and prevent imminent treatment delay in cases where clinical assessment is difficult and immediate neuroimaging is not readily available [7, 9]. In the broadest sense, these stroke biomarkers can be considered as candidate surrogate markers in the diagnostic context [10].

This chapter provides an overview of the biomarkers that are currently the focus of research, enters into the details of clinically promising candidates, and discusses potential areas of their application from a clinical point of view.

8.2 Overview of Emerging Biomarkers for Risk Stratification, Diagnosis, and Etiological Classification in Acute Stroke

There is a wide range of promising candidates that are currently subject to research. Table 8.1 presents an overview of biomarkers with reported potential diagnostic use in a broader or narrower sense without claiming to be exhaustive.

Table 8.1 Overview of biomarkers for risk stratification, diagnosis, and etiological classification in acute stroke (adapted from [7, 9, 11–21])

Biomarker group	Biomarker	Description
Associated with glial cells	S100β (calcium-binding protein-beta)	Calcium-binding protein expressed by astrocytes and oligodendrocytes
	GFAP (glial fibrillary acidic protein)	Intermediate filament protein predominantly expressed by astrocytes

Table 8.1 (continued)

Biomarker group	Biomarker	Description
Associated with neuronal cells	Serum neurofilament light chain (SNfL)	Polypeptide filaments, component of the axonal cytoskeleton
	NSE (neuron-specific enolase)	Dimeric glycolytic isoenzyme in the cytoplasm of neurons/neuroendocrine cells
	HFABP (heart fatty acid-binding protein)	Cytosolic protein that modulates lipid signaling cascades; involved in intracellular fatty acid transport
	MBP (myelin basic protein)	Main proteolipid constituent of myelin, produced by oligodendroglia cells
	Tau	Protein that stabilizes microtubules and assists with axonal maintenance and transport in neurons
	VLP-1 (visinin-like protein-1)	Member of the family of neuronal intracellular calcium sensor visinin-like proteins, part of the calcium-dependent cell signaling involved in the modulation of cAMP (cyclic adenosine monophosphate)
	NMDA-receptor antibodies (NR2A/NR2B subunits of the NMDA receptor)	Excitotoxic receptor
Associated with hemostasis	D-dimer	Fibrin degradation product that reflects global activation of coagulation and fibrinolysis
	vWf (von Willebrand factor)	Adhesive glycoprotein involved in factor VIII platelet adhesion stabilization
	Fibrinogen	Acute-phase protein, involved in leukocyte-endothelial interaction, platelet aggregation, and hemostasis
Associated with inflammation	CRP (C-reactive protein)	Acute-phase protein, part of innate immune response
	Cytokines (TNF-a, interleukin-1b/-6)	Inflammatory cytokines
	Matrix metalloproteinases (MMP-2, MMP-9)	MMP-2/-9: Proteolytic enzymes from the family of gelatinases; possess the ability to activate pro-inflammatory cytokines
	Lipoprotein-associated phospholipase A2 (Lp-PLA2)	Hydrolytic enzyme
	Adhesion molecules (VCAM-1 [vascular cellular adhesion molecule], ICAM-1)	Immunoglobulin superfamily members VCAM-1: Binds monocytes and lymphocytes
	ApoC-1 (apolipoprotein C-1), ApoC-3 (apolipoprotein C-3)	ApoC-1: Associated with LDL and VLDL, involved in plasma lipoprotein remodeling, inhibits CETP ApoC-3: Associated with VLDL, HDL, and LDL; inhibits triglyceride hydrolysis by lipoprotein/hepatic lipase; interferes with normal endothelial function

(continued)

Table 8.1 (continued)

Biomarker group	Biomarker	Description
Associated with cardiac function	Natriuretic peptides (ANP [atrial natriuretic peptide], BNP [brain natriuretic peptide]/NT-proBNP [N-terminal-pro B-type natriuretic peptide])	Myocardial polypeptides with natriuretic, diuretic, and vasodilator activity
Associated with oxidative stress	PARK7	Redox-sensitive molecular chaperone
Other biomarkers	NDKA (nucleoside diphosphate kinase A)	Protein kinase
	Brain-derived neurotrophic growth factor	Neurotrophin superfamily member; growth factor proteins important for neuronal development and function
	Fibrillin-1	Glycoprotein and important component of elastic fibers

8.3 Blood Biomarkers in the Diagnosis of Acute Stroke: A Clinical Perspective

8.3.1 Background

Through a series of large-scale genome, proteome, and metabolome sequencing, a multitude of promising molecules linked to different pathophysiological steps of the stroke cascade were identified (see Table 8.1) [7]. Studies have shown that a small proportion of proteins, albeit to a varying extent, are capable to distinguish between patients with and without stroke [7]. Nevertheless, there are no blood biomarkers for acute stroke used in daily clinical routine for diagnostic purposes to the present day [7, 22].

The reason is that a diagnostic biomarker has to meet different requirements to be used in clinical diagnostics. Ideally, markers should be easily measurable in the course of the first routine point-of-care blood testing, such as blood glucose or the international normalized ratio (INR) [7, 23]. Stroke markers should be quickly released from the brain tissue after neuronal damage occurred, pass the blood-brain barrier rapidly, and be dispensed steadily into the peripheral blood to be detectable soon after stroke onset [16]. A crucial demand for a diagnostic stroke biomarker is its ability to reliably separate affected from healthy individuals. Key indicators in this respect are sensitivity and specificity. A sensitivity of 90% for the detection of an acute ischemic stroke would still mean that 10% of patients with ischemic stroke would mistakenly remain undetected, potentially impeding a rapid initiation of treatment. On the contrary, a specificity of 90% would mean that 10% of the tested healthy individuals would falsely be identified as sick, entailing the risk of over-treatment [7]. Besides the desired high sensitivity to early cerebral damage and the specificity of a stroke biomarker candidate for the brain tissue, the key question in clinical context due to its attached therapeutic implications is: Can the biomarker candidate distinguish between ischemic and hemorrhagic stroke with sufficient reliability [7, 17]? In hemorrhagic stroke, the ability to make this distinction could allow early antagonization of oral anticoagulants and early initiation of antihypertensive therapy [24, 25]. In acute ischemic stroke, a reliable preclinical biomarker-based identification could facilitate the rapid assignment to a stroke center and therefore potentially increase the proportion of patients treated with intravenous thrombolysis and endovascular treatment, respectively, ensuring the most beneficial outcome [9, 18, 24]. Furthermore, in cases of unclear time of symptom onset, which accounts for up to 28% of all patients with acute ischemic stroke, the release kinetics of a diagnostic biomarker or its detection with known delayed release could help to deduce the approximate beginning of the event and help guide therapeutic decision-making [9, 26].

8.3.2 Biomarkers for the Early Differentiation Between Acute Cerebrovascular Events and Mimicking Conditions

8.3.2.1 *N*-Methyl-D-Aspartate (NMDA) Receptor

NMDA receptors bind the neurotransmitter glutamate. Elevated levels of glutamate mediate excitatory effects through the activation of NMDA receptors within the pathophysiologic ischemic stroke cascade, ultimately leading to neuronal damage [27–29]. The NMDA receptor in its basic configuration consists of 4–5 units (2 NR1 and 2–3 NR2), with NR2A and NR2B as the two major subunits of NR2 in adult neocortex [30–32].

In the course of cerebral ischemia, an autoimmune-mediated formation of antibodies against NMDA receptor peptide fractions has been demonstrated in the peripheral blood [29, 33]. NR2A/2B autoantibody concentrations were significantly higher in patients with transient ischemic attack (TIA) and acute ischemic stroke compared to controls [30]. The sensitivities for the diagnosis of ischemic strokes and TIAs within 3 h after symptom onset using a cutoff of 2.0 µg/L were 97% and 95%, respectively. The specificity for both entities was 98% [30].

Differences within the temporal course of NR2A antibody elevations have been demonstrated in cases of ischemic stroke with a concentration peak around 9 h after hospital admission [28]. Interestingly, the antibody concentrations were higher in infarcts involving the brain cortex [28]. As demonstrated by another study, the formation of NMDA receptor antibodies is also detectable in cases of intracranial hemorrhage suggesting that a reliable differentiation from patients with ischemic stroke is not possible through the sole evidence of antibodies in the serum [30]. Nevertheless, regarding the time course of the concentration changes in the serum, peak values were achieved earlier and were lower in patients with intracranial hemorrhage compared to patients with acute ischemic stroke [30]. The latency between symptom onset and the achievement of peak concentrations ranged between 9 and 12 h for patients with acute ischemic stroke and 3 and 5 h for patients with intracranial hemorrhage [30]. The positive predictive value for ischemic strokes was 86% and 91% for TIAs, and the negative predictive value was 98% for both entities [30].

The measurement of NMDA receptor antibodies might be helpful to discriminate between patients with TIAs and stroke mimics [30]. However, the additional informative value of NMDA receptor antibodies in the emergency setting remains uncertain. A study with 120 patients presenting with acute ischemic stroke or TIA within 72 h after symptom onset showed that men and women with a history of stroke in the prior 6 months had elevated NR2 antibody levels compared to controls, potentially reducing its informative significance for the detection of recent ischemic cerebral events in patients with a history of stroke or TIA, respectively [34].

Another issue in the diagnostic context is the expected relatively long latency period between the formation of antibodies and their detectability in the peripheral blood, leading to a shift of interest towards the NR2 peptides, which are thought to be produced earlier after the ischemic event [16].

8.3.2.2 Lipoprotein-Associated Phospholipase A2 (Lp-PLA2)

Lp-PLA2 is an enzyme that catalyzes the conversion of low-density lipoprotein into proinflammatory metabolites and is found to be predominantly expressed in macrophage-containing atherosclerotic lesions [35, 36]. Lp-PLA2 is considered a marker for vascular inflammation [35, 37]. The pathophysiological linkage between Lp-PLA2 and occurrence of ischemic stroke is likely to be that inflammation, as a recognized underlying mechanism for the development of atherosclerosis including the rupture of unstable plaques, may ultimately lead to cerebrovascular events [38–40]. Lp-PLA2 mainly circulates bound to LDL in the peripheral blood with a small fraction binding to HDL [39]. A proof-of-concept trial with individuals with previous ischemic stroke under therapy with statins demonstrated lower Lp-PLA2 mass levels compared to individuals with ischemic stroke without established statin therapy [41]. Nevertheless, Lp-PLA2 and LDL cholesterol levels appear to be independent of each other [39, 42].

Lp-PLA2 activity was demonstrated to predict ischemic stroke and coronary heart disease in the general population [35, 43]. Lp-PLA2 mass and activity showed to be associated with symptomatic large vessel stenosis, but not with cardioembolism [40]. A recent clinical trial investigated the relation between intima-media thickness of the carotids and Lp-PLA2 blood levels in cases of arterioembolic stroke [44]. Although not reaching the threshold of statistical significance, Lp-PLA2 blood levels were correlated with the intima-media thickness in patients with arteriosclerotic ischemic stroke supporting the previously suspected pathophysiological linkage [44].

Additionally, Lp-PLA2 mass levels were shown to predict recurrent stroke in individuals with known stroke history [35]. Although the predictive value of Lp-PLA2 activity for recurrent stroke seems to be limited to individuals with LDL levels below 130 mg/dL, suggesting a possible interaction of the Lp-PLA2 activity and LDL levels, Lp-PLA2 is widely considered as an independent predictor for stroke [35, 38, 39].

Furthermore, Lp-PLA2 proved to add valuable information to the risk stratification in patients with TIAs [40]. Patients with high Lp-PLA2 activity and mass levels exposed a higher risk for subsequent stroke and death, classified as members of the moderate-risk group using the $ABCD_2$ score before [40].

There is still a certain heterogeneity regarding the measurement of Lp-PLA2. This is likely due to different assays that measure either the mass or the activity of Lp-PLA2, causing a variability since Lp-PLA2 mass and activity do not strictly correlate [45]. The main reason for this limited correlation is thought to be that mass tests mainly detect the HDL-associated Lp-PLA2, which represents only a small proportion of the total Lp-PLA2 [45]. Altogether, it remains unclear to which extent the observed incomplete correlation between measurable Lp-PLA2 activity and mass is attributable to the enzymes' biochemical characteristics or technical aspects of the available assays [35]. Further studies investigating the temporal release kinetics of Lp-PLA2 are needed.

8.3.2.3 Heart-Type Fatty Acid-Binding Protein (HFABP)

HFABP belongs to a family of proteins with different tissue distribution patterns [46]. It is found in the brain, but also the heart, the lung, and the kidneys [46]. This family of proteins plays an important role in maintaining cellular homeostasis [46].

A pilot study investigated the ability of HFABP to discriminate between patients with stroke, patients with myocardial infarction, and healthy controls [46]. The specificity and sensitivity of HFABP for the diagnosis of acute stroke were 100% and approximately 68%, respectively [46]. However, no differentiation between hemorrhagic and ischemic stroke was possible [46].

Moreover, there is evidence that HFABP serum levels within the 6 h after stroke onset correlate with the severity of symptoms in patients with acute ischemic stroke [47]. As expected, elevated HFABP serum levels were also observed in patients with acute myocardial infarction, which might pose a diagnostic obstacle in acute clinical situations [46]. The relatively low sensitivity would call for a multi-marker approach in a clinical setting [47].

A potential benefit of HFABP is its relatively fast release into the blood with measurable elevations within a few hours after stroke onset [46, 47]. Overall, the evidence regarding the potential clinical benefit of HFABP is still too limited—only a few studies with a low number of cases exist—to be able to make general statements about possible fields of application in clinical routine.

8.3.2.4 Parkinson Disease Protein 7 (PARK 7)

The gene coding for PARK 7 was discovered as an autosomal recessive gene related to a form of familial Parkinson's disease [48–50]. Although expressed in the cerebral tissue where it is assumed to have a reparative function in cellular damage caused by oxidative stress, PARK 7 does not appear to be specific for the central nervous system [48, 50]. The exact function of PARK 7 and its release mechanisms are not entirely understood [48, 50]. Yet it is plausible to assume that neuronal damage in the context of acute stroke leads to a release of the protein to the systemic circulation through direct penetration of the disrupted blood-brain barrier [48].

This assumption is supported by a large-scale three-center study demonstrating a significant release of PARK 7 into the systemic circulation within 30 min to 3 h after symptom onset in patients with acute ischemic (including TIA) and hemorrhagic stroke [48].

The diagnostic sensitivity for the diagnosis of acute stroke (i.e., hemorrhagic, ischemic, and TIA) varied between 54% and 91%, and the specificity between 80% and 97%, depending on the used cutoffs and the timeframe between symptom onset and time of blood sample collection (range of 30 min to 5 days) [48]. As the previous data implicates, discrimination between stroke subtypes and conditions that may mimic stroke using (serial) PARK 7 measurements is currently not possible [48].

8.3.3 Biomarkers for the Differentiation Between Ischemic and Hemorrhagic Stroke

8.3.3.1 Glial Fibrillary Acidic Protein (GFAP)

One of the most promising markers for stroke diagnosis is GFAP. It is a monomeric filament protein that is relatively specific for astrocytic glial brain cells [51, 52]. Various studies suggest its potential use for the differentiation of stroke subtypes as GFAP serum levels were shown to be elevated in patients with ischemic stroke and intracranial hemorrhage compared to healthy subjects and other neurological conditions [51, 53].

One of the first larger studies including 135 patients with first-time acute stroke, ischemic or hemorrhagic, evaluated the ability of GFAP to differentiate between both stroke entities within 6 h after symptom onset [54]. The analysis of the serum GFAP levels at admission revealed that 81% of patients with intracranial hemorrhage demonstrated measurable GFAP-level elevations, while only 5% of patients with ischemic stroke showed an increase over the detection threshold [54]. The diagnostic specificity of GFAP for the identification of intracranial hemorrhage in this mixed stroke cohort within the first 6 h after symptom onset was 98%, and the sensitivity 79% at a cutoff point of 2.9 ng/L [54]. The overall diagnostic accuracy of GFAP for the differentiation between intracranial hemorrhage and acute ischemic stroke within a timeframe of 3 h after symptom onset was 91% [54].

A subsequent multicenter study with 202 patients with radiologically confirmed acute ischemic stroke or intracranial hemorrhage, who were admitted to the hospital in less than 4.5 h after symptom onset, evaluated the ability of GFAP to differentiate between both stroke entities [24]. Patients with prior ischemic or hemorrhagic stroke or other preexisting neurological disorders were excluded [24]. The diagnostic specificity of GFAP for the differentiation between ischemic stroke and intracranial hemorrhage in this cohort within the first 4.5 h after symptom onset was 96.3%, and sensitivity 84.2% [24]. The GFAP levels in patients with intracranial hemorrhage correlated with the NIHSS (National Institutes of Health Stroke Scale) scores at admission, most likely reflecting the tissue damage-dependent GFAP release into the blood [24, 55].

However, the specifications vary across different studies considering the different times of specimen collections and cutoffs used [25, 54, 56, 57]. A research project further examining the release kinetics of GFAP demonstrated an accuracy of over 80% in the timeframe of 2–6 h after symptom onset, whereby GFAP levels correlated significantly with the hemorrhage volume in cases of intracranial bleeding 2 h after symptom onset [56].

On the contrary, the prolonged release of GFAP into the blood reaches the maximum concentration between 48 and 96 h after event onset in cases of ischemic stroke [54]. Therefore, no correlation between the initial GFAP levels and symptom severity can be seen in cases of ischemic stroke [24, 55]. In this context, it becomes evident why transient hypoperfusion not leading to permanent structural damage does not necessarily translate into elevated GFAP levels in the peripheral blood [24, 55, 58]. It should also be taken into account that GFAP baseline blood levels may vary by age, as there is evidence derived of cerebrospinal fluid samples of 25 subjects with no history or current evidence for neurological disorders that shows an increase with age [59].

As indicated above, the release kinetics are thought to be different depending on the stroke subtype with a suspected faster release of GFAP due to immediate astrocytic damage and a consecutive timely disruption of the blood-brain barrier in cases of intracranial hemorrhage [24, 25, 54]. Consequently, the available upper time limit in which high GFAP levels are likely attributable to intracranial hemorrhage is 6–12 h after the onset of stroke symptoms [24, 25].

A Swedish multicenter study measured several biomarker levels in a mixed stroke cohort of 97 patients within 24 h of symptom onset. Interestingly, the combination of GFAP with another blood biomarker called APC-PCI (activated protein C–protein C inhibitor complex) revealed a negative predictive value of 100% for intracranial hemorrhage in patients with NIHSS scores of more than 3, compared to the previous stated negative predictive value of 91% with GFAP alone [53, 54].

Yet, there is still a fundamental problem concerning the use of GFAP in clinical routine. The knowledge of how concomitant cerebral pathologies potentially leading to cerebral gliosis themselves might influence the release of GFAP into the bloodstream is limited [24]. Moreover, the observation that GFAP was not detectable in the wide majority of patients with acute ischemic stroke within the time window of 6 h after symptom onset reduces its informative value in acute management [54]. It is also noteworthy that data about GFAP concentrations and their temporal release in cases of lacunar ischemic stroke or cerebral microbleeds, especially infratentorial, is still scarce [24]. One study investigated several biomarkers concerning their ability to differentiate vertigo due to posterior circulation stroke from the vertigo of nonvascular origin [60]. The vast majority of patients suffering from vertigo due to an infratentorial hemorrhage did not show elevated GFAP blood levels within the first 24 h after symptom onset [60]. A convincing explanatory approach is the already previously described correlation between GFAP release and lesion size [60].

Even though increases of GFAP concentrations emerge earlier compared to other astroglial markers such as S100β in cases of acute ischemia in the anterior circulation, an important limitation for the use of GFAP as a point-of-care test remains the limited discriminatory power between intracranial hemorrhage and lacunar stroke in cases of unknown time of symptom onset [56, 61]. Given these contradictory findings regarding the sensitivity of GFAP for the early detection of intracranial hemorrhage within a 0–2 h after symptom onset, further studies are needed to clarify the diagnostic accuracy in this timeframe [24, 56].

8.3.3.2 S100 Calcium-Binding Protein β (S100β)

S100β is part of the cytosol of astrocytic glial brain cells, consists of two subunits (α and β), and is specific to the nervous system [52, 62–64]. The history of the name goes back to the 1960s and is derived from its solubility in a saturated ammonium sulfate solution [65]. Interestingly, S100β-expressing cells do not express GFAP, although both being glial typical markers, due to different developmental stages of the brain astrocytes [66]. Mainly intracellularly localized, S100β has a variety of regulatory functions in the calcium homeostasis, cell proliferation, and apoptosis [64, 67].

S100β levels were significantly higher in stroke cohorts compared to healthy controls [64, 68, 69]. However, elevated S100β serum levels have not exclusively been reported in patients with TIAs and ischemic and hemorrhagic stroke, but also in context with other neurological conditions such as traumatic brain injury, migraine, and neurodegenerative diseases [69–73]. Surprisingly, significant differences regarding the temporal course were observed between patients with ischemic stroke, TIA, and traumatic brain injury suggesting different underlying release mechanisms [72].

Whether S100β can distinguish between ischemic and hemorrhagic stroke has been a matter of ongoing debate. A large Spanish study addressed this question using a biomarker-based approach with a total number of 915 patients with confirmed acute ischemic or hemorrhagic stroke [74]. The blood biomarker panel contained, among others, CRP, D-dimer, S100β, sRAGE (soluble receptor for advanced glycation end products), MMP-9, and BNP [74]. Blood samples were collected within 6 h after event onset [74]. As a result, within the tested panel, increased S100β and decreased sRAGE levels were associated with intracranial hemorrhage, emphasizing its potential distinctive ability towards patients with ischemic stroke [74]. Even though the exact release mechanisms are still not understood, the authors assume that an early release in cases of intracranial bleeding as observed with GFAP, another glial marker, is due to faster cell destruction compared to the gradual neuronal demise associated with ischemic damage [74].

Despite these promising results, S100β failed to discriminate between ischemic stroke and intracranial hemorrhage within the first 24 h after symptom onset in an explorative biomarker analysis containing 97 patients with acute stroke [53].

On the other end of the spectrum, a more recent study with a total of 142 stroke patients, including TIAs, came to a different result [69]. Higher S100β serum levels were reported in patients admitted within 48 h after symptom onset in cases of cerebral ischemia compared to patients with intracranial hemorrhage and TIAs [69]. Remarkably, the proportion of individuals with intracranial hemorrhage was relatively high with almost 25%, exceeding the proportion of the previous studies by approximately 10% [69].

To elucidate these seemingly contradictory findings which may partly be due to different times of sample collections, heterogeneous cohorts, or technical measurement aspects, understanding the release kinetics of $S100\beta$ is particularly important.

The half-life of $S100\beta$ is approximately around 30 min, indicating that a measurable elevation over days is associated with an ongoing neuronal injury [70]. Overall, the release kinetics of $S100\beta$ seem to be strongly influenced by the duration of the astrocytic functional disruption as well as the site and the extent of neuronal damage [75]. The first studies to determine the time course of $S100\beta$ levels in the peripheral blood in patients with acute ischemic stroke stated a maximum increase of $S100\beta$ serum levels 2–3 days after symptom onset [68, 76, 77]. Notably, ischemic stroke due to mainstem or multiple branch occlusion lasting for more than 6 h showed significantly higher $S100\beta$ levels than patients with a single branch or smaller artery occlusions [75]. In addition, there is some evidence that cortical infarctions lead to earlier elevations of serum $S100\beta$ levels compared to subcortical or brainstem ischemic events [64]. In patients with ischemic stroke, the $S100\beta$ peak level reflected the NIHSS score at admission as well as the changes in NIHSS score over the first 10 days after symptom onset [72]. Increments of $S100\beta$ plasma levels were shown to be associated with larger infarct volume in cases of ischemic stroke and unfavorable outcomes in cases of ischemic and hemorrhagic stroke [63, 64, 75]. According to a study with a cohort of patients with proximal occlusions of the middle cerebral artery, $S100\beta$ predicted a malignant course defined as the evidence of space-occupying edema with possible subsequent herniation [62]. A large-scale study investigating the initial blood samples of patients that were admitted with acute ischemic stroke and received treatment with rt-PA demonstrated $S100\beta$ elevations within the first 24 h after symptom onset [78]. Interestingly, the serial analysis of blood samples 2 and 24 h after the administration of rt-PA did not show significant differences regarding the concentrations of $S100\beta$ [78]. An almost simultaneously published study confirmed the early elevation of $S100\beta$ after stroke onset [79].

A comparison of the temporal profiles of $S100\beta$ level changes within 3 days after admission showed a significant difference between stroke patients and patients with traumatic brain injuries and TIAs, respectively [72]. Furthermore, no differences of serum $S100\beta$ levels on admission were reported between cases of confirmed stroke when compared to those with TIAs, brain metastasis, or hypertensive emergencies [80]. Despite the uncertainties, this finding suggests different underlying pathophysiological mechanisms of damage in each entity [72].

In contrast to other biomarkers such as GFAP and MMP-9, $S100\beta$ showed the potential to discriminate patients with ischemic and hemorrhagic stroke in the posterior circulation from patients without acute vascular events [60]. A recent study investigated whether $S100\beta$, alone and in combination with copeptin, was able to preclude a cerebrovascular event in patients presenting at the emergency department for newly occurred dizziness [81]. $S100\beta$ levels were shown to be significantly higher in patients with stroke as the suspected underlying cause for the new episode of dizziness [81]. The negative predicate value of S100β alone for stroke was 95% at a diagnostic sensitivity of 54%, and specificity of 97% [81].

8.3.4 Biomarkers for the Prediction of Clinical Severity and Complications in Acute Stroke

8.3.4.1 Matrix Metalloproteinase 9 (MMP-9)

MMP-9 belongs to a group of proteolytic enzymes that are involved in remodeling processes of the extracellular matrix through their ability to cleave collagen and laminin, representing two of the main components of basement membranes [82–84].

The overexpression and capability of MMP-9 to deteriorate components of the basal membrane are widely considered as an explanatory approach for the disruption of the blood-brain barrier entailing perifocal edema, inflammatory response, and ultimately neuronal demise in the context of stroke [82, 83, 85, 86]. Elevated MMP-9 levels were observed in ischemic stroke, treated [82] or not treated with rt-PA [85], as well as in cases of hemorrhagic stroke [83]. High MMP-9 levels seem to be associated with a higher degree of neurological impairment and a larger infarct volume within the first 48 h of acute ischemic stroke [85].

The temporal course of MMP-9 levels was observed in patients with ischemic stroke due to an occlusion of the middle cerebral artery treated with rt-PA within the first 3 h after symptom onset [82]. Consistent with the supposed role of MMP-9 for the preservation of the blood-brain barrier, the pretreatment MMP-9 levels predicted intraparenchymal hemorrhage in acute ischemic stroke after applying thrombolytic therapy in those patients [82].

Apart from the administration of thrombolytic therapy, a study conducted on 250 patients with acute hemispheric ischemic stroke demonstrated an association between elevated MMP-9 levels within the first 24 h after symptom onset and hemorrhagic transformation [87]. The sensitivity and specificity of MMP-9 levels from 140 ng/mL upwards for the prediction of hemorrhagic transformation were around 90%, whereas the negative predictive value was 97% [87]. Unfortunately, it is still not clear whether elevated MMP-9 serum levels during the first 4.5 h after stroke onset are robust predictors of secondary hemorrhage within this critical early phase [87].

Interestingly, a subsequent study of the blood levels of cellular fibronectin (c-Fn), an adhesive protein primarily produced by endothelial cells, in patients with acute ischemic stroke treated with rt-PA showed a significant association with hemorrhagic transformation [86]. Although a positive correlation between c-Fn and MMP-9 blood levels was observed, the sensitivity (100%), specificity (96%), and negative predictive value (100%) of c-Fn for the prediction of hemorrhagic transformation at a cutoff of 3.6 μ/mL were shown to be even higher in comparison to those of MMP-9 [86]. Moreover, the applied logistic regression models only revealed c-Fn levels to be independently associated with hemorrhagic transformation, indicating its potential superiority compared to MMP-9 regarding its diagnostic value in rt-PA-associated intracranial bleedings [86].

A further study examining the temporal profiles of different metalloproteinases including MMP-9 after spontaneous intracranial bleeding showed dynamic changes within the further course [83]. Baseline MMP-9 blood levels were related to the radiologically determined hemorrhage-associated edema and the residual scar volume at 3 months [83].

8.3.4.2 Myelin Basic Protein (MBP)

MBP is a myelin membrane protein with a structural role within the myelin sheaths of Schwann cells and oligodendrocytes [78, 88, 89]. Analogous to S100β, increasing serum MBP concentrations were reported in cases of ischemic stroke within the first 24 h after symptom onset [78]. A comparison of serum MBP levels between patients with radiologically confirmed acute ischemic stroke, obtained within the first 12 h after symptom onset, and a healthy control group did not show a significant difference [88].

A smaller study investigated the admission levels of different stroke biomarkers, including MBP, in a heterogeneous cohort of 28 patients with acute ischemic stroke [90]. Among these patients, 1 had a total anterior circulation stroke, 10 had partial anterior circulation stroke, 8 had lacunar ischemic stroke, 4 had posterior circulation stroke, and 5 had unknown types [90]. Overall, the analysis showed elevated MBP levels on admission in 39% of patients [90].

Although MBP might not qualify as a sufficiently accurate diagnostic biomarker in early stroke, the release kinetics may provide additional information. Higher MBP peak concentrations within the first days were associated with the higher NIHSS baseline scores and larger lesion volume in the CT brain scans [78]. Moreover, smaller changes in MBP levels within the first 24 h were observed in patients demonstrating favorable outcomes [78].

8.3.5 Biomarkers for the Etiological Classification of Ischemic Cerebrovascular Events

8.3.5.1 Natriuretic Peptides (ANP/BNP)

Atrial (ANP) and brain natriuretic peptides (BNP) are co-released mainly by the cardiac atriums and ventricles in response to an increased myocardial wall tension and hemodynamic stress but remarkably also in the course of acute ischemic stroke, promoting vasodilatation and natriuresis [73, 91–96].

Besides being expressed by cardiomyocytes, ANP is also found within the central nervous systems (i.e., hypothalamus and septum) [97]. In recent years, there has been growing interest in the midregional fragment of the precursor hormone of ANP (midregional proANP; MR-proANP) due to its higher sample stability [98]. In a large multicenter study including over 700 patients with acute ischemic stroke high MR-proANP levels were independently associated with cardioembolic stroke etiology and atrial fibrillation [97, 99]. Moreover, high levels of MR-proANP are associated with small vessel infarcts and white matter lesions on MRI [100].

The name BNP is derived from the fact that this peptide was first isolated from porcine brain tissue [92]. ProBNP represents the precursor molecule of BNP, whereby inactive N-terminal peptides (NT-proBNP; N-terminal pro-brain natriuretic peptide) are released in the course of the cleavage process [93]. The fact that the half-life of NT-proBNP is longer compared to that of BNP makes it preferable for measuring purposes [93].

NT-proBNP blood levels were found to be elevated in patients with acute ischemic stroke within the first 24 h after symptom onset independently of echocardiographic parameters [91]. The admission levels were significantly higher in cases of cardioembolic origin [91]. A meta-analysis comparing circulating BNP/NT-proBNP levels across different stroke etiologies with data from over 2800 patients demonstrated significant increments of BNP/NT-proBNP in cardioembolic ischemic stroke within the first 72 h after stroke onset compared to patients with non-cardioembolic stroke [93].

These findings are in line with other reports of an observed strong association between elevated NT-proBNP levels and an increased risk of cardioembolic stroke in the general population [101]. BNP secretion is believed to be induced due to its vasodilatory effect as a counter-regulation mechanism in cases of ischemic stroke [91]. Independent from the occurrence of an ischemic stroke, there is evidence that increased NT-proBNP levels are associated with the presence of atrial fibrillation [93, 101, 102]. In patients with chronic non-valvular atrial fibrillation, BNP represents an independent predictor of thromboembolic complications as BNP blood levels were demonstrated to be higher in patients with thromboembolic events compared to individuals without complications [95]. Following this, high proBNP levels predicted the occurrence of atrial fibrillation within 2 years after cryptogenic stroke [103]. Although the mechanisms are not clear, BNP elevations in the peripheral blood have also been reported in patients with subarachnoid hemorrhage [91].

Overall, data comparing the performance of NT-proBNP and MR-proANP for the prediction of cardioembolic etiology in the context of ischemic stroke are limited.

8.3.5.2 D-Dimer

D-dimer represents a product of plasmin-mediated fibrin degradation and typically indicates thrombus formation [30, 104–106]. Elevated D-dimer levels were found ubiquitously in cardioembolic and atherothrombotic ischemic stroke [107, 108]. Nevertheless, existing research recognizes the potential of D-dimer level measurements in acute stroke to conclude the underlying disease mechanism based on the extent of the value increase [106, 109, 110].

Patients with a cardioembolic cerebral vessel occlusion, most likely caused by atrial fibrillation [103, 111, 112], demonstrated higher D-dimer levels compared to cases with lacunar ischemic events [106]. This is most likely due to the structural differences between fibrin-rich thrombi of cardiac origin and platelet-rich thrombi encountered in cases of arterial blood vessel occlusions [106]. Based on the assumption of a thrombotic small vessel occlusion as the pathophysiological correlate of lacunar ischemic stroke, the small-scale arterial thrombus formation might not be able to create measurable D-dimer level increases [106].

It is noteworthy that D-dimer levels were also significantly elevated in cases of transient cerebral ischemia (i.e., TIA) within the first week after the event as well as 1 and 3 months after the episode [113]. Spontaneous intracerebral hemorrhage may also trigger an early systemic D-dimer elevation [114]. The exact biochemical mechanisms of how a local derangement of the hemostatic equilibrium may lead to a measurable systemic response are unclear [114]. D-dimer levels were also reported to independently predict clinical progression in patients with ischemic stroke within the further course [104, 115].

A vivid example of an established area of application of D-dimer measurements in daily clinical routine is the diagnosis of cerebral venous sinus thrombosis [116]. Cerebral venous thrombosis is a relatively rare but, especially in younger individuals, considerable cause of cerebral infarction or hemorrhage, but may also mimic the clinical picture of stroke itself [116–118]. Rapid diagnosis is crucial to initiate appropriate therapeutic measures involving anticoagulation [116]. Normal D-dimer levels preclude cerebral venous thrombosis with high reliability whereas elevated levels are not reliable enough to establish the diagnosis due to a lack of specificity [116, 119–121].

The underlying cause for the observed elevations in acute ischemic stroke has not been definitively clarified. D-dimer elevations in ischemic stroke may be due to a secondary inflammatory response, potentially depending on the extent of affected brain tissue, or caused by a local dysregulation of the coagulation system [104, 108]. Interestingly, D-dimer itself is suspected of being able to promote inflammatory processes in the context of progressive ischemic stroke [104].

A potential concern regarding the informative value of D-dimer and other elements of the coagulation cascade is that a variety of these markers (e.g., fibrinogen, plasminogen) also represent acute-phase reactants [122, 123]. A multitude of acute and chronic inflammatory conditions, local (e.g., traumatic) or systemic (e.g., infectious, neoplastic), can trigger the release of these markers that might persist elevated prolonged over several days depending on the stimulus [30, 122]. Particularly noteworthy in this respect is that about 5% of patients with embolic stroke of undetermined source show occult malignancies [124]. Conversely, the incidence of stroke among patients with cancer is remarkably high with almost 15%, exceeding that of the general population by far [125]. Elevated blood D-dimer levels and multiple lesions in different vascular territories demonstrated the potential to predict the presence of occult malignancies in patients with ischemic stroke with unknown origin [126]. The pathogenetic relationship between undetected cancer and ischemic stroke has not been fully elucidated but a hypercoagulable state is considered as one of the underlying key mechanisms [124]. Reports addressing the temporal association between both entities vary, with some describing stroke as a phenomenon encountered more frequently in terminal stages of cancer, and others emphasizing the role of ischemic stroke as an early indicator for malignant primary disease [124, 125, 127].

8.3.5.3 Interleukin-6 (IL-6)

IL-6 is a cytokine and is known as a nonspecific marker of inflammation [128]. Within the central nervous system, IL-6 mediates a range of other effects such as demyelination and astrogliosis [129]. There is evidence that, although stroke is often accompanied by infections, cerebral ischemia itself may trigger an inflammatory response and may, therefore, lead to the initiation of an acute-phase reaction [128, 130–132]:

First, the extent of the IL-6 elevation in the blood correlates with the infarct size in the early phase after ischemic stroke [130, 131, 133]. Second, cerebrospinal fluid levels of IL-6 surpass the blood levels in patients with ischemic stroke [130]. Maximum serum values of IL-6 are described to occur within the first 10 days after symptom onset in patients with acute stroke [131]. Third, the IL-6 peak serum concentrations after ischemic stroke correlate with the stroke severity measured by the NIHSS score [131, 133].

Thus, elevations of C-reactive protein, tumor necrosis factor, plasma cortisol, and IL-6 have been demonstrated in the peripheral blood in cohorts of patients with ischemic stroke [128, 130, 131, 134, 135].

In nonvalvular atrial fibrillation, there is evidence for another chronological relationship considering inflammation not as a consequence of cerebral ischemia but as a potential contributing factor to thromboembolism, as it may contribute to a prothrombotic milieu, potentially increasing the risk of thrombogenesis [136]. Although elevated acute-phase proteins in the context of atrial fibrillation may be due to an underlying vascular disease, an abnormal inflammatory condition is believed to be a major contributing factor in the thrombogenesis in the context of nonvalvular atrial fibrillation [136]. This hypothesis is also supported by the observation that patients with a cardioembolic etiology of acute ischemic stroke show significantly higher median blood levels of IL-6 compared to patients with lacunar infarcts [132].

8.3.5.4 Serum Neurofilament Light Chain (SNfL)

SNfL is a neurofilament subunit and represents an essential structural element of the axonal cytoskeleton [13, 137–139]. Neurofilaments are released into the peripheral blood and cerebrospinal fluid in the course of axonal injury [13]. This might be due to a large variety of underlying acute or chronic neurological conditions such as subarachnoid hemorrhage, traumatic brain injury, multiple sclerosis, and normal pressure hydrocephalus [13, 138, 140].

However, serum neurofilament levels in patients with acute ischemic stroke and TIAs with symptom onset within the last 24 h were associated with the clinical severity (measured by the NIHSS score) on admission and the diagnosis of TIAs [13]. Based on its anatomical location, SNfL has proven to be indicative of subcortical axonal damage and constitutes a marker for the severity of white matter lesions [137]. Maximum concentration levels in the cerebrospinal fluid are reached within several days after neuronal damage [141].

A relevant cause of stroke among the 18–50 age group, accounting for approximately 20% of strokes, is cervical artery dissection [142, 143]. The exact pathophysiology has not yet been fully elucidated but hypertension, cervical trauma, and systemic infections are some of the numerous described risk factors [142–144]. As headache and neck pain are the most frequent initial symptoms in cases of cervical artery dissection, cerebrovascular infarction as the first clinical manifestation is observed in not more than approximately one-third of cases [144]. Interestingly, the risk of consecutive ischemic stroke due to cervical artery dissection generally seems to be relatively low, whereby the majority of strokes seem to occur within the first 2 weeks after diagnosis [144]. It is worth noting that the time of treatment initiation in cases of cervical artery dissection seems to play an important role in the prevention of consecutive cerebral infarction. A study including patients with traumatic cervical artery dissection demonstrated that more than 50% of untreated patients presenting without stroke developed stroke subsequently, whereas the stroke rate could be reduced to under 5% with early treatment [144]. Recent evidence suggests that SNfL levels are higher in patients with cervical artery dissection presenting with ischemic stroke compared to patients with TIA and local symptoms [145]. Moreover, SNfL levels are associated with clinical stroke severity (measured by NIHSS score) in this cohort [145]. These findings are in line with those of a more recent study that demonstrated an association between SNfL admission levels and clinical severity on admission in patients with acute ischemic stroke and TIA [13]. In this cohort, the control group showed lower SNfL serum levels than patients with acute cerebrovascular events (i.e., acute ischemic stroke or TIA) [13].

8.3.5.5 Fibrillin-1

Fibrillin-1 is a glycoprotein and a structural component of the vascular wall [12]. The potential clinical relevance in the context of arterial dissections becomes evident since fibrillin-1 gene mutations can cause Marfan syndrome [12, 146]. In turn, hospitalized individuals with Marfan syndrome demonstrate a significantly higher rate of carotid dissections and cerebral aneurysms compared to controls, underlining its physiological function [12, 146].

In young and middle-aged adults dissections of the internal carotid and the vertebral artery account for up to 25% of ischemic strokes [147, 148]. The pathophysiological explanation for the measurable elevations of fibrillin-1 in the blood due to spontaneous acute cerebrocervical arterial dissections is related to suspected subintimal arterial injury as the starting point [12, 147]. Due to the subsequently emerging intramural hematoma, it is hypothesized that fibrillin-1 is released from within the vascular wall due to the rupture of its elastic fibers [12, 147]. Moreover, higher fibrillin-1 blood levels were associated with radiologically more severe cerebrocervical dissections [149]. However, no differences regarding fibrillin-1 elevations have been reported between intra- and extracranial arterial dissections [12].

To date, there have been no detailed investigations of fibrillin-1 serum levels in patients with other vascular comorbidities, such as atherosclerosis or temporal course of its blood concentrations, respectively [12]. Although fibrillin-1 elevations in the blood were described in aortic dissections, it is not yet clear why elevations of fibrillin-1 were also detectable in healthy controls, calling for further research regarding the biological distribution patterns within different types of tissue [12].

8.3.6   Limitations of Biomarkers

The most evident limitations when it comes to biomarker-based stroke diagnosis, at least from a clinical point of view, certainly derive from the complexity of "real" patients out of any standardized study criteria. In clinical routine, physicians frequently encounter stroke mimics and patients with multiple comorbidities including vascular diseases. How certain is it that detected elevations of certain biomarkers are attributable to an acute cerebrovascular event? The currently available data is sobering: different forms of brain tissue damage can potentially lead to elevated biomarker levels [7]. Moreover, biomarkers used for diagnostic purposes might also be released from extracerebral tissue [18].

Another fundamental problem is the heterogeneity of stroke itself with different and complex, yet not fully understood, pathophysiological relationships [7, 14]. Biomarkers are unlikely to differentiate between small and large vessel occlusions or to provide information about the exact location or the tissue at risk, all of which are essential information for guiding therapeutic decisions [17]. Given the pathophysiological alterations in the context of stroke, the blood-brain barrier may hinder or distort the transition of released biomarkers from the brain tissue into the systemic circulation, depending on its functional capacity [7, 19]. Furthermore, frequently encountered restrictions of renal or liver function could interfere with test results and potentially influence the temporal course of biomarker candidates in the blood [70].

A prerequisite for the use of diagnostic biomarkers in clinical practice is the standardization of the measurement techniques and threshold values to enhance comparability. To this date, the different measurement methods used in prior studies still represent a potential confounding factor in the interpretation of the current data [14]. Prospective studies with mixed populations are needed to validate the results of preliminary studies under real-life conditions.

8.3.7   Outlook: The Future of Biomarkers

Given the large quantity of potential diagnostic biomarkers that are subject of current research and the specific field of application of each biomarker candidate with its unique limitations, the development of diagnostic biomarker panels may be sensible to improve the accuracy for the detection of acute stroke [19].

8.4   Conclusion

The past 30 years have seen rapid advances in neuroradiological imaging techniques, especially MRI, which lead to improvements regarding the early, reliable diagnosis of cerebral ischemia and timely treatment initiation. During the last decade, considerable literature around the theme of biomarkers in the context of acute stroke diagnosis has emerged. Although raised public awareness for the time-critical clinical picture of stroke and advances in its treatment has led to the establishment of centers specialized in the management of those patients, the heterogeneity and diversity of its clinical presentation with possible subtle initial symptoms still pose a challenge in everyday routine. To address this issue, a multitude of biomarker candidates targeting specific steps of the pathophysiological cascade were studied. Due to the complexity of the underlying and not yet fully understood mechanisms, numerous mimicking conditions, and various comorbid conditions, every marker reflects only a partial aspect of the whole disease picture and is unlikely to provide sufficient information to guide therapeutic decisions. Yet, there still is a need for further diagnostic strategies in a significant proportion of cases where the etiology of ischemic stroke remains unclear after a completed search for potential sources of embolism.

A point-of-care blood marker differentiating an ischemic from hemorrhagic stroke can inform—in the prehospital setting—the decision for or against thrombolysis, e.g., complementing prehospital brain imaging.

A blood-borne biomarker approach might be able to yield valuable information to guide further secondary prophylaxis and provide clarity on the issue to the patient with reliable statements regarding the risk of recurrence. As this chapter has demonstrated, every single biomarker candidate has its unique limitations and potential fields of application. To a large extent, this is because it reflects only a small element of the pathophysiological cascade and therefore only provides limited conclusiveness. To facilitate the distinction between cerebrovascular events and mimicking conditions and accelerate the preclinical management, a multi-biomarker panel combining different strengths and target points seems to be the most promising and practical way.

Nevertheless, before the admission for clinical use several obstacles must be overcome: first, the standardization of the measurement techniques as the basis for the comparability of results; second, the composition of a biomarker set with sufficient discriminative capacity between cerebrovascular events and mimicking conditions; and third, biomarker sets must be validated in a large international cohort with a wide range of comorbidities.

References

1. Donkor ES. Stroke in the 21st century: a snapshot of the burden, epidemiology, and quality of life. Stroke Res Treat. 2018; https://doi.org/10.1155/2018/3238165.
2. Lo EH, Dalkara T, Moskowitz MA. Mechanisms, challenges and opportunities in stroke. Nat Rev Neurosci. 2003; https://doi.org/10.1038/nrn1106.
3. Aroor S, Singh R, Goldstein LB. BE-FAST (balance, eyes, face, arm, speech, time): reducing the proportion of strokes missed using the FAST mnemonic. Stroke. 2017; https://doi.org/10.1161/STROKEAHA.116.015169.
4. Yew KS, Cheng E. Acute stroke diagnosis. Am Fam Physician. 2009;80:33–40.
5. Bustamante A, García-Berrocoso T, Rodriguez N, Llombart V, Ribó M, Molina C, Montaner J. Ischemic stroke outcome: a review of the influence of post-stroke complications within the different scenarios of stroke care. Eur J Intern Med. 2016; https://doi.org/10.1016/j.ejim.2015.11.030.

6. Ragoschke-Schumm A, Walter S, Haass A, et al. Translation of the "time is brain" concept into clinical practice: focus on prehospital stroke management. Int J Stroke. 2014; https://doi.org/10.1111/ijs.12252.

7. Jickling GC, Sharp FR. Blood biomarkers of ischemic stroke. Neurotherapeutics. 2011; https://doi.org/10.1007/s13311-011-0050-4.

8. Strimbu K, Tavel JA. What are biomarkers? Curr Opin HIV AIDS. 2010;5:463–6.

9. Glushakova O, Glushakov A, Miller E, Valadka A, Hayes R. Biomarkers for acute diagnosis and management of stroke in neurointensive care units. Brain Circ. 2016; https://doi.org/10.4103/2394-8108.178546.

10. Katz R. Biomarkers and surrogate markers: an FDA perspective. NeuroRx. 2004;1:189–95.

11. Larpthaveesarp A, Ferriero DM, Gonzalez FF. Growth factors for the treatment of ischemic brain injury (growth factor treatment). Brain Sci. 2015;5:165–77.

12. Jickling GC, Lorenzano S. Finding fibrillin in cerebral artery dissection. Neurology. 2018;90:399–400.

13. De Marchis GM, Katan M, Barro C, et al. Serum neurofilament light chain in patients with acute cerebrovascular events. Eur J Neurol. 2018;25:562–8.

14. Makris K, Haliassos A, Chondrogianni M, Tsivgoulis G. Blood biomarkers in ischemic stroke: potential role and challenges in clinical practice and research. Crit Rev Clin Lab Sci. 2018; https://doi.org/10.1080/10408363.2018.1461190.

15. Pase MP, Himali JJ, Aparicio HJ, Romero JR, Satizabal CL, Maillard P, DeCarli C, Beiser AS, Seshadri S. Plasma total-tau as a biomarker of stroke risk in the community. Ann Neurol. 2019; https://doi.org/10.1002/ana.25542.

16. Saenger AK, Christenson RH. Stroke biomarkers: progress and challenges for diagnosis, prognosis, differentiation, and treatment. Clin Chem. 2010; https://doi.org/10.1373/clinchem.2009.133801.

17. Kernagis DN, Laskowitz DT. Evolving role of biomarkers in acute cerebrovascular disease. Ann Neurol. 2012; https://doi.org/10.1002/ana.22553.

18. Katan M, Elkind MS. The potential role of blood biomarkers in patients with ischemic stroke. Clin Transl Neurosci. 2018; https://doi.org/10.1177/2514183x18768050.

19. Kim SJ, Moon GJ, Bang OY. Biomarkers for stroke. J Stroke. 2013; https://doi.org/10.5853/jos.2013.15.1.27.

20. Stein BC, Levin RI. Natriuretic peptides: physiology, therapeutic potential, and risk stratification in ischemic heart disease. Am Heart J. 1998;135:914–23.

21. Kurzepa J, Kurzepa J, Golab P, Czerska S, Bielewicz J. The significance of matrix metalloproteinase (MMP)-2 and MMP-9 in the ischemic stroke. Int J Neurosci. 2014;124:707–16.

22. Hinman JD, Rost NS, Leung TW, Montaner J, Muir KW, Brown S, Arenillas JF, Feldmann E, Liebeskind DS. Principles of precision medicine in stroke. J Neurol Neurosurg Psychiatry. 2017; https://doi.org/10.1136/jnnp-2016-314587.

23. Riley RS, Rowe D, Fisher LM. Clinical utilization of the international normalized ratio (INR). J Clin Lab Anal. 2000;14:101–14.

24. Foerch C, Niessner M, Back T, et al. Diagnostic accuracy of plasma glial fibrillary acidic protein for differentiating intracerebral hemorrhage and cerebral ischemia in patients with symptoms of acute stroke. Clin Chem. 2012; https://doi.org/10.1373/clinchem.2011.172676.

25. Stanca DM, Mărginean IC, Soriţău O, Dragoş C, Mărginean M, Mureşanu DF, Vester JC, Rafila A. GFAP and antibodies against NMDA receptor subunit NR2 as biomarkers for acute cerebrovascular diseases. J Cell Mol Med. 2015;19:2253–61.

26. Tsai JP, Albers GW. Wake-up stroke: current understanding. Top Magn Reson Imaging. 2017;26:97–102.

27. Wu QJ, Tymianski M. Targeting NMDA receptors in stroke: new hope in neuroprotection. Mol Brain. 2018;11:15.

28. Dambinova SA, Khounteev GA, Skoromets AA. Multiple panel of biomarkers for TIA/stroke evaluation. Stroke. 2002;33:1181–2.

29. Kalev-Zylinska ML, Symes W, Little KCE, Sun P, Wen D, Qiao L, Young D, During MJ, Barber PA. Stroke patients develop antibodies that react with components of N-methyl-d-aspartate receptor subunit 1 in proportion to lesion size. Stroke. 2013;44:2212–9.
30. Dambinova SA, Khounteev GA, Izykenova GA, Zavolokov IG, Ilyukhina AY, Skoromets AA. Blood test detecting autoantibodies to N-methyl-D-aspartate neuroreceptors for evaluation of patients with transient ischemic attack and stroke. Clin Chem. 2003;49:1752–62.
31. Gascón S, Sobrado M, Roda JM, Rodríguez-Peña A, Díaz-Guerra M. Excitotoxicity and focal cerebral ischemia induce truncation of the NR2A and NR2B subunits of the NMDA receptor and cleavage of the scaffolding protein PSD-95. Mol Psychiatry. 2008;13:99–114.
32. Massey PV, Johnson BE, Moult PR, Auberson YP, Brown MW, Molnar E, Collingridge GL, Bashir ZI. Differential roles of NR2A and NR2B-containing NMDA receptors in cortical long-term potentiation and long-term depression. J Neurosci. 2004;24:7821–8.
33. Carvajal FJ, Mattison HA, Cerpa W. Role of NMDA receptor-mediated glutamatergic signaling in chronic and acute neuropathologies. Neural Plast. 2016;2016:2701526.
34. Weissman JD, Khunteev GA, Heath R, Dambinova SA. NR2 antibodies: risk assessment of transient ischemic attack (TIA)/stroke in patients with history of isolated and multiple cerebrovascular events. J Neurol Sci. 2011;300:97–102.
35. Elkind MSV, Tai W, Coates K, Paik MC, Sacco RL. Lipoprotein-associated phospholipase A2 activity and risk of recurrent stroke. Cerebrovasc Dis. 2009; https://doi.org/10.1159/000172633.
36. Thompson A, Gao P, Orfei L, et al. Lipoprotein-associated phospholipase A2 and risk of coronary disease, stroke, and mortality: collaborative analysis of 32 prospective studies. Lancet. 2010; https://doi.org/10.1016/S0140-6736(10)60319-4.
37. Suchindran S, Rivedal D, Guyton JR, Milledge T, Gao X, Benjamin A, Rowell J, Ginsburg GS, McCarthy JJ. Genome-wide association study of Lp-PLA(2) activity and mass in the Framingham Heart Study. PLoS Genet. 2010;6:e1000928.
38. Gorelick PB. Lipoprotein-associated phospholipase A2 and risk of stroke. Am J Cardiol. 2008;101:34F–40F.
39. McConnell JP, Hoefner DM. Lipoprotein-associated phospholipase A2. Clin Lab Med. 2006;26:679–vii.
40. Cucchiara BL, Messe SR, Sansing L, MacKenzie L, Taylor RA, Pacelli J, Shah Q, Kasner SE. Lipoprotein-associated phospholipase A 2 and C-reactive protein for risk-stratification of patients with TIA. Stroke. 2009; https://doi.org/10.1161/STROKEAHA.109.553545.
41. Alkuraishy HM, Al-Gareeb AI, Waheed HJ. Lipoprotein-associated phospholipase A2 is linked with poor cardio-metabolic profile in patients with ischemic stroke: a study of effects of statins. J Neurosci Rural Pract. 2018;9:496–503.
42. Ballantyne CM, Hoogeveen RC, Bang H, Coresh J, Folsom AR, Heiss G, Sharrett AR. Lipoprotein-associated phospholipase A2, high-sensitivity C-reactive protein, and risk for incident coronary heart disease in middle-aged men and women in the Atherosclerosis Risk in Communities (ARIC) study. Circulation. 2004;109:837–42.
43. Oei HHS, Van Der Meer IM, Hofman A, Koudstaal PJ, Stijnen T, Breteler MMB, Witteman JCM. Lipoprotein-associated phospholipase A2 activity is associated with risk of coronary heart disease and ischemic stroke: the Rotterdam study. Circulation. 2005; https://doi.org/10.1161/01.CIR.0000154553.12214.CD.
44. Huang L, Yao S. Carotid artery color Doppler ultrasonography and plasma levels of lipoprotein-associated phospholipase A2 and cystatin C in arteriosclerotic cerebral infarction. J Int Med Res. 2019;47:4389–96.
45. Zhuo S, Wolfert RL, Yuan C. Biochemical differences in the mass and activity tests of lipoprotein-associated phospholipase A(2) explain the discordance in results between the two assay methods. Clin Biochem. 2017;50:1209–15.
46. Zimmermann-Ivol CG, Burkhard PR, Le Floch-Rohr J, Allard L, Hochstrasser DF, Sanchez J-C. Fatty acid binding protein as a serum marker for the early diagnosis of stroke: a pilot study. Mol Cell Proteomics. 2004;3:66–72.

47. Park S-Y, Kim M-H, Kim O-J, Ahn H-J, Song J-Y, Jeong J-Y, Oh S-H. Plasma heart-type fatty acid binding protein level in acute ischemic stroke: comparative analysis with plasma S100B level for diagnosis of stroke and prediction of long-term clinical outcome. Clin Neurol Neurosurg. 2013;115:405–10.

48. Allard L, Burkhard PR, Lescuyer P, Burgess JA, Walter N, Hochstrasser DF, Sanchez J-C. PARK7 and nucleoside diphosphate kinase A as plasma markers for the early diagnosis of stroke. Clin Chem. 2005;51:2043–51.

49. Nagakubo D, Taira T, Kitaura H, Ikeda M, Tamai K, Iguchi-Ariga SM, Ariga H. DJ-1, a novel oncogene which transforms mouse NIH3T3 cells in cooperation with ras. Biochem Biophys Res Commun. 1997;231:509–13.

50. Bonifati V, Rizzu P, van Baren MJ, et al. Mutations in the DJ-1 gene associated with autosomal recessive early-onset parkinsonism. Science. 2003;299:256–9.

51. Rozanski M, Waldschmidt C, Kunz A, et al. Glial fibrillary acidic protein for prehospital diagnosis of intracerebral hemorrhage. Cerebrovasc Dis. 2017;43:76–81.

52. Ehrenreich H, Kastner A, Weissenborn K, et al. Circulating damage marker profiles support a neuroprotective effect of erythropoietin in ischemic stroke patients. Mol Med. 2011;17:1306–10.

53. Undén J, Strandberg K, Malm J, Campbell E, Rosengren L, Stenflo J, Norrving B, Romner B, Lindgren A, Andsberg G. Explorative investigation of biomarkers of brain damage and coagulation system activation in clinical stroke differentiation. J Neurol. 2009; https://doi.org/10.1007/s00415-009-0054-8.

54. Foerch C, Curdt I, Yan B, Dvorak F, Hermans M, Berkefeld J, Raabe A, Neumann-Haefelin T, Steinmetz H, Sitzer M. Serum glial fibrillary acidic protein as a biomarker for intracerebral haemorrhage in patients with acute stroke. J Neurol Neurosurg Psychiatry. 2006; https://doi.org/10.1136/jnnp.2005.074823.

55. Xiong L, Yang Y, Zhang M, Xu W. The use of serum glial fibrillary acidic protein test as a promising tool for intracerebral hemorrhage diagnosis in Chinese patients and prediction of the short-term functional outcomes. Neurol Sci. 2015;36:2081–7.

56. Dvorak F, Haberer I, Sitzer M, Foerch C. Characterisation of the diagnostic window of serum glial fibrillary acidic protein for the differentiation of intracerebral haemorrhage and ischaemic stroke. Cerebrovasc Dis. 2009; https://doi.org/10.1159/000172632.

57. Llombart V, Garcia-Berrocoso T, Bustamante A, Giralt D, Rodriguez-Luna D, Muchada M, Penalba A, Boada C, Hernandez-Guillamon M, Montaner J. Plasmatic retinol-binding protein 4 and glial fibrillary acidic protein as biomarkers to differentiate ischemic stroke and intracerebral hemorrhage. J Neurochem. 2016;136:416–24.

58. Katsanos AH, Makris K, Stefani D, et al. Plasma glial fibrillary acidic protein in the differential diagnosis of intracerebral hemorrhage. Stroke. 2017; https://doi.org/10.1161/STROKEAHA.117.018409.

59. Lamers KJB, Vos P, Verbeek MM, Rosmalen F, van Geel WJA, van Engelen BGM. Protein S-100B, neuron-specific enolase (NSE), myelin basic protein (MBP) and glial fibrillary acidic protein (GFAP) in cerebrospinal fluid (CSF) and blood of neurological patients. Brain Res Bull. 2003;61:261–4.

60. Purrucker JC, Herrmann O, Lutsch JK, Zorn M, Schwaninger M, Bruckner T, Auffarth GU, Veltkamp R. Serum protein S100β is a diagnostic biomarker for distinguishing posterior circulation stroke from vertigo of nonvascular causes. Eur Neurol. 2014;72:278–84.

61. Herrmann M, Vos P, Wunderlich MT, de Bruijn CH, Lamers KJ. Release of glial tissue-specific proteins after acute stroke. Stroke. 2000;31:2670–7.

62. Foerch C, Otto B, Singer OC, Neumann-Haefelin T, Yan B, Berkefeld J, Steinmetz H, Sitzer M. Serum S100B predicts a malignant course of infarction in patients with acute middle cerebral artery occlusion. Stroke. 2004; https://doi.org/10.1161/01.STR.0000138730.03264.ac.

63. Alatas OD, Gurger M, Atescelik M, Yildiz M, Demir CF, Kalayci M, Ilhan N, Acar E, Ekingen E. Neuron-specific enolase, S100 calcium-binding protein B, and heat shock protein 70 levels in patients with intracranial hemorrhage. Medicine (Baltimore). 2015;94:e2007.

64. Fassbender K, Schmidt R, Schreiner A, Fatar M, Muhlhauser F, Daffertshofer M, Hennerici M. Leakage of brain-originated proteins in peripheral blood: temporal profile and diagnostic value in early ischemic stroke. J Neurol Sci. 1997;148:101–5.
65. Moore BW. A soluble protein characteristic of the nervous system. Biochem Biophys Res Commun. 1965;19:739–44.
66. Raponi E, Agenes F, Delphin C, Assard N, Baudier J, Legraverend C, Deloulme J-C. S100B expression defines a state in which GFAP-expressing cells lose their neural stem cell potential and acquire a more mature developmental stage. Glia. 2007;55:165–77.
67. Sorci G, Bianchi R, Riuzzi F, Tubaro C, Arcuri C, Giambanco I, Donato R. S100B protein, a damage-associated molecular pattern protein in the brain and heart, and beyond. Cardiovasc Psychiatry Neurol. 2010; https://doi.org/10.1155/2010/656481.
68. Missler U, Wiesmann M, Friedrich C, Kaps M. S-100 protein and neuron-specific enolase concentrations in blood as indicators of infarction volume and prognosis in acute ischemic stroke. Stroke. 1997;28:1956–60.
69. Kumar H, Lakhotia M, Pahadiya H, Singh J. To study the correlation of serum S-100 protein level with the severity of stroke and its prognostic implication. J Neurosci Rural Pract. 2015;6:326–30.
70. Sedaghat F, Notopoulos A. S100 protein family and its application in clinical practice. Hippokratia. 2008;12:198–204.
71. Yilmaz N, Karaali K, Ozdem S, Turkay M, Unal A, Dora B. Elevated S100B and neuron specific enolase levels in patients with migraine-without aura: evidence for neurodegeneration? Cell Mol Neurobiol. 2011;31:579–85.
72. Elting JW, de Jager AE, Teelken AW, Schaaf MJ, Maurits NM, van der Naalt J, Sibinga CT, Sulter GA, De Keyser J. Comparison of serum S-100 protein levels following stroke and traumatic brain injury. J Neurol Sci. 2000;181:104–10.
73. Laskowitz DT, Kasner SE, Saver J, Remmel KS, Jauch EC. Clinical usefulness of a biomarker-based diagnostic test for acute stroke: the biomarker rapid assessment in ischemic injury (BRAIN) study. Stroke. 2009; https://doi.org/10.1161/STROKEAHA.108.516377.
74. Montaner J, Mendioroz M, Delgado P, et al. Differentiating ischemic from hemorrhagic stroke using plasma biomarkers: the S100B/RAGE pathway. J Proteome. 2012;75:4758–65.
75. Wunderlich MT, Wallesch C-W, Goertler M. Release of neurobiochemical markers of brain damage is related to the neurovascular status on admission and the site of arterial occlusion in acute ischemic stroke. J Neurol Sci. 2004;227:49–53.
76. Buttner T, Weyers S, Postert T, Sprengelmeyer R, Kuhn W. S-100 protein: serum marker of focal brain damage after ischemic territorial MCA infarction. Stroke. 1997;28:1961–5.
77. Kim JS, Yoon SS, Kim YH, Ryu JS. Serial measurement of interleukin-6, transforming growth factor-beta, and S-100 protein in patients with acute stroke. Stroke. 1996;27:1553–7.
78. Jauch EC, Lindsell C, Broderick J, Fagan SC, Tilley BC, Levine SR (2006) Association of serial biochemical markers with acute ischemic stroke: the National Institute of Neurological Disorders and Stroke recombinant tissue plasminogen activator stroke study. Stroke 37:2508–2513.
79. Rainer TH, Wong KS, Lam W, Lam NYL, Graham CA, Lo YMD. Comparison of plasma beta-globin DNA and S-100 protein concentrations in acute stroke. Clin Chim Acta. 2007;376:190–6.
80. González-García S, González Quevedo A, Peña Sánchez M, Menéndez Saínz C, Fernández Carriera R, Arteche-Prior M, Pando-Cabrera A, Fernández-Concepción O. Serum neuron-specific enolase and S100 calcium binding protein B biomarker levels do not improve diagnosis of acute stroke. J R Coll Physicians Edinb. 2012; https://doi.org/10.4997/JRCPE.2012.302.
81. Deboevere N, Marjanovic N, Sierecki M, Marchetti M, Dubocage M, Magimel E, Mimoz O, Guenezan J. Value of copeptin and the S-100b protein assay in ruling out the diagnosis of stroke-induced dizziness pattern in emergency departments. Scand J Trauma Resusc Emerg Med. 2019;27:72.

82. Montaner J, Molina CA, Monasterio J, Abilleira S, Arenillas JF, Ribó M, Quintana M, Alvarez-Sabín J. Matrix metalloproteinase-9 pretreatment level predicts intracranial hemorrhagic complications after thrombolysis in human stroke. Circulation. 2003; https://doi.org/10.1161/01.CIR.0000046451.38849.90.

83. Alvarez-Sabin J, Delgado P, Abilleira S, Molina CA, Arenillas J, Ribo M, Santamarina E, Quintana M, Monasterio J, Montaner J. Temporal profile of matrix metalloproteinases and their inhibitors after spontaneous intracerebral hemorrhage: relationship to clinical and radiological outcome. Stroke. 2004;35:1316–22.

84. LeBleu VS, Macdonald B, Kalluri R. Structure and function of basement membranes. Exp Biol Med (Maywood). 2007;232:1121–9.

85. Montaner J, Alvarez-Sabín J, Molina C, Anglés A, Abilleira S, Arenillas J, González MA, Monasterio J. Matrix metalloproteinase expression after human cardioembolic stroke: temporal profile and relation to neurological impairment. Stroke. 2001; https://doi.org/10.1161/01.STR.32.8.1759.

86. Castellanos M, Leira R, Serena J, Blanco M, Pedraza S, Castillo J, Dávalos A. Plasma cellular-fibronectin concentration predicts hemorrhagic transformation after thrombolytic therapy in acute ischemic stroke. Stroke. 2004; https://doi.org/10.1161/01.STR.0000131656.47979.39.

87. Castellanos M, Leira R, Serena J, Pumar JM, Lizasoain I, Castillo J, Davalos A. Plasma metalloproteinase-9 concentration predicts hemorrhagic transformation in acute ischemic stroke. Stroke. 2003; https://doi.org/10.1161/01.STR.0000046764.57344.31.

88. Can S, Akdur O, Yildirim A, Adam G, Cakir DU, Karaman HIO. Myelin basic protein and ischemia modified albumin levels in acute ischemic stroke cases. Pak J Med Sci. 2015;31:1110–4.

89. Marty MC, Alliot F, Rutin J, Fritz R, Trisler D, Pessac B. The myelin basic protein gene is expressed in differentiated blood cell lineages and in hemopoietic progenitors. Proc Natl Acad Sci. 2002;99:8856–61.

90. Hill MD, Jackowski G, Bayer N, Lawrence M, Jaeschke R. Biochemical markers in acute ischemic stroke. CMAJ. 2000;162:1139–40.

91. Giannakoulas G, Hatzitolios A, Karvounis H, Koliakos G, Charitandi A, Dimitroulas T, Savopoulos C, Tsirogianni E, Louridas G. N-terminal pro-brain natriuretic peptide levels are elevated in patients with acute ischemic stroke. Angiology. 2005;56:723–30.

92. Hunt PJ, Yandle TG, Nicholls MG, Richards AM, Espiner EA. The amino-terminal portion of pro-brain natriuretic peptide (pro-BNP) circulates in human plasma. Biochem Biophys Res Commun. 1995;214:1175–83.

93. Llombart V, Antolin-Fontes A, Bustamante A, et al. B-type natriuretic peptides help in cardio-embolic stroke diagnosis: pooled data meta-analysis. Stroke. 2015;

94. Minamino N, Aburaya M, Ueda S, Kangawa K, Matsuo H. The presence of brain natriuretic peptide of 12,000 daltons in porcine heart. Biochem Biophys Res Commun. 1988;155:740–6.

95. Shimizu H, Murakami Y, Inoue SI, et al. High plasma brain natriuretic polypeptide level as a marker of risk for thromboembolism in patients with nonvalvular atrial fibrillation. Stroke. 2002; https://doi.org/10.1161/hs0402.105657.

96. Sudoh T, Kangawa K, Minamino N, Matsuo H. A new natriuretic peptide in porcine brain. Nature. 1988;332:78–81.

97. De Marchis GM, Schneider J, Weck A, et al. Midregional proatrial natriuretic peptide improves risk stratification after ischemic stroke. Neurology. 2018;90:e455–65.

98. Katan M, Fluri F, Schuetz P, et al. Midregional pro-atrial natriuretic peptide and outcome in patients with acute ischemic stroke. J Am Coll Cardiol. 2010;56:1045–53.

99. Schnabel RB, Wild PS, Wilde S, et al. Multiple biomarkers and atrial fibrillation in the general population. PLoS One. 2014;9:e112486.

100. Katan M, Moon Y, von Eckardstein A, Spanaus K, DeRosa J, Gutierrez J, DeCarli C, Wright C, Sacco R, Elkind M. Procalcitonin and midregional proatrial natriuretic peptide as biomarkers of subclinical cerebrovascular damage: the Northern Manhattan Study. Stroke. 2017;48:604–10.

101. Cushman M, Judd SE, Howard VJ, Kissela B, Gutiérrez OM, Jenny NS, Ahmed A, Thacker EL, Zakai NA. N-terminal pro-B-type natriuretic peptide and stroke risk: the reasons for geographic and racial differences in stroke cohort. Stroke. 2014; https://doi.org/10.1161/STROKEAHA.114.004712.
102. Nakagawa K, Yamaguchi T, Seida M, Yamada S, Imae S, Tanaka Y, Yamamoto K, Ohno K. Plasma concentrations of brain natriuretic peptide in patients with acute ischemic stroke. Cerebrovasc Dis. 2005; https://doi.org/10.1159/000083249.
103. Rodriguez-Yanez M, Arias-Rivas S, Santamaria-Cadavid M, Sobrino T, Castillo J, Blanco M. High pro-BNP levels predict the occurrence of atrial fibrillation after cryptogenic stroke. Neurology. 2013;81:444–7.
104. Barber M, Langhorne P, Rumley A, Lowe GDO, Stott DJ. Hemostatic function and progressing ischemic stroke: D-dimer predicts early clinical progression. Stroke. 2004; https://doi.org/10.1161/01.STR.0000126890.63512.41.
105. Haapaniemi E, Soinne L, Syrjälä M, Kaste M, Tatlisumak T. Serial changes in fibrinolysis and coagulation activation markers in acute and convalescent phase of ischemic stroke. Acta Neurol Scand. 2004;110:242–7.
106. Ageno W, Finazzi S, Steidl L, Biotti MG, Mera V, D'Eril GVM, Venco A. Plasma measurement of D-dimer levels for the early diagnosis of ischemic stroke subtypes. Arch Intern Med. 2002; https://doi.org/10.1001/archinte.162.22.2589.
107. Altès A, Mbellán MT, Mateo J, Avila A, Martí-Vilalta JL, Fontcuberta J. Hemostatic disturbances in acute ischemic stroke: a study of 86 patients. Acta Haematol. 1995;94:10–5.
108. Lip GY, Blann AD, Farooqi IS, Zarifis J, Sagar G, Beevers DG. Abnormal haemorheology, endothelial function and thrombogenesis in relation to hypertension in acute (ictus <12 h) stroke patients: the West Birmingham Stroke Project. Blood Coagul Fibrinolysis. 2001;12:307–15.
109. Isenegger J, Meier N, Lämmle B, Alberio L, Fischer U, Nedeltchev K, Gralla J, Kohler HP, Mattle HP, Arnold M. D-dimers predict stroke subtype when assessed early. Cerebrovasc Dis. 2009; https://doi.org/10.1159/000256652.
110. Montaner J, Perea-Gainza M, Delgado P, Ribó M, Chacón P, Rosell A, Quintana M, Palacios ME, Molina CA, Alvarez-Sabín J. Etiologic diagnosis of ischemic stroke subtypes with plasma biomarkers. Stroke. 2008; https://doi.org/10.1161/STROKEAHA.107.505354.
111. Kumagai K, Fukunami M, Ohmori M, Kitabatake A, Kamada T, Hoki N. Increased intracardiovascular clotting in patients with chronic atrial fibrillation. J Am Coll Cardiol. 1990;16:377–80.
112. Danese E, Montagnana M, Cervellin G, Lippi G. Hypercoagulability, D-dimer and atrial fibrillation: an overview of biological and clinical evidence. Ann Med. 2014;46:364–71.
113. Fon EA, Mackey A, Cote R, Wolfson C, McIlraith DM, Leclerc J, Bourque F. Hemostatic markers in acute transient ischemic attacks. Stroke. 1994;25:282–6.
114. Fujii Y, Takeuchi S, Harada A, Abe H, Sasaki O, Tanaka R. Hemostatic activation in spontaneous intracerebral hemorrhage. Stroke. 2001;32:883–90.
115. Barber M, Langhorne P, Rumley A, Lowe GDO, Stott DJ. D-dimer predicts early clinical progression in ischemic stroke: confirmation using routine clinical assays. Stroke. 2006;37:1113–5.
116. Cucchiara B, Messe S, Taylor R, Clarke J, Pollak E. Utility of D-dimer in the diagnosis of cerebral venous sinus thrombosis. J Thromb Haemost 2005;3:387–9.
117. Talbot K, Wright M, Keeling D. Normal d-dimer levels do not exclude the diagnosis of cerebral venous sinus thrombosis. J Neurol. 2002;249:1603–4.
118. Saposnik G, Barinagarrementeria F, Brown RD Jr, Bushnell CD, Cucchiara B, Cushman M, deVeber G, Ferro JM, Tsai FY. Diagnosis and management of cerebral venous thrombosis. Stroke. 2011;42:1158–92.
119. Kosinski CM, Mull M, Schwarz M, Koch B, Biniek R, Schläfer J, Milkereit E, Willmes K, Schiefer J. Do normal D-dimer levels reliably exclude cerebral sinus thrombosis? Stroke. 2004;35:2820–5.

120. Lalive PH, de Moerloose P, Lovblad K, Sarasin FP, Mermillod B, Sztajzel R. Is measurement of D-dimer useful in the diagnosis of cerebral venous thrombosis? Neurology. 2003;61:1057–60.
121. Tardy B, Tardy-Poncet B, Viallon A, Piot M, Garnier P, Mohamedi R, Guyomarc'h S, Venet C. D-dimer levels in patients with suspected acute cerebral venous thrombosis. Am J Med. 2002;113:238–41.
122. Kushner I. The phenomenon of the acute phase response. Ann N Y Acad Sci. 1982;389:39–48.
123. Cem Gabay IK. Correction: acute-phase proteins and other systemic responses to inflammation. N Engl J Med. 1999;340:1376.
124. Cocho D, Gendre J, Boltes A, Espinosa J, Ricciardi AC, Pons J, Jimenez M, Otermin P. Predictors of occult cancer in acute ischemic stroke patients. J Stroke Cerebrovasc Dis. 2015;24:1324–8.
125. Taccone FS, Jeangette SM, Blecic SA. First-ever stroke as initial presentation of systemic cancer. J Stroke Cerebrovasc Dis. 2008;17:169–74.
126. Gon Y, Sakaguchi M, Takasugi J, Kawano T, Kanki H, Watanabe A, Oyama N, Terasaki Y, Sasaki T, Mochizuki H. Plasma D-dimer levels and ischaemic lesions in multiple vascular regions can predict occult cancer in patients with cryptogenic stroke. Eur J Neurol. 2017;24:503–8.
127. Ryu J-A, Bang OY, Lee G-H. D-dimer levels and cerebral infarction in critically ill cancer patients. BMC Cancer. 2017;17:591.
128. Laskowitz DT, Grocott H, Hsia A, Copeland KR. Serum markers of cerebral ischemia. J Stroke Cerebrovasc Dis. 1998;7:234–41.
129. Van Wagoner NJ, Benveniste EN. Interleukin-6 expression and regulation in astrocytes. J Neuroimmunol. 1999;100:124–39.
130. Acalovschi D, Wiest T, Hartmann M, Farahmi M, Mansmann U, Auffarth GU, Grau AJ, Green FR, Grond-Ginsbach C, Schwaninger M. Multiple levels of regulation of the Interleukin-6 system in stroke. Stroke. 2003;34:1864–9.
131. Smith CJ, Emsley HCA, Gavin CM, et al. Peak plasma interleukin-6 and other peripheral markers of inflammation in the first week of ischaemic stroke correlate with brain infarct volume, stroke severity and long-term outcome. BMC Neurol. 2004; https://doi.org/10.1186/1471-2377-4-2.
132. Tuttolomondo A, Di Sciacca R, Di Raimondo D, et al. Plasma levels of inflammatory and thrombotic/fibrinolytic markers in acute ischemic strokes: relationship with TOAST subtype, outcome and infarct site. J Neuroimmunol. 2009;215:84–9.
133. Orion D, Schwammenthal Y, Reshef T, Schwartz R, Tsabari R, Merzeliak O, Chapman J, Mekori YA, Tanne D. Interleukin-6 and soluble intercellular adhesion molecule-1 in acute brain ischaemia. Eur J Neurol. 2008;15:323–8.
134. Lynch JR, Blessing R, White WD, Grocott HP, Newman MF, Laskowitz DT. Novel diagnostic test for acute stroke. Stroke. 2004; https://doi.org/10.1161/01.STR.0000105927.62344.4C.
135. Fornage M, Chiang YA, O'Meara ES, Psaty BM, Reiner AP, Siscovick DS, Tracy RP, Longstreth WTJ. Biomarkers of inflammation and MRI-defined small vessel disease of the brain: the cardiovascular health study. Stroke. 2008;39:1952–9.
136. Lip GYH, Patel JV, Hughes E, Hart RG. High-sensitivity C-reactive protein and soluble CD40 ligand as indices of inflammation and platelet activation in 880 patients with nonvalvular atrial fibrillation: relationship to stroke risk factors, stroke risk stratification schema, and prognosis. Stroke. 2007;38:1229–37.
137. Hjalmarsson C, Bjerke M, Andersson B, Blennow K, Zetterberg H, Aberg ND, Olsson B, Eckerstrom C, Bokemark L, Wallin A. Neuronal and glia-related biomarkers in cerebrospinal fluid of patients with acute ischemic stroke. J Cent Nerv Syst Dis. 2014;6:51–8.
138. Zanier ER, Refai D, Zipfel GJ, Zoerle T, Longhi L, Esparza TJ, Spinner ML, Bateman RJ, Brody DL, Stocchetti N. Neurofilament light chain levels in ventricular cerebrospinal fluid after acute aneurysmal subarachnoid haemorrhage. J Neurol Neurosurg Psychiatry. 2011;82:157–9.

139. Van Geel WJA, Rosengren LE, Verbeek MM. An enzyme immunoassay to quantify neurofilament light chain in cerebrospinal fluid. J Immunol Methods. 2005;296:179–85.
140. Rosengren LE, Karlsson JE, Karlsson JO, Persson LI, Wikkelso C. Patients with amyotrophic lateral sclerosis and other neurodegenerative diseases have increased levels of neurofilament protein in CSF. J Neurochem. 1996;67:2013–8.
141. Nylen K, Csajbok LZ, Ost M, Rashid A, Karlsson J-E, Blennow K, Nellgard B, Rosengren L. CSF—neurofilament correlates with outcome after aneurysmal subarachnoid hemorrhage. Neurosci Lett. 2006;404:132–6.
142. Ekker MS, Boot EM, Singhal AB, Tan KS, Debette S, Tuladhar AM, de Leeuw F-E. Epidemiology, aetiology, and management of ischaemic stroke in young adults. Lancet Neurol. 2018;17:790–801.
143. Micheli S, Paciaroni M, Corea F, Agnelli G, Zampolini M, Caso V. Cervical artery dissection: emerging risk factors. Open Neurol J. 2010;4:50–5.
144. Morris NA, Merkler AE, Gialdini G, Kamel H. Timing of incident stroke risk after cervical artery dissection presenting without ischemia. Stroke. 2017;48:551–5.
145. Traenka C, Disanto G, Seiffge DJ, et al. Serum neurofilament light chain levels are associated with clinical characteristics and outcome in patients with cervical artery dissection. Cerebrovasc Dis. 2015;40:222–7.
146. Kim ST, Cloft H, Flemming KD, Kallmes DF, Lanzino G, Brinjikji W. Increased prevalence of cerebrovascular disease in hospitalized patients with Marfan syndrome. J Stroke Cerebrovasc Dis. 2018;27:296–300.
147. Engelter ST, Traenka C, Von Hessling A, Lyrer PA. Diagnosis and treatment of cervical artery dissection. Neurol Clin. 2015;33:421–41.
148. Engelter ST, Traenka C, Lyrer P. Dissection of cervical and cerebral arteries. Curr Neurol Neurosci Rep. 2017;17:59.
149. Zhu Z, Tang W, Ge L, Han X, Dong Q. The value of plasma fibrillin-1 level in patients with spontaneous cerebral artery dissection. Neurology. 2018;90:e732–7.

Future Application: Prognosis Determination

9

Svetlana Lorenzano

9.1   Introduction

Important and crucial challenges need to be faced in the field of cerebrovascular diseases over the next years, including the individuation of novel and more specific factors for prognosis determination [1]. A new milestone has been recently reached in the acute stroke management; indeed, besides the continuing implementation of intravenous (IV) thrombolysis in the real-world setting, the recently published randomized clinical trials (RCTs) on endovascular treatment have undoubtedly increased the therapeutic armamentarium available for acute ischemic stroke [2]. As a consequence, the search for factors to predict endovascular treatment response and outcome has been further implemented. However, although dramatic efforts have been invested to reduce the time from stroke onset to treatment and arrival-to-puncture time and particularly to improve patient selection based on the potential prognosis, it should be considered that in the reperfusion/recanalization era, the number of patients with ischemic stroke that could benefit from acute treatment is still relatively small for reasons related to the therapeutic window and logistics.

Furthermore, stroke is not only ischemic but also hemorrhagic, it is not only acute but also subacute and chronic, and cerebrovascular diseases include several peculiar conditions and have important implications in terms of cognitive functions. As a new paradigm which can have impact on patient prognosis determination on an individual basis, cerebrovascular diseases should be considered as a *continuum*. Indeed, brain damage from vascular alterations of different etiopathogenesis—wherever they occur, in large, medium, or small vessels—can be progressive and lead to a slow, sneaky, and insidious neuro- and vascular degeneration which can start with apparently normal white and gray matter alterations or silent lesions (e.g., lacunar lesions, white matter hyperintensities, cerebral microbleeds), and culminate

S. Lorenzano (✉)
Department of Human Neurosciences, Sapienza University of Rome, Rome, Italy

© Springer Nature Switzerland AG 2021

A. C. Fonseca, J. M. Ferro (eds.), *Precision Medicine in Stroke*,
https://doi.org/10.1007/978-3-030-70761-3_9

in acute events such as transient ischemic attacks (TIA), and ischemic or hemorrhagic strokes, or with the increase of vascular and brain lesion burden up to mild cognitive impairment or dementia.

At admission to the hospital for a stroke, the first question asked by patients and relatives regards prognosis. Accurate prognosis is relevant not only for patients and relatives but also for physicians who need to be guided in their decision-making process for an optimal patient management and allocation of healthcare resources.

Despite the improvement of our knowledge in the pathophysiology of cerebrovascular diseases, several clinical studies focused on the search of molecular biomarkers to improve outcome prediction of clinical scores, and despite the advances in research technology, translation of this evidence into the development of novel prognostic markers, including novel advanced neuroimaging markers, to be used in routine clinical practice in every hospital or stroke center around the world is challenging and complicated for different reasons: (1) the extraordinary complexity of brain physiology and pathophysiology of stroke and other cerebrovascular diseases that involves multiple and different biochemical processes; (2) the heterogeneity of stroke phenotypes and their *continuum* that need further insight; and (3) the lack of proper, well-designed, large collaborative studies across preclinical and clinical research.

Because of the abovementioned complexity and phenotypic heterogeneity of cerebrovascular diseases, in routine clinical practice several specific questions regarding individualized patient selection for acute treatments and functional and cognitive outcome prediction remain unanswered. Identification and analysis of the multitude of variables obtained from each patient to tailor the most adequate treatment based on the potential prognosis for each individual patient are the guiding principles of precision medicine.

Precision medicine represents the future for improving outcome determination; it has been initially focused on oncology where important advances in this direction have already been made and have led to the development of effective individualized treatments with important implications for patient outcome [3]. Expanding precision medicine to the stroke area in order to identify prognostic markers is therefore crucial although challenging.

In order to achieve this goal, new approaches and strategies along with novel technologies, informatics, and identification of practical clinical paradigms need to be implemented [4, 5]. Similarly to oncology, the great amount of data coming from clinical trials; routine care; databases; registries, including clinical, cognitive, and neuroimaging data; omics (genomics/transcriptomics/proteomics/metabolomics), and other molecular biomarkers from biological samples, i.e., serum/cerebrospinal fluid [CSF]; clot composition analysis; and brain biopsy data, should be shared across centers, collected using standardized methods and a high-quality big data approach, and made available as a fertile ground for future studies. Furthermore, the use of artificial intelligence could allow the development of algorithms that, if validated, may guide stroke physicians in more precisely tailoring decision-making process regarding patient selection and outcome prediction for each individual patient [4, 6–8].

This obviously needs expertise and a multidisciplinary approach including stroke clinicians and both clinical and basic researchers, but also data scientists, omics specialists, biostatisticians for adopting and implementing adequate statistical methodologies, epidemiologists, computer scientists, engineers, and experts in advanced analytics and artificial intelligence.

In this chapter, we focus on the potential future applications of precision medicine for prognosis determination in cerebrovascular diseases.

9.2 Phenotyping of Cerebrovascular Diseases

The correct ascertainment of phenotypes of cerebrovascular disease represents the basis for an adequate and optimal patient management and outcome prediction.

- *Ischemic stroke.* Ischemic stroke is characterized by a highly etiopathogenetic and phenotypic heterogeneity along with imprecise therapeutic window for acute intervention. The call of precision medicine is particularly for specific strategies to define a personalized therapeutic window that can take into account individual variability in the treatment response even in those subjects arriving beyond the standard time window, and to allow the development of novel prognosis prediction models in terms of survival, functional recovery, and recurrence [9].
- *TIA.* In patients with TIA, precision medicine could help to build tailored prognostic models regarding the risk of stroke in the short and long terms and to better understand the molecular signature of the ischemic preconditioning characteristic of this condition and its potential protective role as well as therapeutic implications.
- *Hemorrhagic stroke.* In hemorrhagic stroke, the challenge for precision medicine is mainly represented by the identification of specific demographics and clinical, radiological, and molecular markers for defining the individual risk of hematoma expansion in the first hours after symptom onset and the implications for arterial blood pressure management, the risk of survival, of poor functional outcome, and of recurrency in case it is needed to resume prevention antithrombotic medications due to the presence of specific cardiovascular comorbidities.
- *Chronic cerebral small vessel-related cerebrovascular conditions.* White matter hyperintensities, silent cortical and subcortical lacunar infarcts, cerebral microbleeds, superficial siderosis, and dilated perivascular spaces represent some of the radiological signs which are characteristics of chronic cerebral small vessel-related cerebrovascular conditions such as amyloid angiopathy, vascular dementia, or well-established genetic diseases. Cerebral small vessel disease as a chronic condition has important and variable implications on patient prognosis particularly in terms of cognitive function. In this setting, precision medicine could help in reducing the variability in outcome determination by tailoring the risk of developing and progressing vascular cognitive impairment, the risk of functional dependence and stroke occurrence and recurrence, and the hemorrhagic risk related to antithrombotic treatments.

9.3 Clinical Data

The use of clinical data represents in general the basics for the development of prognosis prediction models in stroke patients. However, because clinical variables could be identified by different criteria, they should be well defined a priori in order to preserve their value for future studies. In the era of precision and individualized medicine, there is the urgent need to standardize the definition and/or quantification methods of clinical variables, the clinical data collection, and the adjudication methods. The development of common data elements to use in clinical trials could allow stroke clinicians and researchers to speak the same language and to have homogeneous clinical data to be reliably analyzed for outcome prediction across studies and, hence, larger sample size to reach an adequate power for investigating clinical outcomes in specific subgroups [4, 10]. These common data elements, from basic to more complex and larger set of clinical variables in addition to imaging and physiological/biological data, obviously require adequate logistics, infrastructure, and technology that could make these data easily available for future studies on prognosis determination in stroke [4]. Furthermore, while local assessments of clinical data are important for generalizability, central assessments/adjudications are crucial for reliability. The indication of the precise time when clinical data are ascertained along with serial data collection allows to better define temporal aspects of outcome prediction. The possibility of a long-term storage of clinical data through the adoption of specific novel software in association with the implementation of clinical trial network, neuroimaging libraries, or biobanks could allow to have a huge number of archived repository clinical data to use for future analyses in order to identify novel clinical determinants of prognosis in stroke [4, 10, 11].

9.4 Molecular Biomarkers

The identification of molecular biomarkers that are hallmarks of the natural course of neurovascular diseases could help in better and more in-depth understanding of the pathophysiology of these conditions and this will certainly improve prognosis.

Concerning acute stroke, several studies have been conducted so far to find the "troponin" of stroke with all its diagnostic and prognostic implications. However, the search for the "holy grail" of specific, rapid, sensitive, easily measurable in accessible tissue, reproducible, relatively stable, and non-expensive surrogate peripheral molecular biomarkers in stroke in general and, particularly, for prognosis determination has been disappointing [12]. The reasons are several and, besides the abovementioned complexity of brain biology and stroke pathophysiology and the heterogeneity of stroke phenotypes, they are also related to (1) the use of non-standardized assays; (2) the difficulties and caution in collecting CSF or to perform brain biopsy in stroke patients for safety issues (e.g., increased risk of spinal and subdural cerebral hematoma, herniation syndrome, and infection) and time constraints; and, therefore, (3) the need to detect and measure the levels of biomarkers peripherally, in the circulating blood.

The use of blood biomarkers in stroke and their relevance for prognosis determination have important limitations. Indeed, while biomarkers measured in CSF have undoubtful advantages because they can be more brain specific, blood biomarkers are strongly influenced by the presence and degree of blood-brain barrier (BBB) disruption, the time when BBB changes occur after stroke onset in respect to the time of blood withdrawal, the brain lesion size, and the actual specificity for the central nervous system and the index cerebrovascular disease, given the potential relationship between the peripheral levels of molecular biomarker/s and other concurrent acute or chronic diseases or physiological processes related for example to aging and disease-induced stress.

Studies have been focused on investigating biomarkers of stroke underlying pathophysiological processes that impact clinical outcome, such as inflammation, apoptosis, oxidative stress, immune system and coagulation/fibrinolysis alterations, tissue remodeling, and heart damage [13].

The technologies of "omics," based on large screening processes of entire sets of molecules expressed in the course of a specific condition, represent novel methods for searching prognostic biomarkers in stroke.

In the last years, relevant progresses have been made in genomics, transcriptomics, proteomics, and metabolomics which have given a crucial contribution to the discovery and identification of prognostic stroke biomarkers. The next step and challenge would be to combine this knowledge and techniques through integromics and system biology to give a boost to the use of molecular biomarkers in clinical practice in the very next future and to lead towards a more precise and individualized prognosis determination, the individuation of novel therapeutic targets, and therefore a personalized therapy [13].

9.4.1 Genomics

Genetics and genomics probably represent the main and the most immediately understandable reflection of the precision medicine concept. However, it should be taken into account that cerebrovascular conditions are in general complex genetic traits characterized by the combined influence of several genes having a small effect size which have been identified so far, and environmental risk factors modulating the genetic effects and family inheritance [4, 14]. It is likely that the genetic contribution on prognosis determination is larger in younger patients, in hemorrhagic stroke, and in non-cardioembolic stroke particularly in small vessel and atherosclerotic large vessel stroke subtypes [15, 16]. Specific genes for stroke have not been individuated yet while there are cerebrovascular conditions that are known to be "genetic" such as CADASIL (cerebral autosomal dominant arteriopathy with subcortical infarcts and leukoencephalopathy), the most common form of hereditary disorders thought to be caused by mutations of the *Notch 3* gene on chromosome 19; MELAS (mitochondrial encephalomyopathy, lactic acidosis, and stroke-like episodes) which is mainly caused by defects in the mitochondrial genome that is inherited purely from the female parent; or Fabry disease, which is a rare genetic disease of the group of lysosomal storage diseases, inherited in an X-linked manner, where the genetic mutation interferes with the function of the alpha-galactosidase enzyme [17]. Genomics has changed the approach in the management of some of these conditions, even up to the putting in place of enzyme replacement therapy like in Fabry disease, and consequently in their prognosis [14, 17, 18].

Genetic architecture of stroke prognosis is not fully understood and determined yet. Molecular hallmarks of ischemic stroke subtypes need to be identified in order to make patient selection for acute treatment as well as personalized risk stratification, prognosis determination, and hence long-term secondary prevention strategies more rapid and accurate [18].

In particular, the individuation of genetic associations with stroke implies the investigation of molecular mechanisms underlying stroke risk and therefore stroke outcome.

In most cases, the issue is that genetic risk variants contribute to a multifactorial predisposition to stroke and singular genetic variation is responsible for only modest increase in the risk of stroke. In order to individuate reliable genetic associations, there is the need of large studies including thousands of subjects to achieve a sufficient statistical power. This has been overcome by the use of high-throughput genotyping and the creation of large international consortia such as the International Stroke Genetics Consortium (ISGC). The largest genome-wide association study (GWAS) in stroke derived from the MEGASTROKE initiative which includes 72,147 patients with stroke and 823,869 healthy controls [19, 20].

Table 9.1 reports the main genetic loci which have been found specifically associated with stroke outcome.

To date, 42 loci with a robust significant association with stroke (all strokes, specific types—ischemic or hemorrhagic—or subtypes) and potentially implicated in prognosis determination have been identified, mainly in European ancestry populations [13]. Of these, 22 are associated with any ischemic stroke and 2 with intracerebral hemorrhage (ICH); 1 locus is associated with both ischemic and deep ICH related to cerebral small vessel disease which indeed could lead to both ischemic and hemorrhagic stroke [21]. Furthermore, 12 loci have been associated with specific etiopathogenetic subtypes of ischemic stroke: 6 with large vessel-related stroke, 4 with cardioembolic stroke, and 2 with small vessel stroke [19]. Two loci were specifically associated with ischemic stroke in the young and with cervical artery dissection [15, 22].

Nevertheless, it should be considered that genetic associations at a lower significance threshold could also be helpful to better understand the genetic contribution to stroke. These associations could indicate a *continuum* between monogenic and multifactorial stroke. Interestingly, it has been found that common variants in the same genes associated to Mendelian forms of stroke (monogenic stroke), for example, *COL4A1/COL4A2* and *HTRA1*, are also associated with complex forms of ischemic stroke and ICH [16, 19, 23].

The genetic architecture of stroke etiologies has not been in-depth investigated. In the last years, large genetic studies have been complemented by smaller studies conducted on stroke subtypes where it has been observed that genes associated with

Table 9.1 Potential optimal candidate genetic loci identified in genomics studies which resulted to be specifically associated with stroke outcome for future application of precision medicine in prognosis determination

SNP	Chromosome/location	Affected genes	Risk allele (frequency)	Associated stroke subtype	Application in prognosis determination	Odds ratio (p value)	Reference
rs1842681	18/Intronic	*LOC105372028*	A (23%)	IS	Clinical outcome	1.40 (5.27 × 10^{-9})	[13]
rs76221407	1/Intronic	*PATJ*	G (3%)	IS	Clinical outcome	0.4 (1.72 × 10^{-9})	[13]
rs11655160	17/Intergenic	*PIRT*	G (76%)	ICH	Increased volume of ICH	0.82 (2.5 × 10^{-9})	[13]

any stroke could present a strong association also with specific subtype of stroke such as *HDAC9* and *PITX2* loci with large vessel and cardioembolic stroke, respectively. These variants probably are involved in biological pathways that influence the risk of most types of stroke, for example genes that predispose to vascular risk factors such as hypertension, or to vessel fragility, thrombosis, or bleeding, or genes that are implicated in the resilience and tolerance to brain injury, i.e., how much the brain adapts and recovers [19]. One study showed that in a polygenic risk score, genetic variants associated with atrial fibrillation are associated also with cardioembolic stroke and stroke of undetermined origin [24].

These results could allow a better insight into the biological and pathophysiological mechanisms underlying stroke in general and the multitude of its subtypes, and the identification of novel therapeutic targets. In the setting of precision medicine, the goal is to develop and validate polygenic risk score for stroke in order to identify those subjects who have a risk of stroke like it is possible with monogenic stroke.

Interesting results have been obtained also in genetic studies specifically investigating genetic associations with stroke prognosis. Two large meta-analyses of GWAS from the Genetics of Ischemic Stroke Functional Outcome (GISCOME) network and the ISGC have identified common and low-frequency genetic variants at two distinct loci that resulted to be associated with functional outcome in terms of modified Rankin Scale (mRS) score at 3 months [25]. An intergenic region on chromosome 17p12 has resulted to be associated with hematoma volume, neurological severity, and functional outcome in patients with non-lobar ICH [26]. Genetic imbalance in terms of copy number variations has also been found to be associated with 3-month unfavorable outcome in patients with ischemic stroke [27].

Although the genetic variations associated with stroke risk and stroke severity are different, there are some loci that have been found associated with both, particularly if they have a role in modulating the underlying pathogenetic mechanism like in cerebral small vessel diseases [24, 28]. This is the case of *APOE* locus, which is associated with small vessel disease and resulted to be associated also with mean volume of ICH. In particular, patients who are carriers of the *APOE*ε2* allele are more likely to have larger ICH volumes [29]. In addition, in patients with lobar ICH, presence of *APOE* gene mutation (ε2 or ε4 allele) has been found to be associated with an increased risk of hematoma recurrence and this may guide physicians in individualizing the selection of antithrombotic treatments if indicated, in case of concomitant prothrombotic vascular risk factors [17]. Furthermore, the *FOXF2* locus, which is involved in the development of cerebral vessel and associated with an increased risk of stroke, has been found to be associated with a higher risk of death from stroke [24].

There is an increasing knowledge development in the specific field of ***pharmacogenomics*** where studies have led to important results in investigating genetic variations in drug response with relevant implications in routine clinical practice and modification of patient prognosis [30]. In particular, regarding antithrombotic treatment, the following findings are of interest: (1) variability in response to oral anticoagulant therapy with warfarin has been shown to be related with common genetic variants in *VKORC1* and *CYP2C9* genes; (2) the *CYP2C19*2* variant is associated with reduced blood concentrations of clopidogrel and a consequent increase of cardiovascular thrombotic events; (3) a polymorphism *CES1* (rs2244613) is associated with the reduction by 15% of the direct thrombin inhibitor dabigatran and, consequently, with a decreased risk of bleeding by 33% [31]; (4) similarly, other genetic variants have been found to relate with response to specific drugs used in stroke treatment such as statins or antihypertensive drugs [30]; and (5) regarding the acute setting, the response to alteplase in terms of hemorrhagic transformation and in-hospital death seems to be influenced by variants in *A2M* (rs669) and *F12* (rs181020) [32].

In some cases, these findings have been specifically reflected in the drug labels and therefore they directly influence clinical practice. In the next future, it is expected that genetic tests could guide in selecting the type or dose of medication or avoiding drug adverse effects or drug resistance.

Genetic correlates of neuroimaging findings and their influence on prognosis have also been investigated. For example, experimental studies showed genetic variability of collateral circulation and its response following acute ischemic stroke [33].

Genetic studies on leukoaraiosis/white matter hyperintensity, a radiological sign known to be associated with increased risk of stroke and poor post-stroke outcome, could allow a more in-depth understanding of the pathophysiological mechanisms involved in the brain susceptibility to acute ischemia and modify patient prognosis in terms of stroke occurrence and recovery [34]. WMH are highly heritable and associated with small artery ischemic stroke. Data on the genetic architecture of white matter hyperintensities are still controversial and not conclusive yet. A systematic assessment of 19 candidate gene polymorphisms—mostly involved in lipid metabolism, control of vascular tone, or blood pressure regulation—in 46 studies on 19,000 subjects found that there was no association between apolipoprotein E (ε4+/−), methylenetetrahydrofolate reductase (677 cytosine/thymine polymorphism [C/T]), or angiotensinogen (Met235Thr) and WMH. For the angiotensin-converting enzyme insertion/deletion polymorphism (I/D) there appeared to be a significant association, but this was partly attributed by the authors to the small studies and other biases [35]. A more recent genome-wide meta-analysis of cerebral WMH volume (WMHV) in 3670 patients with stroke found no association at genome-wide significance with WMHV in stroke patients and observed that genetic associations with WMHV are shared in otherwise healthy individuals and patients with stroke. In particular, in a meta-analysis of the genome-wide significant and suggestive loci from community populations (15 single-nucleotide polymorphisms in total) and from stroke patients, six independent loci were associated with WMHV in both populations. Four of these are novel associations at the genome-wide level (rs72934505 [*NBEAL1*]; rs941898 [*EVL*]; rs962888 [*C1QL1*]; rs9515201 [*COL4A2*]) [34]. Genetic variation in *PLEKHG1* (a Rho guanine nucleotide exchange factor that is involved in reorientation of cells in the vascular endothelium) is associated with WMH and ischemic stroke, more strongly with the small vessel subtype, suggesting it to act by promoting small vessel arteriopathy [36]. These findings indicate common genetic susceptibility in cerebral small vessel disease. A recently published study on 8395 subjects from a general population cohort reported a statistically significant association between *APOE* ε4 genotype and increased WMH volumes which is a marker of poor cerebrovascular health, confirming the promise of *APOE* ε4 as one of the molecular biomarkers with potential link between cerebrovascular impairment and cognitive aging [37]. In another study using GWAS data on 2336 patients with ischemic stroke, the authors found that a significant proportion of the variance of WMH volume was attributable to common SNPs after adjustment for significant risk factors and the SNP heritability estimates were higher among hypertensive individuals, while they were lower and nonsignificant in nonhypertensive subjects. Therefore, it seems that the genetic architecture of WMH in ischemic stroke differs between hypertensives and nonhypertensives [38]. Further larger studies are needed to better understand how genetics modulate the influence of WMH on stroke outcome.

Of great interest is the use of genomics and also of transcriptomics to identify molecular signature of specific neuroimaging findings such as ischemic penumbra that have an important impact on patient outcome (see below Sect. 9.4.2) [39].

Conversely to genetic factors which are fixed, ***epigenetic modifications*** such as DNA methylation which regulate gene expression are dynamic and tissue specific [13]. Epigenetic factors can have an influence on the development and the course of complex diseases like stroke. Indeed, DNA methylation could impact underlying stroke mechanisms by modulating genetic and environmental risk factors and could have a role as a biomarker of stroke, even indirectly, by helping to assess biological age which independently predicts the outcome in ischemic stroke more than chronological age [40]. There are still few epigenome-wide association studies in stroke; one of these have shown that methylation of *PPM1A*, which encodes protein phosphatase 1A, has been associated with vascular recurrence in patients treated with aspirin [41].

In conclusion, most studies on stroke genetics have investigated common or low-frequency single-nucleotide polymorphisms, which can partially explain the heritability of stroke. Furthermore, very rare single-nucleotide variants or variations related to copy numbers have not been fully studied yet [42]. Despite the multitude and variety of published studies on genetics in stroke, a direct translation of their results into clinical practice for prognosis determination has not systematically occurred yet. This is one of the challenges of precision medicine in stroke that would require the conduction of more and larger scale studies specifically and systematically investigating genetic associations with clinical outcomes in the setting of genetic consortia, inclusion of groups of non-European ancestry, accurate stroke phenotype ascertainment, and advanced methodology including genome-wide genotyping, whole-genome (and/or exome) sequencing, and gene expression studies [4]. The goal should be using strategies and models incorporating genetics and genomics for a personalized outcome prediction and, hence, implementation of therapeutic strategies on individual basis.

In particular, the individuation of genetic associations with stroke implies the investigation of molecular mechanisms underlying stroke risk and therefore stroke outcome, which can provide information for the development of novel therapeutic targets [13], by (1) identifying the most likely causal genes and variants in the associated locus implicated in the occurrence of stroke, its severity, and outcome through bioinformatics, to be used as promising biotargets with potential therapeutic implications [24]; (2) determining the potential enrichment of stroke-associated genes in known drug targets; (3) using genetic variants that mimic the effects of a drug by increasing or reducing the expression of drug target gene, to support clinical trials investigating specific drug effects; (4) facilitating the classification of stroke into more homogeneous subtypes that might have distinct responses to specific treatment and different outcomes; and (5) identifying individuals who have a high risk of stroke and tailoring early preventive interventions and outcome prediction models.

9.4.2 Transcriptomics

Stroke transcriptomics allows the study of RNAs in the peripheral blood as potential biomarkers. Microarray and RNA sequencing or PCR with reverse transcription (RT-PCR) are used to assess both coding and noncoding RNA transcripts in the circulating blood as prognostic biomarkers. Stroke research in this field is still at the beginning; there is initial evidence that some micro-RNAs (miRNAs) (i.e., short [18–23 nucleotides] noncoding RNA) and long noncoding RNAs (lncRNAs) have the potential to become stroke biomarkers for patient stratification and outcome definition [13]. Table 9.2 reports some of the potential candidate transcriptomics biomarkers usable for outcome determination in stroke.

A more precise identification of stroke etiology with implications in prognosis could benefit from the development of RNA panels, like it has been found for cardioembolic, large vessel, or small vessel subtypes [43, 44, 54]. In particular, some genes included in panels seem to distinguish stroke subtypes in terms of inflammation and clot formation: one 40-gene panel has been found to be helpful to discriminate cardioembolic from large vessel stroke with sensitivity and specificity of >95%; a 37-gene panel, to differentiate cardioembolic stroke due to atrial fibrillation from that without atrial fibrillation with sensitivity and specificity of 90%; and a 41-gene panel, to differentiate lacunar from non-lacunar stroke with sensitivity and specificity of >90% [43, 44]. Interestingly, the use of these RNA panels in patients with stroke of unclear origin suggested that 27% of them had stroke related to atrial fibrillation and 18% to large vessel stenosis/occlusion [55]. However, these results and their actual biological plausibility need to be confirmed in larger studies in order to also assess whether patients identified by these panels as having cardioembolic or large vessel stroke could benefit from specific therapies.

In the last decade, a number of studies have been performed on miRNA and their dysregulation in stroke for their important potential signaling role [56–59]. Since many cell types express a set of miRNAs, circulating miRNAs seem to be tissue specific and, hence, a signature of their original source. Some of these studies have observed changes in extracellular miRNA that derived from the ischemic brain but also from other organs/tissues/cells and this can obviously confound the results. Intracellular miRNAs found to be changed, mostly in terms of downregulation, in

Table 9.2 Potential optimal candidate biomarkers identified in transcriptomic studies for future application of precision medicine in prognosis determination in stroke

RNA transcript	Application in prognosis determination	Reference
Micro-RNAs (mRNAs)		
mRNA panels	Identification of stroke etiology Gene panels discriminating: • Cardioembolic from large vessel stroke (40-gene panel, with sensitivity and specificity of >95%) • Cardioembolic stroke due to atrial fibrillation from that without atrial fibrillation (37-gene panel, with sensitivity and specificity of 90%) • Lacunar from non-lacunar stroke (41-gene panel, with sensitivity and specificity of >90%)	[43, 44]
mi424, mi200c (decreased and increased levels, respectively)	Ischemic brain injury	[45, 46]
mRNA panel	• t-PA-related hemorrhagic transformation at 24 h (6-gene panel [SMAD4, INPP5D, VEGI, AREG, MCFD2, and MARCH7], with sensitivity of 80% and specificity of 70.2%)	[47]
miR-199b-3p, miR-27b-3p, miR-130a-3p, miR-221-3p, miR-24-3p, miR-29c, and miR200 (increased levels)	• Carotid disease progression and carotid plaque instability	[48]
mRNA panel	• Molecular identification of ischemic penumbra, as defined by MRI perfusion (PWI)-diffusion (DWI) mismatch in acute ischemic stroke (5-gene panel, CORO1A, HCAR2, HCAR3, IL1B, PF4)	[39]
Long noncoding RNA (lnc-RNA)		
lnc-RNAs encoding lipoprotein, lipoprotein(a)-like2, prostaglandin I2 synthase, α-adducins, and the ABO blood group (transferase A, α1-3-*N*-Acetylgalactosaminyltransferase; transferase B, α1-3-galactosyltransferase)	• Associated with stroke risk genes and hence potentially influencing prognosis determination	[49]
Upregulated and downregulated lnc-RNAs linc-DHFRL1-4, SNHG15, and linc-FAM98A-3	• Identification of some stroke subtypes like large vessel stroke with consequent prognostic implications	[50–53]

stroke patients are miR-122, mi-148a, let-7i, miR-19a, miR-320d, miR-4429, miR-363, and miR-487b [60]. Furthermore, mi424 levels were decreased in animal model of stroke and in acute stroke patients while post-stroke increases of miRNA-200c contributed to ischemic brain injury by inhibiting reelin expression, and its inhibition increases cell survival [45, 46]. The roles of these miRNAs include the regulation of Toll-like receptor signaling, nuclear factor-κB (NF-κB) signaling, leukocyte extravasation signaling, and prothrombin activation pathway [45]. All these processes are involved in the immune response to ischemic brain damage with consequent implications for neuroprotection and therefore for stroke prognosis; however, further studies are needed to confirm these associations. Interestingly, an mRNA expression panel comprising six genes (SMAD4, INPP5D, VEGI, AREG, MCFD2, and MARCH7) measured within 1.5 h of stroke onset could identify patients that developed t-PA-related hemorrhagic transformation at 24 h with 80% sensitivity and 70.2% specificity [47]. The increased levels of the following miRNA may also inform on the risk of stroke in patients with carotid atherosclerosis, disease progression, and carotid plaque instability: miR-199b-3p, miR-27b-3p, miR-130a-3p, miR-221-3p, miR-24-3p, miR-29c, and miR200; most of them are implicated in inflammation, angiogenesis, endothelial and smooth muscle cell proliferation, migration, and differentiation [48].

Regarding the lnc-RNAs, these are molecules of RNA longer than the miRNA that do not have a coding role but contribute to gene expression. Studies on lnc-RNA have been more focused on stroke diagnosis more than on prognosis. Indeed, differences in lnc-RNAs were found between stroke patients and healthy controls. However, lnc-RNAs resulted to be also associated with stroke risk genes potentially influencing prognosis determination, for example those that encode lipoprotein, lipoprotein(a)-like 2, prostaglandin I2 synthase, α-adducins, and ABO blood group (transferase A, α1-3-*N*-acetylgalactosaminyltransferase; transferase B, α1-3-galactosyltransferase) [49]. Other studies have found the association between both upregulated and downregulated lnc-RNAs (e.g., linc-DHFRL1-4, SNHG15, and linc-FAM98A-3) not only with ischemic stroke diagnosis and Moyamoya disease, but also with the identification of some stroke subtypes like large vessel stroke with consequent prognostic implications [50–53].

As mentioned above, of great interest is the recent attempt to find molecular signatures of penumbra. A recently published pilot study on 23 patients has attempted to find molecular signatures of penumbra, as defined by MRI perfusion (PWI)-diffusion (DWI mismatch in acute ischemic stroke) [39]. The authors observed that PWI-DWI mismatch volume is associated with a specific gene expression profile in the peripheral blood characterized by overlap of inflammatory and neuroprotective pathways that are regulated by lipopolysaccharide inhibition. In particular, mismatch was found to significantly correlate with the expression of 34 genes including those related to inflammation, SUMOylation (small ubiquitin-like modifier protein-related pathways), and coagulation, while lipopolysaccharide inhibition was identified to be a candidate upstream regulator of these processes for five genes (*CORO1A, HCAR2, HCAR3, IL1B, PF4*). Most of these genes are involved in immune response and inflammation. Inhibition of these genes in the blood in association with penumbra might be another indicator of biological plausibility as inflammation promotes cytotoxicity in acute cerebral ischemia. Although all these proinflammatory and prothrombotic genes were inhibited except *CORO1A*, upregulation of this gene can be associated with both autoimmunity and immune deficiency. These findings may help in acute patient management and prognosis determination through the identification at individual level of those patients who are more susceptible to the presence of ischemic penumbra and to its progression into infarction.

We are still far from using RNA transcripts into clinical practice. Therefore, large studies and validation in independent cohorts are needed to allow the translation from their research to routine use as prognostic biomarkers in precision medicine.

9.4.3 Proteomics

Proteomics is a truly promising tool for the molecular determination of prognosis in stroke because proteins are actually the most widely used biomarkers and can also be easily measured by point-of-care devices. This approach mainly uses mass spectrometry-based techniques covering a large number of proteins in the serum or plasma [4, 61].

Since early outcome prediction represents a key priority for improving stroke management, finding specific protein markers as determinants of prognosis would allow to make this management with therapeutic and prevention interventions more appropriate and accurate for each single individual. However, this is challenging also with proteomics because, given the extreme complexity of stroke pathophysiology and heterogeneity of stroke phenotypes, outcome in stroke patients is influenced by several clinical factors such as age, stroke severity, comorbidities, and specific complications such as cerebral edema, hemorrhagic transformation, and post-stroke infections. Appropriate and easy-to-obtain blood molecular biomarkers, such as proteins, may reduce this variability in outcome prediction. Nevertheless, an ideal biomarker to be helpful in prognosis determination in clinical practice should improve the outcome predictive performance of an already well-established clinical model. Indeed, further research would be required for validation, data integration, and translation of specific algorithms into clinical practice. In addition, the lack of common criteria for the definition of an outcome endpoint (e.g., post-stroke pneumonia) makes the individuation of proper blood molecular protein biomarkers more complicated than expected. Subsequently to their identification and validation of their performance in predicting outcome in stroke patients, prognostic proteomic biomarkers could also be tested as surrogate biomarkers for their link with a specific intervention in semi-interventional trials [62].

In the last decades, in a large number of studies a remarkable amount of proteins have been identified in both ischemic and hemorrhagic stroke patients and proposed as prognostic biomarkers. However, only some of them can be considered promising candidates and potentially usable for future application in the setting of stroke precision medicine (Table 9.3).

Table 9.3 Potential optimal candidate molecular protein biomarkers identified in proteomics and non-proteomics studies for future application of precision medicine in prognosis determination in ischemic stroke and/or intracerebral hemorrhage

Molecular biomarkers	Description	Source	Levels	Application in prognosis determination	Reference
Brain tissue					
Copeptin	C-terminal of pro-vasopressin, agent of stress response (neuroendocrine marker released by the hypothalamus in equimolar concentrations to vasopressin, which is a hormone involved in the response to sympathetic activation and therefore to stress)	Human blood	High	*Ischemic stroke*: Neurological severity (NIHSS); poor 90-day functional outcome and mortality; post-stroke infection; stroke recurrence	[63–69]
				Intracerebral hemorrhage: Positively correlated with hematoma volume and negatively with GCS score; neurological deterioration; 30-day and 1-year mortality; 90-day and 1-year poor functional outcome	[70, 71]
MMP-9 (also inflammatory biomarker)	Protease which plays a key role in microvascular and BBB integrity and in neuroinflammatory response	"	High	*Ischemic stroke*: Hemorrhagic transformation (with a gradient response when measured prior to IV thrombolytic treatment and also in non-thrombolyzed ischemic stroke patients); baseline neurological severity (NIHSS); poor outcome; infarct growth; radiologic sign of BBB disruption (e.g., the hyperintense acute reperfusion injury marker, HARM sign)	[12, 72–80]
				Intracerebral hemorrhage: Perihematomal edema development and extent; hematoma growth; neurological worsening	[81]

(continued)

Table 9.3 (continued)

Molecular biomarkers	Description	Source	Levels	Application in prognosis determination	Reference
S100B	Calcium-binding protein, marker of glial activation and brain injury in general	Human CSF or blood	High	*Ischemic stroke*: Malignant infarction and cerebral edema; brain damage; infarct volume; stroke severity; poor functional outcome	[82, 83]
				Intracerebral hemorrhage: Early mortality (1-week mortality); poor functional outcome at discharge	
NSE	Enzyme found in mature neurons and cells of neuronal origin	Human blood	High	*Ischemic stroke*: Poor outcome	[84]
Excitotoxic					
Glutamate	Neurotransmitter	Human blood	High	*Ischemic stroke*: Early neurological deterioration	[85]
Oxidative stress					
F2-isoPs	Products of non-cyclooxygenase free radical-induced neuronal arachidonic acid peroxidation of membrane phospholipids and lipoproteins	Human blood	High	*Ischemic stroke*: Ischemic penumbra (independently predicted radiographic evidence of MRI PWI-DWI mismatch >20% and mismatch salvage); infarct growth occurrence; infarct growth volume	[86, 87]
ORAC	Measure of the blood antioxidant capacity	"	High	*Ischemic stroke*: Ischemic penumbra (independently predicted radiographic evidence of MRI PWI-DWI mismatch >20% and mismatch salvage)	[86]

Inflammatory					
hs-CRP	Acute-phase protein, nonspecific inflammation marker	Human blood	High	*Ischemic stroke*: Early neurological deterioration; plaque instability; poor functional outcome; increased mortality	[12, 48, 72, 85, 88–92]
				Intracerebral hemorrhage: Early hematoma growth; stroke severity; 30-day mortality	[70, 93–97]
Homocysteine	Non-proteinogenic α-amiro acid	"	High	*Ischemic stroke*: Early neurological deterioration	[85]
LpPLA2	Serine lipase that circulates in the peripheral blood linked to low-density lipoproteins (LDL) and metabolizes LDL to form free fatty acids and other proinflammatory molecules	"	High	*Ischemic stroke*: Stroke recurrence; plaque instability; mortality	[4, 48, 92, 98, 99]
ADAMTS13	Protease	"	Low	*Ischemic stroke*: Poor response to IV thrombolysis; mortality, poor 90-day functional outcome	[48, 100]
IL-6	Cytokine	"	High	*Ischemic stroke*: Poor outcome; post-stroke infection	[72]
				Intracerebral hemorrhage: Early hematoma growth; severity of stroke; poor functional outcome; mortality	[70, 93–97]
IL-10	Cytokine	"	High	*Intracerebral hemorrhage*: Stroke severity; poor functional outcome; rebleeding	[70, 93–97]
IL-11	Cytokine	"	High	*Intracerebral hemorrhage*: Stroke severity; mortality	[70, 96]

(continued)

Table 9.3 (continued)

Molecular biomarkers	Description	Source	Levels	Application in prognosis determination	Reference
HMGB-1	Chromatin protein secreted by immune cells (like macrophages, monocytes, and dendritic cells), proinflammatory protein	"	High	*Intracerebral hemorrhage*: Poor 3-month functional outcome	[70, 97]
CD34+ progenitor cells	Bone marrow-derived progenitor cells	"	High	*Intracerebral hemorrhage*: Neurological improvement; good 3-month functional outcome	[101]
VEGF	Growth factors in angiogenesis	"	High	*Intracerebral hemorrhage*: 3-month neurological improvement; good functional outcome	[102]
Ang-1	Growth factors in angiogenesis	"	High	*Intracerebral hemorrhage*: 3-month neurological improvement; good functional outcome	[102]
G-CSF	Growth factors in angiogenesis	"	High	*Intracerebral hemorrhage*: 3-month neurological improvement; good functional outcome	[102]
TNF-α	Cytokine	"	High	*Ischemic stroke*: Poor outcome (particularly in lacunar stroke)	[72, 103]
				Intracerebral hemorrhage: Early hematoma growth; mortality; future bleeding	[70, 93–97]
sICAM-1	Leukocyte-endothelial adhesion molecules	"	High	*Ischemic stroke*: Poor outcome	[72]
				Intracerebral hemorrhage: Early hematoma growth; poor functional outcome; future bleeding	[70, 93–97]
sVCAM-1	Leukocyte-endothelial adhesion molecules	"	High	*Ischemic stroke*: Poor outcome	[72]
sE-selectin	Soluble cell adhesion molecule	"	High	*Ischemic stroke*: Poor outcome	[72]
sP-selectin	Soluble cell adhesion molecule	"	High	*Ischemic stroke*: Poor outcome	[72]

Leptin/adiponectin ratio	Cytokine	"	High	*Ischemic stroke*: >1.16 measured at the first day of hospital admission has been associated with good 90-day functional outcome (mRS 0–2) in patients with atherothrombotic acute ischemic stroke	[48]
Mannose-binding lectin	Component of the complement activation cascade	"	High	*Ischemic stroke*: Mortality; poor 90-day functional outcome	[48]
IL-6, Th1/Th2 profile, copeptin, procalcitonin, serum amyloid A	Cytokine and serum acute-phase reactants	"	High	*Ischemic stroke*: Post-stroke infections	[104]
GFAP	Type III intermediate filament (IF) protein that is expressed by numerous cell types of the central nervous system (CNS), including astrocytes; related to astrogliosis	Brain homogenate; human blood	High	*Ischemic stroke*: Infarct core; brain damage; poor outcome	[13, 105, 106]
Monocytic expression of the human leukocyte antigen gene HLA-DR	–	Human blood	High	*Ischemic stroke*: Independent predictor of an individual's ability to overcome post-stroke infections	[107]
Lysophosphatidylcholine	Phospholipids in the cell membrane	"	High	*Ischemic stroke*: Stroke recurrence	[48]
Soluble CD40L	Marker of atherosclerotic plaque instability	"	High	*Ischemic stroke*: Stroke recurrence	[48]
Omentin-1	Protein regulating vascular inflammation	"	High	*Ischemic stroke*: Plaque instability	[48]
Complement complex C5b-9	Complement complex	"	High	*Ischemic stroke*: Plaque instability; plaque burden and degree of carotid stenosis	[48]
Free ferritin	Free iron released after erythrocyte lysis	"	High	*Intracerebral hemorrhage*: Stroke severity; increased edema volume; poor outcome	[108]

(continued)

Table 9.3 (continued)

Molecular biomarkers	Description	Source	Levels	Application in prognosis determination	Reference
Hemostatic/hematological					
Fibrinogen	Acute-phase protein participating in clot formation	Human blood	High	*Ischemic stroke*: Early neurological deterioration	[85]
				Intracerebral hemorrhage: Neurological deterioration	[109, 110]
Hemoglobin	–	"	Low	*Ischemic stroke*: Early neurological deterioration	[85]
Fibronectin	Glycoprotein of the extracellular matrix	"	High	*Ischemic stroke*: Hemorrhagic transformation after IV thrombolysis	[111, 112]
PAI1	Fibrinolytic inhibitor	"	Low	*Ischemic stroke*: Poor response to IV thrombolysis in terms of recanalization	[113]
TAFI	Fibrinolytic inhibitor	"	High	*Ischemic stroke*: Poor response to IV thrombolysis in terms of recanalization	[113]
α2-Antiplasmin	Serine protease inhibitor inactivating plasmin (an important enzyme that participates in fibrinolysis and degradation of various other proteins)	"		*Ischemic stroke*: Poor response to IV thrombolysis in terms of recanalization	[114]
D-dimer		"	High	*Intracerebral hemorrhage*: 30-day mortality; GCS score, midline shift, and subarachnoid extension of the hemorrhage	[109, 110]
Factor XIII	Factor agent of blood formation	"	High	*Intracerebral hemorrhage*: Hematoma growth	[109, 110]

Metabolic					
Glucose	–	Human blood	High	*Ischemic stroke*: Early neurological deterioration	[85]
				Intracerebral hemorrhage: 30-day and long-term mortality	[115]
Glycosylated hemoglobin	–	"	High	*Ischemic stroke*: Early neurological deterioration; mortality; poor 90-day functional outcome	[48, 85]
LDL cholesterol	Low-density lipoprotein cholesterol	"	High	*Ischemic stroke*: Early neurological deterioration	[85]
			Low	*Intracerebral hemorrhage*: Early neurological deterioration; hematoma growth; 3-month mortality	[116]
Total cholesterol	–	"	High	*Ischemic stroke*: Early neurological deterioration	[85]
Triglycerides	–	"	High	*Ischemic stroke*: Early neurological deterioration	[85]
Urea	–	"	High	*Ischemic stroke*: Early neurological deterioration	[85]
Albumin	–	"	Low	*Ischemic stroke*: Early neurological deterioration	[85]
Glycated albumin		"	High	*Ischemic stroke*: Stroke recurrence	[48]
25-Hydroxyvitamin D	Vitamin	"	Low	*Ischemic stroke*: Mortality and/or 90-day functional outcome	[48]
Calcium levels		"	Low	*Intracerebral hemorrhage*: ≤2.41 mmol/L could predict both death and 90-day major disability	[70]

(continued)

Table 9.3 (continued)

Molecular biomarkers	Description	Source	Levels	Application in prognosis determination	Reference
Miscellaneous					
Gelsolin	Actin-binding protein	Human brain homogenate and blood	High	*Ischemic stroke*: Poor outcome	[13, 117]
DRP2	Dihydropyrimidinase-related protein	"	Low	*Ischemic stroke*: Poor outcome	[13, 117]
Cystatin A	Cysteine protease inhibitor	"	High	*Ischemic stroke*: Poor outcome	[13, 117]
NSF ATPase	Involved in membrane trafficking in neurons	"		*Ischemic stroke*: Target to avoid ischemia-reperfusion injury	[105]
SAHH2	Neuronal specific	Neuron and vessel microdissection and blood	Low	*Ischemic stroke*: Neurological improvement at 24 and 4 h from symptom onset	[13, 118]
CaMK2B	Protein kinase	Rat and human CSF and blood	High	*Ischemic stroke*: Poor outcome at 3 months from symptom onset	[13, 119]
CMPK	Protein kinase	"	High	*Ischemic stroke*: Poor outcome at 3 months from symptom onset	[13, 119]
VAP-1	Part of the semicarbazide-sensitive amine oxidases which are involved in the process of immune cell migration and can be found on the cell surface or soluble in serum	Human blood	High	*Ischemic stroke*: Hemorrhagic transformation after IV thrombolysis	[120]
Progranulin	Multipotent growth factor	"	High	*Ischemic stroke*: Mortality and/or poor 90-day functional outcome	[48]
YKL-40	Glycoprotein associated with acute and chronic inflammation	"	High	*Ischemic stroke*: Mortality and/or poor 90-day functional outcome	[48]

Neurofilament light	Neuronal scaffolding protein	"	High	*Ischemic stroke*: Mortality and/or poor 90-day functional outcome; infarct volume; recurrent stroke	[48]
BNP, NT-proBNP	Natriuretic peptides; hormones secreted by the cardiac smooth muscle cells when stretched	"	High	*Ischemic stroke*: Stroke risk; cardioembolic; stroke recurrence; poor outcome	[121–125]
				Intracerebral hemorrhage: Brain injury; poor outcome	[126]
s-Fas	Soluble molecules, variant molecular splicing products of the Fas-receptor/ligand apoptosis signaling pathway and they are part of the TNF receptor family. Some of these molecules seem to be potential inhibitors of the Fas-apoptosis system	"	Low	*Intracerebral hemorrhage*: Neuronal death; perihematomal edema growth	[127, 128]
HSP-70	Involved in the process of protein folding and has a role in protecting cells from stressors such as hypoxia	"	High	*Intracerebral hemorrhage*: Survival	[70]
Microparticles	Small membrane particles released by cells under stress conditions having a role in coagulation (procoagulant activity) and inflammation and therefore in neuronal damage	"	High	*Intracerebral hemorrhage*: Presence of intraventricular hemorrhage; greater hematoma volume; stroke severity (GCS score); early mortality (7-day mortality)	[70]
Fibulin-5	Extracellular matrix protein	"	High	*Intracerebral hemorrhage*: 90-day functional outcome; mortality	[129]

(continued)

Table 9.3 (continued)

Molecular biomarkers	Description	Source	Levels	Application in prognosis determination	Reference
Panels					
IL-6 and NT-proBNP	Cytokine/hormone secreted by the cardiac smooth muscle cells when stretched	Human blood	High	*Ischemic stroke*: Poor outcome	[130]
Osteopontin, neopterin, and myeloperoxidase	Extracellular structural proteins/marker of immune system activation/peroxidase enzyme most abundantly expressed in neutrophil granulocytes	"	High	*Ischemic stroke*: Stroke recurrence	[48]
sIL-10 levels ≥23 pg/mL and glutamate ≥130 µmol/L	Cytokine/neurotransmitter	"	High	*Ischemic stroke*: Clinical-diffusion mismatch	[131]
TNF-α, IL-6	Cytokine	"	High	*Intracerebral hemorrhage*: Early hematoma growth	[70]
TNF-α, IL-6, ICAM-1	Cytokine	"	High	*Intracerebral hemorrhage*: Hematoma growth; hematoma size; poor outcome	[70]

ADAMTS13 disintegrin and metalloproteinase with thrombospondin motifs 13, *Ang-1* angiopoietin-1, *CaMK2b* calmodulin-dependent protein kinase II subunit-β, *CMPK* cytidine monophosphate kinase, *CSF* cerebrospinal fluid, *DRP2* dihydropyrimidinase-related protein 2, *F2-isoPs* F2-isoprostanes, *G-CSF* granulocyte colony-stimulating factor, *GCS* Glasgow Coma Scale, *GFAP* glial fibrillary acid protein, *HMGB-1* high mobility group box 1, *hs-CRP* high-sensitivity C-reactive protein, *HSP-70* heat-shock protein 70, *IL* interleukin, *LDL* low-density lipoprotein, *LpPLA2* lipoprotein-associated phospholipase A2, *MMP* matrix metalloproteinase, *NSE* neuron-specific enolase, *NSF* N-ethylmaleimide-sensitive factor (NSF) ATPase, *NIHSS* National Institutes of Health Stroke Scale, *NT-proBNP* N-terminal brain natriuretic peptide, *ORAC* oxygen radical absorbance capacity, *PAI1* plasminogen activator inhibitor, *SAHH2* adenosylhomocysteinase 2, *sICAM-1* soluble intercellular adhesion molecule, *sVCAM-1* soluble vascular cell adhesion molecule, *TAFI* thrombin activable fibrinolysis inhibitor, *TNF-α* tumor necrosis factor-alpha, *VAP-1* vascular adhesion protein 1, *VEGF* vascular endothelial growth factor

9.4.3.1 Ischemic Stroke

In ischemic stroke, all proteomic biomarkers of inflammation, immune system, apoptosis, oxidative stress, coagulation and fibrinolysis, tissue remodeling, and heart damage have been investigated for their potential impact on clinical outcome [13, 48, 72].

Some of these biomarkers have been identified centrally in humans through proteomic technology in experimental studies using whole-brain proteasome, laser microdissection, and cerebral microdialysis or from CSF and then investigated at peripheral levels in circulating blood.

Biomarkers indicating the severity of brain damage would be helpful in guiding prognosis determination. Studies on whole-brain proteasome after ischemic stroke using 2D differential gel electrophoresis-based approach have served to show that actin levels resulted to be the biomarker with the most decreased levels in the infarct core compared with the contralateral areas while albumin levels increased the most. Interestingly, ischemic penumbra had an intermediate protein expression profile between that observed in ischemic core and the apparently intact contralateral area, confirming the potential of penumbra tissue as salvageable [61].

High levels of glial fibrillary acid protein (GFAP), which relate to astrogliosis, have been observed in infarct core. Specific proteins such as N-ethylmaleimide-sensitive factor (NSF) ATPase, which is involved in membrane trafficking in neurons, could become targets to avoid ischemia-reperfusion injury [105]. Peripheral levels of molecules like gelsolin, dihydropyrimidinase-related protein 2 (DRP2), and cystatin A were found to be independent predictors of poor outcome [117].

Studies using laser microdissection to isolate components of neurovascular unit (neurons or BBB components) of ischemic core or contralateral areas have identified neuronal specific adenosylhomocysteinase 2 (SAHH2) as a potential blood biomarker that could be used for early stroke prognosis. Indeed, its low circulating levels have been associated with neurological improvements after ischemic stroke. However, while the sensitivity of this biomarker for the discrimination of stroke outcomes was high (89%) its specificity resulted as moderate (58%). Therefore, probably a combination of SAHN2 with another prognostic biomarker as a panel might be more helpful in the assessment of stroke outcome [118].

Studies on human cerebral microdialysis have allowed in vivo investigations of changes in the composition of brain extracellular fluid from the ischemic core, the penumbra, and the contralateral hemisphere. Overall, 53 proteins have been identified which are highly expressed in the ischemic core and penumbra compared with the contralateral hemisphere. Among these, glutathione S-transferase P1 (GSTP1) and peroxiredoxin 1 (PRDX1), which seem to be involved in redox protective mechanisms, and protein S100B were proposed as blood biomarkers of stroke because circulating levels of these proteins were also higher in stroke patients than in healthy controls [132].

Additional biological data that had the potential to implement precision medicine for stroke prognosis determination can come from CSF and brain biopsy samples. However, as mentioned above, CSF extraction or brain biopsy cannot be routinely performed in stroke patients; therefore, for example most studies on CSF proteome have been performed postmortem when a massive brain injury occurs and this obviously can introduce a confounding effect in the findings and their interpretation. Nevertheless, once biomarkers are determined in CSF-based studies, their circulating levels could be investigated in terms of outcome prediction. The results of these studies showed that CSF levels of fatty acid-binding protein (FABP) were high after death [133]. Other proteins such as protein/nucleic acid glycase DJ-1, also known as PARK7, along with S100B and GFAP, have been identified as biomarkers of brain damage [134]. Further biomarkers from nonclinical studies on CSF samples obtained in rats after hyperacute middle cerebral artery occlusion (MCA)-related infarct have been measured in the blood of ischemic stroke patients and some of them seem to be promising in predicting functional outcome, such as calcium-calmodulin-dependent protein kinase II subunit-α (CaMK2A) and uridine monophosphate–cytidine monophosphate kinase (CMPK) [119].

Other potential prognostic biomarkers have been directly and systematically investigated in peripheral blood in humans.

These studies have shown that peripheral biomarkers may allow to evaluate ***response to acute treatments*** such as IV thrombolysis or endovascular treatment with mechanical thrombectomy, *in terms of prediction of early neurological deterioration, hemorrhagic transformation (in particular symptomatic hemorrhagic transformation), or recanalization*. Indeed, a number of different proteins have been considered and found to be associated with the response to treatment or prognosis of ischemic stroke in general and of treatment-related complications leading to poor outcome.

A meta-analysis of 82 studies, mostly on ischemic stroke, reporting a blood/CSF/urine biomarker measurement within 24 h of acute stroke and at least 2 serial assessments of clinical neurological status (<24 h and 7 days), showed that biomarkers associated with increased risk of early neurological deterioration were metabolic (glucose, glycosylated hemoglobin, low-density lipoprotein, cholesterol, triglycerides, urea, decreasing albumin), inflammatory, and excitotoxic (plasma glutamate, homocysteine, high-sensitivity C-reactive protein), and coagulation related/hematological (fibrinogen, decreasing hemoglobin) [85]. These biomarkers may identify groups of patients particularly at risk of vulnerability to tissue ischemia and brain damage progression, of plaque rupture/complications or thrombus progression, and, hence, of having a poor outcome. However, most of these biomarkers are not brain tissue or stroke specific but could be considered within panels including more specific biomarkers to increase their outcome predictive performance.

Matrix metalloproteinase-9 (MMP-9), a protease which plays a key role in microvascular and BBB integrity and in neuroinflammatory response, represents an optimal candidate biomarker for the prediction of hemorrhagic transformation with a gradient response when measured prior to IV thrombolytic treatment and also in non-thrombolysed ischemic stroke patients [73–75]. A meta-analysis including 12 clinical studies showed that levels of MMP-9 had a high sensitivity (85%) but suboptimal specificity (79%) in predicting hemorrhagic transformation after acute ischemic stroke [76]. Fibronectin and vascular adhesion protein 1 (VAP-1, part of the semicarbazide-sensitive amine oxidases which are involved in the process of immune cell migration and can be found on the cell surface or soluble in serum) may be considered additional potential candidates for hemorrhagic transformation; however, studies combining these biomarkers are lacking [111, 112, 120].

Low baseline levels of plasminogen activator inhibitor 1 (PAI1) or high baseline levels of thrombin activatable fibrinolysis inhibitor (TAFI), which are fibrinolytic inhibitors, have been associated with a poor response to IV thrombolysis with recombinant tissue plasminogen activator (rt-PA) [113]. Finally, low peripheral concentrations of disintegrin and metalloproteinase with thrombospondin motifs 13 (ADAMTS13) have also been associated with a poor response after recanalization therapies, either IV rt-PA or mechanical thrombectomy [100].

Levels of α2-antiplasmin resulted to be predictive of recanalization in patients treated with thrombolysis [114].

All these biomarkers could be helpful in the future in the prehospital setting or in centers where endovascular treatment is not available in order to well manage and speed the transfer of patients to comprehensive stroke centers in case of poor response, in terms of recanalization, to IV thrombolysis. The challenge is to find panels of biomarkers to use in clinical practice for predicting both the efficacy and safety of systemic thrombolysis and endovascular treatments [13].

Many candidate biomarkers specifically resulted to have an independent ***association with poor outcome*** [72]. Among these, there are inflammatory or astroglial and neuronal biomarkers. For inflammatory biomarkers such as C-reactive protein (CRP), interleukin-6 (IL-6), tumor necrosis factor-α (TNF-α), leukocyte-endothelial adhesion molecules (sICAM-1, sVCAM-1, sE-selectin, sP-selectin), and MMP-9, in most cases, data are still controversial. In particular, a large ($n = 160,309$) meta-analysis, the Northern Manhattan Study, and a systematic review showed that high levels of CRP were a significant predictor of poor outcome and they were associated with increased mortality, even nonvascular, after ischemic stroke [12, 88, 89]. Overall, based on the results of large epidemiological studies, CRP is more likely to represent biomarker of general illness rather than a reliable prognostic biomarker. Only some studies reported an association between high levels of TNF-α and poor outcome, in particular in patients with lacunar stroke [103]. MMP-9 has been found to be associated with measures influencing clinical outcomes in ischemic stroke patients, such as baseline neurological severity (i.e., NIHSS [National Health Institutes Stroke Scale]), infarct growth volume, and radiologic sign of BBB disruption (e.g., the hyperintense acute reperfusion injury marker, HARM sign) [77–80].

Regarding astroglial biomarkers, a systematic review including 18 studies and a total of 1643 patients found that high serum concentrations of protein S100B correlate with infarct volume, stroke severity, and functional outcome [82]. Among the neuronal biomarkers, neuron-specific enolase (NSE) and GFAP resulted to be associated with clinical outcome [84, 106].

Among other biomarkers, leptin/adiponectin ratio >1.16 measured at the first day of hospital admission has been associated with good 90-day functional outcome (mRS 0–2) in patients with atherothrombotic acute ischemic stroke. High serum levels of mannose-binding lectin (MLB), a component of the complement activation cascade, were associated with mortality and poor 90-day functional outcome [48].

Other biomarkers associated with mortality and/or 90-day functional outcome were low levels of 25-hydroxyvitamin D (25-OHD); high serum levels of progranulin, a multipotent growth factor; YKL-40, a glycoprotein associated with acute and chronic inflammation; neurofilament light, a neuronal scaffolding protein, also correlated with infarct volume and recurrent ischemic lesions; high levels of glycated hemoglobin or HbA1c; and low activity of ADAMTS13 [48]. All these biomarkers improved at a certain level the performance of the NIHSS and other traditional risk factor models for the prediction of poor functional outcome and mortality. However, further studies are still needed to validate these results and clarify their clinical implications.

Despite several attempts, no specific relevant panels of prognostic biomarkers for ischemic stroke have been identified; the panel of IL-6 and NT-proBNP (N-terminal fragment of the brain natriuretic peptide, a hormone secreted by the cardiac smooth muscle cells when stretched) resulted to be significantly associated with poor outcome. However, it seems that they do not consistently add accuracy of poor outcome prediction to models including simply measurable clinical variables [130].

Different results have been obtained with copeptin, a neuroendocrine marker released by the hypothalamus in equimolar concentrations to vasopressin, which is a hormone involved in the response to sympathetic activation and therefore to stress. Blood concentrations of copeptin have been found to be associated with stress levels in different conditions [135]. The addition of copeptin to neurological severity measured by NIHSS predicted both outcome and mortality at 90 days with a net reclassification improvement for functional outcome by 40% and for mortality by 50% suggesting a relevant incremental value of this blood biomarkers for risk stratification [63]. These results were confirmed by other studies [64–66].

It should be pointed out that the assessment of peripheral molecule levels has not been investigated for association only to general measures of outcome, such as disability or death, but also to all those ***complications that can lead to a poor outcome***. Indeed, besides hemorrhagic transformation, early prediction of cerebral edema, malignant infarction, post-stroke infections, seizures, stroke recurrence, or plaque instability by using biological data in combination with clinical and imaging data could undoubtedly allow to improve stroke management and prognosis determination.

Few biomarkers have been actually rigorously specifically investigated in this setting and independently validated in more than one cohort; therefore, further research is needed to implement the use of peripheral blood prognostic biomarkers in stroke precision medicine.

S100B values of >0.35 g/L measured at 12 h and a cutoff value of >1.03 g/L at 24 h after stroke onset had a sensitivity of 75% and 94% and a specificity of 80% and 83%, respectively, in predicting the development of a malignant infarction and cerebral edema [83].

Biomarkers such as IL-6, Th1/Th2 profile, copeptin, procalcitonin (used as a diagnostic marker of bacterial infections in hospitalized patients), or serum amyloid A (an acute-phase reactant) have been found to be associated with post-stroke infections [104]. Monocytic expression of the human leukocyte antigen gene *HLA-DR* resulted to be an independent predictor of an individual's ability to overcome post-stroke infections [107]. However, their accuracy, sensitivity, and specificity are still not adequate for implementing their use in clinical practice. Of note, regarding procalcitonin, the STRAWINSKI trial showed that antibiotic therapy guided by this biomarker after stroke was not superior to conventional management [136].

The identification of patients at higher risk of stroke recurrence would make the triage more efficient in the emergency setting, particularly in case of TIA. CRP, lipoprotein-associated phospholipase A2 (LpPLA2), and copeptin could be potential candidates for this purpose; however, different studies showed conflicting results [89–92]. Indeed, since CRP is an acute-phase reactant, its levels have been found to increase in linear correlation with the stroke severity and the number of comorbidities. Therefore, CRP tends to be more associated with mortality than stroke risk; however, its predictive value for stroke recurrence seems to be more apparent among lacunar stroke patients where the brain injury is smaller compared with other stroke subtypes and the consequent inflammatory reaction is lower [137]. LpPLA2 is a serine lipase that circulates in the peripheral blood linked to low-density lipoproteins (LDL) and metabolizes LDL to form free fatty acids and other proinflammatory molecules. It has been found to be independently associated not only to mortality and to first-ever stroke but also to stroke recurrence in population-based studies and independent cohorts [4, 92, 98, 99]. Indeed, LpPLA2 has been approved by FDA to predict the risk of both first-ever and recurrent strokes in healthy subjects. Therefore, this biomarker is helpful for establishing a proper prevention strategy in high-risk patients. Other biomarkers have been found to be associated with recurrent ischemic events in TIA patients where low plasma levels of lysophosphatidylcholine, which seem to add predicting value to the ABCD2 score, high levels of soluble CD40L (marker of atherosclerotic plaque instability), and increased levels of glycated albumin [48].

Different studies have shown an incremental value of copeptin levels for event recurrence over well-established clinical risk stratification models in patients with TIA and stroke [67–69]. Recently, a novel panel of three biomarkers, osteopontin, neopterin, and myeloperoxidase, has been investigated with promising results in terms of prediction of stroke recurrence, showing improved risk classification when added to a clinical model with a continuous net reclassification improvement of 29.1% [48].

In patients with large artery atherosclerotic stroke the following biomarkers resulted to be correlated with plaque instability although the specificity of these biomarkers for carotid atherosclerosis is uncertain since they may also reflect the inflammatory response to brain ischemia: serum levels of omentin-1, a protein regulating vascular inflammation; serum levels of complement complex C5b-9, also associated with plaque burden and degree of carotid stenosis; high-sensitivity CRP; and Lp-PLA2 [48].

Some biomarkers specific for ***ischemic stroke etiology*** could help in improving stroke prognosis through the choice of the correct prevention treatment strategy.

Since inflammation-related processes are shared by large vessel atherosclerosis and small vessel disease, inflammatory biomarkers, such as CRP, IL-6, IL-1b, and TNF-α, might be useful candidates for both stroke subtypes related to these etiopathogenetic mechanisms [72]. However, in the acute phase they are also elevated in cardioembolic stroke patients. Furthermore, intracellular adhesion molecule-1 (ICAM-1), soluble receptor for advanced glycation end products (sRAGE), fibrinogen, P-selectin, adiponectin, and Lp-PLA2 have also been associated with large vessel disease. In cardioembolic stroke, the natriuretic peptides have been extensively studied and the evidence is high. Several studies have found and confirmed that levels of B-type natriuretic peptides (BNP and NT-proBNP) have been found to be high in stroke of cardioembolic origin and in those patients with embolic stroke of undetermined source (ESUS) of ascertained cardioembolic source, and to be associated with stroke risk [121–123]. In addition, a relationship was observed between higher NT-proBNP levels and a relative benefit of warfarin compared with aspirin for prevention of recurrent stroke [124]. Given these findings, there is an ongoing clinical trial that has the objective to investigate whether anticoagulants can prevent recurrent strokes in patients who had a cryptogenic stroke and have high levels of natriuretic peptides [125]. Hence, these biomarkers seem to very likely become usable to implement precision medicine in clinical practice with implications on patient outcome.

With the inclusion of thrombectomy in the standard armamentarium of acute ischemic stroke management, the collection of samples of clots or endothelial cells retrieved during thrombectomy could become even more common (see the section below) [138]. The ***clot/thrombus composition and the histological and proteomic analysis of clots*** could provide important information on the potential stroke etiopathogenesis with implications for short- and long-term outcome. Furthermore, an in-depth knowledge of clot composition could allow a better definition of the corresponding imaging aspects of vessel occlusion, the identification of specific biological/imaging patterns, and the use of this information to evaluate and predict response to acute treatment.

Regarding the ***molecular signature of neuroimaging findings***, as mentioned above, great interest is rising in searching blood molecular biomarkers of *ischemic penumbra* which are even more affordable and easier to measure compared with genomics or transcriptomics. A recently published study on 216 patients from a large prospective study on biomarkers in acute ischemic stroke within 9 h of symptom onset found that elevated hyperacute plasma levels of oxidative stress biomarkers, such as F2-isoprostanes (F2-isoPs: products of non-cyclooxygenase free radical-induced neuronal arachidonic acid peroxidation of membrane phospholipids and lipoproteins) and oxygen radical absorbance capacity (ORAC: a measure of the blood antioxidant capacity), independently predicted radiographic evidence of MRI PWI-DWI mismatch >20% and mismatch salvage [86]. Interestingly, baseline F2-isoP levels also resulted to independently predict *infarct growth* occurrence and infarct growth volume which in turn positively correlates with mismatch volume [87]. Overall, these findings suggest that oxidative stress biomarkers are likely to have a role in predicting that part of ischemic penumbra which is prone to evolve toward infarction in the absence of an efficient spontaneous or pharmacological/mechanical recanalization/reperfusion [86]. In a previous study, serum IL-10 levels ≥23 pg/mL and glutamate ≥130 μmol/L were found to predict clinical-diffusion mismatch in patients with acute ischemic stroke [131]. If validated, these biomarkers may help in patient stratification in terms of response to treatment and outcome prediction for acute treatment decision-making processes and may serve as optimal targets for novel therapeutic interventions with neuroprotective effects.

Despite all these promising findings in the field of proteomics in ischemic stroke, it should be considered that with 250,000 proteins in addition to 20,000 coding genes, noncoding genes, metabolites, and lipids which represent a huge flood of information, the molecular and namely the proteomic signature of prognosis of ischemic stroke is still being determined. The subsequent step would be to compare well-established clinical models for risk stratification and prognosis including blood biomarkers to the same models without the biomarkers. After that, it would be necessary that biomarkers or biomarker panels that are potentially optimal and meaningful candidates for being the molecular fingerprints of outcome prediction should be taken to the next level of validation and translation into clinical practice.

9.4.3.2 Intracerebral Hemorrhage

Several biomarkers have been associated with different pathophysiological pathways in ICH (markers involved in coagulation processes [e.g., D-dimers], neuroendocrine markers (e.g., copeptin), systemic metabolic markers [e.g., blood glucose levels], markers of inflammation [e.g., IL-6], as well as growth factors [e.g., VEGF], and others [e.g., glutamate]) [70].

Some of those blood biomarkers are agents of pathologic processes associated with hemorrhagic stroke but also other diseases, whereas others play more distinct pathophysiological roles and help in understanding the basic mechanisms of brain damage and/or recovery in ICH. These last biomarkers seem to be promising in the management of ICH and in contributing additional information to the current models for risk stratification, early intervention, and prognosis determination. Furthermore, like for ischemic stroke also for ICH, prognostic molecular biomarkers could be useful for reliably discriminating the risk of rebleeding to guide intervention triage, for the choice of the most adequate late interventions, such as rehabilitation, but also as therapeutic targets for the development of novel treatments.

MMP-9 as a protease induced by thrombin can have a harmful role by increasing capillary permeability, disrupting BBB, and being neurotoxic by degrading the endothelial basal lamina and extracellular matrix. However, this biomarker can also have a beneficial role since it promotes angiogenesis, remodeling, and cell migration. In ICH, MMP-9 is significantly associated with edema development and extent, hematoma growth ($r = 0.64$), and neurological worsening [81]. If validated in independent cohorts, MMP-9 as a marker of hematoma growth could become relevant in selecting patients for hemicraniectomy.

BNP plays a role in the disease progression of brain injury including ICH [139], although the underlying mechanism is unknown, and has been found to independently predict outcome at discharge [126].

Low levels of VAP-1 independently predicted neurological improvement after 48 h from ICH symptom onset (OR = 6.8) probably through the reduction of brain cell injury [140]. Further studies are required in order to better determine whether this biomarker could be an optimal outcome predictor like other imaging variables such as hematoma volume and early hematoma growth.

Soluble Fas (s-Fas) are variant molecular splicing products of the Fas-receptor/ligand apoptosis signaling pathway and they are part of the TNF receptor family. Some of these molecules seem to be potential inhibitors of the Fas-apoptosis system and to correlate with neuronal death [127]; however, this role should be further elucidated. Low levels of s-Fas at baseline have been independently associated with perihematomal edema growth (OR = 0.125) [128].

S100B protein correlates with disease progression by inducing neuronal death and promoting inflammatory stress with the release of IL-1, IL-6, and TNF-α [141, 142]. Levels of S100B increased in patients with ICH reaching a peak at 3 days. Small studies found S100B as an independent predictor of early mortality and functional outcome at discharge. The predictive value of S100B (AUC = 0.88) resulted to be slightly lower than that of clinical (Glasgow Coma Scale [GCS] score) (AUC = 0.94) and imaging (ICH volume) (AUC = 0.93) variables [126, 143]. Demonstration of the incremental value of this biomarker for prognosis determination in larger prospective studies is needed.

In patients with ICH, observational and case-control studies showed that inflammatory biomarkers (TNF-α, ICAM-1, IL-6, IL-10, IL-11) play a relevant role in the rupture of vessels, further bleeding and necrosis, and severity of stroke in the acute phase, predicting mortality (TNF-α, IL-6, CRP), early hematoma growth (IL-6), poor functional outcome (IL-6, IL-10, ICAM-1, HMGB-1 [high mobility group box 1]), and rebleeding (IL-10 with a 75% sensitivity and 72% specificity). It should be considered that inflammatory biomarkers may contribute to neurological damage in the beginning but may contribute to recovery in late ICH [93–97].

CD34+, which are progenitors of endothelial cells, along with vascular endothelial growth factors [VEGF], Ang-1 (angiopoietin-1), and granulocyte colony-stimulating factor (G-CSF), have been found to be valuable prognostic biomarkers during the recovery phase more than during the acute phase since they play a crucial role in angiogenesis with implication on neurological improvement and functional outcome [101, 102].

Glutamate, an important neurotransmitter released by necrotic astrocytes, is involved in the excitotoxicity process, and consequently associated with poor neurological outcome [70].

Biomarkers easily measurable in routine clinical practice such as blood glucose or serum cholesterol levels, which are probably involved in the integrity of vessel walls, can also be helpful in outcome determination. Indeed, high levels of blood glucose and low levels of LDL cholesterol and total cholesterol levels have been associated with outcome measures like mortality after ICH (blood glucose levels: adjusted HR 1.10, 95% CI 1.01–1.19; LDL cholesterol levels: OR 6.34) [115]. Low levels of LDL cholesterol predict hematoma growth (OR 4.24) and early neurological deterioration (OR 8.27) and pretreatment with statin seem not to have an influence [116]. However, blood glucose levels are found increased also in other critically ill patients and LDL cholesterol levels do not provide information on the additive value compared to other prognostic scores.

Coagulation markers such as D-dimer, fibrinogen, and factor XIII may add prognostic information. In ICH, their blood concentrations change as the hemostatic system is activated and have been independently associated with relevant outcome measures: D-dimer, with 30-day mortality (sensitivity of 70% and specificity of 60%), GCS score, midline shift, and subarachnoid extension of the hemorrhage; fibrinogen, with neurological deterioration (OR 5.6); and factor XIII, with hematoma growth. Unfortunately, at the best cutoff levels, these biomarkers have a relatively moderate specificity [109, 110].

Free ferritin is found in the brain after ICH due to the escaped erythrocytes. The release of iron can lead to delayed brain edema through neuronal injury mediated by oxidative stress, glutamate-induced excitotoxicity, and inflammatory response. A high correlation has been found between free serum levels of ferritin and poor outcome in terms of edema volumes and ICH severity ($r > 0.60$) [108].

As it has been observed with ischemic stroke, copeptin, as a neuroendocrine stress marker, can help in risk stratification. Its levels, measured within 72 h from symptom onset, were found to positively correlate with hematoma volume and negatively with GCS score. Furthermore, it resulted as an independent predictor of neurological deterioration, 30-day mortality (AUC 0.88), and 90-day poor functional outcome (AUC 0.68) [71].

Heat-shock protein-70 (HSP-70) is involved in the process of protein folding and has a role in protecting cells from stressors such as hypoxia. It has been found higher in non-survivors than in survivors after ICH. Although this marker has the potential to become a prognostic marker, it seems not to add value to ICH outcome clinical models [70].

Plasma microparticle concentrations are small membrane particles released by cells under stress conditions like ICH, having a role in coagulation and inflammation and therefore in neuronal damage after ICH. This biomarker levels were found elevated in patients with intraventricular hemorrhage, lower GCS score, or greater ICH volumes, and predicted early mortality (7-day mortality) with a 91% sensitivity and 69% specificity. Future studies should be focused on the origin of plasma microparticles in plasma in order to understand which cell types are involved in ICH-related cerebral injury [70].

Other potential prognostic protein biomarkers for ICH are serum fibulin-5, an extracellular matrix protein which predicts mortality and 90-day functional outcome and has been found associated with disease severity, and admission serum levels of calcium ≤ 2.41 mmol/L which could predict both death and 90-day major disability [70, 129].

If we try to select the most interesting candidates among the above-indicated prognostic biomarkers for ICH, we should consider that one of the most important issues in ICH is to individuate those patients at risk of further hematoma expansion that could benefit from intensive blood pressure lowering, pharmacological hemostatic treatments, or surgical interventions (e.g., hemicraniectomy or minimally invasive procedures). Plasma biomarkers predicting further bleeding, such as low LDL and high MMP-9, factor XIII, TNF-α, IL-6, and IL-10, could help to detect this group of patients and individualize therapeutic interventions. However, only randomized trials comparing algorithms with and without the additional information from blood biomarker values could address these issues. Of the abovementioned biomarkers, only few were investigated in studies with large sample size (i.e., blood glucose levels, S100/RAGE, fibrinogen, CRP, GFAP); however, they still need to be further validated in at least similarly large studies [70].

Since blood biomarkers could follow dynamic changes over time, there is the need to take into account the time from symptom onset to withdrawal and perform serial measurements at predefined time points in order to adequately interpret the results on the outcome predictive biomarker value at given time points. This was done in the studies on the following biomarkers: S100B, TNF-α, IL-11, HSP-70, microparticles, and ferritin.

Only S100B has shown a predictive performance for 7-day mortality close to that of a clinical model including GCS and ICH score or imaging data; however, it seems not to add value to this model.

As mentioned above, since some of these biomarkers could serve as links to better understand the pathophysiology of ICH, they could represent potential therapeutic targets for the development of novel treatment. For example, copeptin could be a key player for the development of cerebral edema as shown by the effects of arginine vasopressin (AVP) V1 in mice models, which seems to decrease the leukocyte migrations into the injured area. Similarly, studies in rats showed a neuroprotective effect of s-Fas and deferoxamine, an iron chelant, in reducing cell death and post-ICH edema, confirming the detrimental role of ferritin in disease progression. Animal models of traumatic brain injury or ICH treated with BNP showed a decrease of inflammatory markers (TNF-α and IL-6) and reduction of neuronal damage. Translation of these results to humans is still unclear because conversely with studies in animals, in ICH patients, high levels of BNP have been found to be associated with unfavorable outcome [70].

Although promising prognostic biomarkers in ICH have been individuated, development of further research hypotheses and studies in the setting of precision medicine are urgently needed for this devastating cerebrovascular condition.

9.4.4 Metabolomics

The complex biochemical processes underlying brain damage in stroke include changes in local and systemic metabolism, such as in cellular energy metabolism pathways and systemic stress response. Therefore, some studies have tried to understand whether circulating levels of metabolites can be used as biomarkers in stroke. Metabolites are small molecules and can be lipids, amino acids, carbohydrates, and nucleotides; the technology used for their identification is based on NMR spectroscopy and mass spectrometry. The blood metabolome is simply the expression of genes and is related to environmental aspects such as diet, life habits, and gut microbiota [13]. Therefore, the metabolome profile in stroke patients could allow to have information on system biology and pathophysiological mechanisms underlying stroke. The majority of the studies on metabolomics in stroke have been focused on ischemic stroke and particularly on stroke diagnosis, stroke risk definition, and differentiation of stroke etiologies while the specific role of metabolomics in the prediction of stroke outcome has not been systematically investigated. However, metabolomics of stroke risk and etiology could already serve to provide information helpful for assessing stroke prognosis (Table 9.4). Indeed, the individuation of a metabolomic profile of the stroke risk could be used for putting in place the right preventive strategies, particularly secondary, for each single-stroke patient, including pharmacological treatments and dietary intake. Data on approximately 70,000 patients coming from 30 observational studies have suggested an association between the levels of linoleic acid (one of the polyunsaturated fatty acids) and a lower risk of cardiovascular risk in general and of stroke [148]. Other studies found that levels of triacylglycerols and cholesterol esters with low carbon numbers and double-bond content resulted to be predictors of a cardiovascular risk including stroke and to add predictive performance to a clinical model including classic risk factors [144]. These results could have important implications in stroke precision medicine in terms of personalized dietary counselling and lipid management, which instead is currently focused on cholesterol levels alone, thus contributing to modification of patient prognosis. Data on the metabolic profiles from the Atherosclerosis Risk in Communities (ARIC) study on the metabolomic profiles of patients showed that higher levels of products of the ω-oxidation of fatty acids, such as long-chain dicarboxylic acids tetradecanedioate and hexadecanedioate, resulted to be associated with the risk of ischemic cardioembolic stroke but the biological rationale

Table 9.4 Potential optimal candidate metabolites identified in metabolomics studies for future application of precision medicine in prognosis determination in stroke

Metabolite	Description	Evidence and application in prognosis determination	Reference
Linoleic acid	ω-6 Polyunsaturated fatty acid	Predictors of a cardiovascular risk including stroke and add predictive performance to a clinical model including classic risk factors	[13, 144]
Tetradecanedioate Hexadecanedioate	ω-Oxidation-derived long-chain dicarboxylic acids	Higher levels associated with risk of ischemic cardioembolic stroke	[13, 145]
Free fatty acids, tricarboxylic acid cycle intermediates succinate, α-ketoglutarate, and malate	Lipids Succinate: Tricarboxylic acid cycle	Higher levels in patients with cardioembolic stroke compared with patients with non-cardioembolic stroke; succinate was also associated with left atrial enlargement and subclinical atrial dysfunction	[13, 146, 147]

underlying this association has not been established yet [145]. Levels of free fatty acids, tricarboxylic acid cycle intermediates succinate, α-ketoglutarate, and malate were higher in patients with cardioembolic stroke compared with patients with non-cardioembolic stroke and succinate was also associated with left atrial enlargement and subclinical atrial dysfunction [146, 147].

In conclusion, similarly with genomics, transcriptomics, and proteomics, also for metabolomics, inconsistencies in the results on the associations of different metabolites with stroke risk and etiologies could be related to study design flaws. Small sample sizes do not help to achieve the adequate statistical power to detect the actual differences between large numbers of metabolites. Furthermore, there is a wide across-study heterogeneity in terms of inclusion/exclusion criteria and time from stroke onset to blood sample collection. Different techniques for metabolite detection have been used and this could further confound the results. Therefore, there is the need to overcome these limitations to make data on the association between metabolites and stroke risk and etiologies more reliable and closer to clinical application [13]. Finally, specific studies to investigate the association between peripheral metabolites and stroke outcome and their role in prognosis determination should be performed.

9.4.5 Other Molecular Biomarkers

Caveolin-1 is a membrane protein and the main component of caveolae which are 50–100 nm cell surface plasma membrane invaginations that are abundant in endothelial cells and play a major role in the regulation of endothelial vesicular trafficking and signal transduction and seems to be involved in the pathogenesis of vascular diseases [149]. Therefore, caveolin-1 could be a promising candidate stroke biomarker and target for novel treatments. Recent studies show that caveolin levels are decreased in the serum of patients with Moyamoya [150]. Furthermore, the caveolin-1 expression is crucial for vascular endothelial growth factor-induced angiogenesis [151].

Chemokines (stromal cell-derived factor 1α [SDF-1α]) are among other potential emerging prognostic stroke biomarkers and their levels have been found to be increased in the infarcted brain during the acute phase of stroke as a consequence of neurorestorative processes, and to decrease over time [151].

Extracellular vesicles (EVs) are small vesicles with a diameter of 0.1–1 μm that can include genetic information (e.g., miRNA) as well as proteins and may play a crucial role in cell communications. For example, stem cell-derived EVs may impact neurovascular plasticity and functional recovery [152]. Methods for analyzing EVs are complicated due to the very small size of these molecular biomarkers; therefore studies investigating the role of EVs in stroke in general and in stroke prognosis are currently at a rudimentary state of development [152].

9.4.6 Cellular Markers

Significant progress in understanding the pathobiology of circulating peripheral blood cells in stroke has been made. Not only the innate immune system but also the adaptive immune system mediated by lymphocytes may also be involved in stroke prognosis. Increased count of monocyte expressing Toll-like receptor-4 (TLR-4) was independently associated with large infarct volume in multivariable model [153]. Increased number of CD4+ CD28− cells in acute phase of stroke was reported to be associated with higher risk of stroke recurrence and was an independent predictor of death [154].

Higher levels of endothelial progenitor cells (EPC), a marker of vascular injury, have been found to be independently associated with smaller acute infarction and final infarct volumes, less infarct growth, and less poor clinical outcome after adjustments for major factors influencing EPC [155]. Similar results were obtained in different studies; therefore, although larger prospective studies are needed to confirm the role of EPC in stroke prognosis as well as there is the need of a consensus regarding the definition of EPC, EPC levels might be considered as a potential prognostic candidate for stroke.

Overall, despite these findings, thus far no single-cell population was identified that fully meets biomarker definition. Methodologically robust prospective studies with a priori sample size calculations and predefined endpoints, in addition to systematic evaluation of accuracy, are required.

9.4.7 Integromics

If we take into account that the risk of stroke, its occurrence, and severity depend on an interrelation between environmental risk factors and extraordinarily complex molecular aspects including DNA, epigenetic changes, RNA transcripts, proteins, and metabolites, then it is obvious to conclude that a better and an in-depth understanding of the biology and pathophysiology of stroke and stroke outcome will derive by the combination of all this information.

In order to achieve a more precise approach to diagnosis, risk stratification, choice of tailored safe and effective treatments, and clinical outcome prediction which can reflect into an overall improved patient prognosis, the next future application of stroke precision medicines in terms of molecular prognostic biomarkers would be to integrate all information derived from each level of omics (i.e., genomics, transcriptomics, proteomics, and metabolomics). The objective is to have a better understanding of the interactions between processes at different molecular levels, of their biological role in the pathophysiological mechanisms underlying cerebrovascular diseases, and of their clinical relevance. This will bring our knowledge of system biology to the next levels to increase the reliability and plausibility of data coming from omics and our ability to personalize outcome prediction and consequent treatment and management of stroke patients. The integromics approach has not been used yet so far in the stroke research field. Integromics studies will need to use specific statistical methods in order to correctly eliminate the noise derived by the number and variability of molecular and clinical data, and from the possible biological irrelevance of some of the investigated molecules. Furthermore, they should take into account that the biomarker/s with large or at least moderate changes and association with stroke prognosis will be the best candidate/s for translating its/their use into clinical practice and for being the best therapeutic target/s [13].

Some initiatives of particular interest, such as the Trans-Omics for Precision Medicine (TOPMed) program initiative, are being put in place and are very promising [156].

9.4.8 System Biology

System biology is a very sophisticated approach to integromics that combines data at different molecular levels with computational modeling and considers the system as a whole to make easier the identification of biomarkers with an actual prognostic and therapeutic value [13]. This approach also enables to assess the dynamic of molecular biomarker interaction over time. Therefore, it allows to better evaluate for each single individual which is the time point of the stroke disease course when those specific biomarkers should be measured or to better define the therapeutic window for particular treatments [13]. The system biology approach is still at an embryonal state in the stroke field where heterogeneity and biological complexity make its application more difficult. Bioinformatics is necessary to properly integrate molecular and clinical data and provide a global view of cerebrovascular diseases as well as new methods. Indeed, bidirectional Mendelian randomization is used to differentiate biomarkers that are most likely to be causal from those that are most likely a consequence of stroke [157]. For example, the use of this method has suggested that higher peripheral levels of lipids, homocysteine, and CC-chemokine ligand 2 (CCL2, also known as MCP1) are associated with an increased risk of stroke [158–161]. Furthermore, bidirectional Mendelian randomization could enable the assessment of the effects of a drug on a specific risk factor by investigating how genetic variants that modulate the expression of drug target are associated with the disease. This could lead to improvement of study design on stroke treatment, including combined therapies, and on stroke prognosis. A similar approach can be used to predict outcome in terms of adverse events.

Integromics and system biology represent the future of stroke personalized medicine through the development of experimental disease models including simulation of MCA occlusion-related stroke effects by decreasing uptake levels of metabolites into the brain leading to change in glutamate levels. These models could allow comparisons of biomarkers and molecular pathways, the so-called diseasome which could guide the investigations of novel therapeutic options [13].

9.4.9 Conclusions

Despite the tremendous progress in the technology of omics in the last years, the translatability of the results from basic and clinical studies to clinical practice of these technologies as an approved standardized tool to predict prognosis in stroke is a challenge. The main issue is represented by the misconception that in neurological diseases a biomarker or a panel of biomarkers can fit all, but instead particularly patients with neurovascular diseases respond differently to treatments and have different prognosis as a consequence of several factors including specific genomic and proteomic profiles. Furthermore, clinical implementation of omics is slowed by the need to perform large studies with very expensive technology to employ and to validate the results in similarly large independent cohorts.

Therefore, precision medicine is the new and ultimate frontier of the prognostic molecular biomarker research in stroke because it can take into account the interindividual variability. Strategies for increasing the probability to detect protein in picogram or nanogram concentration in the peripheral blood would be the use of antibodies to enrich cerebrovascular proteins. This would be possible using extracellular vesicles, including exosome and microparticles, which are specific to their cells of origin and, therefore, those deriving from brain endothelial cells are likely to be a good source of protein biomarkers potentially associated with changes occurring after stroke and to be helpful for prognosis determination. Another future approach to increase the specificity and sensitivity of prognostic molecular biomarkers and to overcome the stroke heterogeneity as much as possible would be to combine different promising biomarkers in a unique panel. This would increase their individual performance in patient stratification and outcome prediction along with clinical parameters such as age, sex, neurological severity measured by NIHSS, or vascular risk factors. The challenge is to combine the correct biomarkers based on their association with specific complex pathophysiological aspects of stroke and investigate them in large clinical studies.

In any case, in order to allow omics to transform the current clinical general practice in the field of cerebrovascular diseases into personalized stroke medicine and tailored prognosis determination with the objective to dramatically improve patient management and outcome, it is of utmost importance that efforts are put in place for future studies to adequately validate specific findings and before they are integrated into clinical practice.

9.5   Markers Related to Clot Histopathological Composition

After mechanical thrombectomy has become part of the standard of care for patients with acute large vessel occlusion-related ischemic stroke, investigations on clot composition have surged renewed interest. The objective is to find on an individual basis a biological plausibility and correlation with corresponding imaging characteristics and stroke etiology to improve prediction of response to IV thrombolysis and thrombectomy, thrombectomy speed, and completeness, to choose the best and most adequate secondary prevention treatment, and therefore to improve patient outcome. Indeed, high rates of clot fragmentation and failure to remove the clot resulting in poor neurological outcomes indicate that further advance in acute stroke endovascular treatment may benefit from a better understanding of the clot science.

A recently published review on histopathological composition of acute ischemic stroke clot pointed out the need to better differentiate the composition of different types of clots in terms of omics and not only based on their histopathological and immunohistochemical characteristics that distinguish red blood cell-rich, fibrin-rich, fibrin/platelet-rich, and mixed thrombi, including the presence of calcifications [162]. The definition of clot features and a complete understanding of the across-individual distribution of clot phenotypes could also help to study resistance to and, hence, the outcome of thrombectomy also depending on the use of different types of devices.

Red blood cell-rich clots seem to be associated with significantly higher recanalization rates, reduced number of maneuvers, and a shorter mean recanalization time than fibrin-rich clots. Calcifications, high percentage of white blood cells, high platelet-to-lymphocyte ratio as a marker of inflammation, increased levels of factor von Willebrand and low ADAMTS13, and low amount of neutrophil elastase-positive cells are associated with a poor revascularization outcome, extended mechanical revascularization time, and a poorer clinical outcome [162].

Precision medicine could also help to address all the issues and controversial findings regarding the associations between clot histology/immunohistology and stroke etiology: for example, between red blood cell-rich emboli and cardioembolic vs. large artery atherosclerosis; between fibrin/platelet-rich emboli or embolus rich of white blood cells and cardioembolic stroke; and between the presence of neutrophil extracellular traps (NET, fibrous networks of extracellular DNA released by neutrophils) and emboli of cardiac origin vs. any etiologies, or the presence of immune cells as components of erythrocytic and red clot more than white and mixed clot and the uncertainties of their role in the pathogenesis of stroke. The mechanisms by which blood cells, coagulation factors, and immune cells interact in the different types of clots and their influences on prognosis are not well and completely understood yet. Precision medicine through the omics technology could allow a better understanding of the molecular mechanism of thrombus formation and inform for a consequent more adequate and correct definition of stroke phenotypes, particularly in the group of patients with stroke of undetermined source. Some studies have identified several proteins mostly related to inflammation; however, larger studies and validation in independent cohorts are needed. In the next future, the use of artificial intelligence with machine learning could become an important tool for the analysis and quantification of histological and immunohistochemically stained clot images. Machine learning-based image analysis software packages can allow for quick and accurate quantification of tissue components by using automated segmentation algorithms combined with trainable cell/tissue classification. These techniques will undoubtedly increase the accuracy and reproducibility of quantitative clot histopathology which will be crucial for a personalized determination of clot cellular composition in acute ischemic stroke patients [162].

Clear recommendations on how to apply the continuing increasing knowledge in clot composition in stroke precision medicine are yet to come; however, they should be always considered in the context of individual arterial anatomy and collaterals characteristics of stroke patients.

9.6   Neuroimaging Markers

In stroke precision medicine, similarly to a molecular profile, there is an imaging profile for each or some phenotype/s of cerebrovascular diseases that should be taken into account. In relation to the importance of data, neuroimaging prognostic biomarkers should not be considered the last in the hierarchy after molecular prognostic biomarkers. Indeed, advances in neuroimaging technologies have allowed to better evaluate the pathophysiology of stroke in general and particularly cerebral hemodynamics, intracranial vessel status, and possible degree of reversibility of ischemic damage [9, 163, 164].

The wider availability of advanced imaging is increasing the amount of data available and therefore the size of the dataset to analyze.

It should be considered that neuroimaging is usually acquired only when symptoms of neurovascular disorders become overt while, since cerebrovascular diseases can be considered a *continuum*, as mentioned above, the brain damage from vascular alterations can be progressive and lead to neuro- and vascular degeneration that could culminate with acute events such as transient attacks, ischemic or hemorrhagic strokes, or mild cognitive impairment/dementia. The ideal would be to monitor with longitudinal serial neuroimaging at different time points the chronic impact of microvascular disorders and risk factor modification or response to certain treatment.

9.6.1   Neuroimaging in Ischemic Stroke

The severity of neurovascular changes detectable on neuroimaging with prognostic implications is mainly represented by vessel narrowing, symptomatic or silent lesion size, brain atrophy, parenchyma perfusion, and collateral circulation status.

First of all, neuroimaging is fundamental for the definition of *stroke etiopathogenesis* and, hence, a more precise determination of stroke phenotype which should be a prerequisite for properly predicting stroke outcome and for a correct interpretation and application of the results of genetic studies on prognosis. Imprecise ischemic stroke subtyping could occur, for example, in the case of large vessel occlusion (large artery atherosclerosis) related stroke. Indeed, TOAST classification does not distinguish between extracranial and intracranial carotid artery disease, which are two distinct conditions with different epidemiology and prevalence in Caucasians, Asians, Hispanics, and Blacks; different pathophysiology of related stroke; and different rate of recurrence and response to the available treatment options [4, 165]. In fact, angioplasty/stenting has been proved to be effective for extracranial artery disease while it was found to be inferior to medical treatment in intracranial artery disease [4]. Similarly, if an adequate neuroimaging diagnostic workup is not performed, a small infarct related to artery-to-artery thromboembolism from large artery atherosclerosis may be classified as a lacunar infarct related to small vessel disease [4].

Advanced neuroimaging can help in defining the dynamics of cerebrovascular diseases in terms of tissue perfusion, collaterals, cerebral autoregulation, and infarct expansion. These properties have served in clinical trials on acute ischemic stroke to investigate highly selected and more homogeneous patient populations and hence to increase the precision and efficiency of clinical trials. Although this obviously can lead to a reduction of eligible patients and slower enrolment rate, studies on reperfusion treatment using imaging selection methods showed larger benefit than the studies without imaging selection, as it has been observed for in the trials on tenecteplase and endovascular thrombectomy [2, 166–171]. Patients with a favorable penumbra pattern can have improved outcomes and smaller infarct volumes and infarct growth compared with patients without a penumbral pattern.

Imaging of Infarct Core and Ischemic Penumbra

In the emergency setting, in ischemic stroke, imaging data may elucidate pathophysiology and help in _selecting eligible patients who are more likely to respond to acute treatments_ (IV thrombolysis and/or endovascular treatment with thrombectomy which has been recently officially included in the stroke therapeutic armamentarium) _and to have a favorable outcome outside the therapeutic window_ from 6 to 24 h since the last time the patient had been seen in good health or patients with wake-up stroke. Examples derive from the last two RCTs DAWN, DEFUSE-3, and WAKE-UP where the use of neuroimaging was crucial to investigate the timing of the pathophysiology of acute ischemic stroke, by calculating the volume of the ischemic core (central area of tissue irreversibly damaged) and/or ischemic penumbra (area surrounding the infarct core where neural cells are electrically silent but structurally viable and, therefore, still salvageable) [172–174]. Therefore, a transition from "temporal window" to "cerebral tissue" window has definitely taken place, mainly based on different individual neuroanatomical and physiological parameters that have an impact on the determination of response to brain ischemic damage. This is true when it is considered that patients receiving reperfusion therapy within 6 h but without good collateral circulations may have a rapid progression of ischemic penumbra into infarction, which defines the "fast progressors," while those patients with good collateral are more likely to preserve the salvageability/reversibility of the ischemic penumbra for a longer time, which defines the "slow progressors" [175].

The neuroimaging methods used for selecting acute stroke patients on an individual basis for tailoring the right treatment are CT perfusion (CTP), triphasic angioscopy, MRI with DWI, PWI, and FLAIR sequence. Infarct core is generally identified by DWI lesion and significantly reduced cerebral blood flow (CBF) or cerebral blood volume (CBV) on CT perfusion (CTP) while potentially viable tissue is defined by hypoperfusion which is identified as tissue with prolonged contrast transit but with normal DWI on MRI (PWI-DWI mismatch) or normal CBF or CBV on CTP. In particular [176]:

1. *Infarct core on DWI*: DWI lesion volume is a relatively well-established independent predictor of unfavorable outcome despite the reperfusion/recanalization therapy, as confirmed by the recent large clinical trials on endovascular treatment (including DEFUSE 2, DEFUSE 3, SWIFT-PRIME, and EXTEND-IA) [177].
2. *Infarct core on CTP*: Various parameters derived from CTP have been used to define ischemic core, including CBF, CBV, and delay time (DT). However, the optimal parameter and threshold for defining ischemic core have not yet been established (CBF thresholds range from 4.8 to 8.4 mL/100 g/min or absolute CBV of 2.0 mL × 100/g, or DT $\geq$2 s, or the combination of relative CBF [rCBF] $\leq$30% and DT $\geq$3 s). Interestingly, CBV ASPECTS resulted to have a predictive value of neurological outcome better than ASPECTS on NCCT, particularly at the cutoff of 9 [176].
3. *Imaging of ischemic penumbra*: Perfusion-weighted imaging (PWI) can semi-quantitatively or quantitatively reflect hemodynamic information using the various parameters, including CBF, CBV, mean transit time (MTT), and time to maximum of tissue residue function (Tmax) with high spatial and temporal resolution. Data from the DEFUSE trial demonstrated that, in patients with DWI-PWI mismatch ratio of 2.6, reperfusion was associated with a favorable response (sensitivity, 90%; specificity, 83%). Furthermore, in patients with early reperfusion, the frequency of favorable clinical response increased with increasing mismatch ratio, while in patients without reperfusion, larger mismatch ratios were related with negative outcomes. In addition, clinical outcome of acute ischemic stroke patients with comparable DWI-PWI mismatch is time dependent, which was confirmed by several large trials (DEFUSE 2, DEFUSE 3, SWIFT-PRIME, EXTEND-IA) [177].

Finally, combining quantitative DWI and MTT with NIHSS had powerful prognostic value. Indeed, lesion volumes of DWI and MTT predicted outcome better than mismatch or percentage mismatch. All patients with a large DWI volume and a high NIHSS score had poor outcomes, whereas patients with a small MTT volume and a low NIHSS score had good outcomes. Combination of clinical and imaging thresholds improved predictive value (70%) over sole clinical (43%) or imaging thresholds (54%) [176].

CTP penumbra volume, defined as time to peak (TTP)-CBV mismatch, was demonstrated to be an independent predictor of clinical outcome, especially in patients achieving recanalization.

Unfortunately, there is not full agreement on which time metrics (mean transit time, time to peak, delay time, or time to the maximal tissue) and which cutoffs should be considered optimal for indication of the presence of ischemic penumbra [178]. In some cases, specific software, like RAPID, that enable automated calculations of volumes can be used for support and for speeding imaging reading and assessment. It is still unknown which is the best method selection for these patients in the acute setting.

Criteria of the DEFUSE 3 trial for treating thrombectomy patients between 6 and 16 h from the last known well include DWI and PWI MRI and the corresponding mismatch PWI-DWI while criteria of the DAWN trial for the longer therapeutic window between 6 and 24 h include TC perfusion or DWI [172, 173]. A different neuroimaging approach, the so-called DWI-FLAIR mismatch, is used for the selection of wake-up stroke patients, for which the presence of areas of altered diffusion restriction in DWI sequences associated with a corresponding area of absent or tenuous hyperintensity in FLAIR is indicative of symptom onset within 4.5 h, which is the therapeutic window approved for IV thrombolysis [174].

Given the above, the use of advanced imaging allows to define an individualized temporal, clinical, and radiological profile of a patient with ischemic stroke, which supports the physicians not only in the decision-making process for tailored acute treatment but also in the prediction of the single patient short- and long-term outcome.

The next challenges are first of all to further improve the selection of patients by achieving a standardization of image acquisition parameters and of specific automated software in order to make the patient stratification by revascularization and clinical outcome reproducible and reliable, and by reducing the time of acquisition minimizing the delays to treatment. The second challenge is to make wider the availability of advanced neuroimaging in order to guarantee recommended treatment to a large as possible number of patients. Furthermore, other unanswered questions should be addressed, such as whether complete or partial occlusions are identical, and whether patients with pure clot are the same as those with atherosclerotic stenosis plus clot, and the same for those with or without collaterals. Finally, the next step would be trying to change the current practice from performing advanced neuroimaging at a single time point to a serial imaging acquisition that could be helpful for a better determination of prognosis in terms of functional recovery [179].

The following other neuroimaging markers can be considered valuable for the determination of clinical outcome on individual basis in ischemic stroke, may play a guiding or referential role in therapy and clinical recovery, and therefore could be included in the artificial intelligence algorithm for personalized prognostication.

Early parenchymal abnormalities: It was demonstrated that, in acute MCA occlusion, early parenchymal abnormalities were significantly associated with subsequent infarct location and extension. In particular, the presence of two or three signs (attenuation of lentiform nucleus, loss of the insular ribbon, or hemispheric sulci effacement) was significantly associated with extended infarction and could predict poor outcome [176].

Other Imaging of the Infarct Core

1. *Alberta Stroke Program Early CT score (ASPECTS)*: Strong predictor of neurological functional outcome at 3 months (sensitivity 0.78 and specificity 0.96) in patients with acute ischemic stroke regardless of the treatment with IV thrombolysis [176].

2. *Fractional anisotropy (FA) of corticospinal tract*: Diffusion tensor imaging (DTI), an imaging technique for assessing the integrity of the white matter, enables visualization and quantification of microstructural damage to white matter tracts in vivo. Studies of subacute and chronic stroke patients showed that the FA of corticospinal tract decreased due to anterograde degeneration of axons and myelin sheaths of affected tracts, also known as Wallerian degeneration. However, it offered minimal predictive value of motor outcomes at 3 months when applied in an acute phase. More evidence from specific studies is needed [176].

3. *Imaging of corticospinal tract lesion on DWI*: This marker could predict motor impairment in the long term (at 3 months) better than clinical assessment ($R^2 = 0.47$ vs. $R^2 = 0.11$, $p = 0.03$) [176].

4. *Early infarct growth*: It is due to the expansion of cerebral infarction from penumbra to core and cytotoxic edema as a consequence of vessel occlusion, reperfusion, collateral flow patterns, vasogenic edema, or different stroke etiology. It is an independent predictor of clinical outcome at 3 months [176].

5. *Other imaging of ischemic penumbra*: See Sect. 9.6.1.3.

6. *BBB alterations on CTP*: Used for prediction of the risk of hemorrhagic transformation of the index infarct after reperfusion/recanalization treatment.

7. *Imaging of draining veins*: The appearance of asymmetric deep medullary vein sign (ADMVS) on susceptibility-weighted imaging (SWI) (probably related to the increase of deoxyhemoglobin levels consequent to blood flow reduction) in patients with MCA occlusion could be an independent predictor of poor outcome. The prognostic evaluation based on cortical vein score difference in stroke (PRECISE) score of 4–8 could reliably predict poor clinical outcome [176].

9.6.1.1 Metabolic Imaging

Novel precision neuroimaging technology is needed to be developed to even better define the precise therapeutic window for the treatment of individual ischemic stroke patients.

Precision neuroimaging on brain metabolism could represent an effective tool for the identification of salvageable brain tissue in individual stroke cases independent of time and, hence, for the selection of stroke patients for acute treatment and personalized prognosis prediction. In this setting, the following techniques have the potential to be used for future applications having positron-emission tomography (PET) as a reference standard for metabolic imaging [180]: (1) proton MR spectroscopy (MRS) (applicable as surrogate marker in clinical trials to confirm a tissue effect from investigational medicinal products); (2) sodium imaging (potentially applicable for patient selection for reperfusion/recanalization therapies with the optimal imaging profile being a PWI-DWI mismatch without any significant changes seen on a sodium imaging; sodium imaging may further refine the definition of core and distinguish regions of DWI lesions that are penumbral while they are already core); (3) MR images sensitive to deoxyhemoglobin, oxygen challenge imaging (potentially applicable for detecting salvageable tissue within the DWI lesion), or MRI measured of $CMRO_2$ (cerebral metabolic rate of oxygen; could allow to delineate the ischemic penumbra with high predictive ability); and (4) pH imaging (the addition of pH-weighted imaging data to a model to predict tissue outcome seems to be superior to the use of PWI DWI data alone; indeed, pH imaging may help to define the ischemic penumbra whereby hypoperfused tissue with normal ADC and pH represents benign oligemia, and hypoperfused tissue with normal ADC and low pH may represent ischemic penumbra).

Further studies are need for better understanding of how metabolic imaging would fit into current imaging protocols and precisely what information on prognosis determination can be added that cannot already be inferred from existing techniques [180].

9.6.1.2 Intra-arterial Thrombus/Clot Imaging

The following imaging parameters suggestive of the presence of intra-arterial thrombus/clot can be considered valuable markers of response to reperfusion/recanalization treatment and clinical outcome on individual basis [162, 176]:

1. *Hyperdense artery sign*: Both hyperdense MCA and internal carotid signs, likely indicating the presence of a red blood cell-rich clot, have been found to be independently associated with poor outcomes at 3 months despite the thrombolytic treatment. Distal FLAIR hyperintensity vessel (FHV), probably caused by slow blood flow and decreased oxyhemoglobin, can also serve as prognostic biomarkers. Distal FHV resulted in an independent predictor of favorable outcome at 3 months in patients with MCA occlusion who did not receive thrombolytic therapy. Basilar artery FHV was also found as a negative outcome predictor and associated with high risk of mortality [162, 176].
2. *Clot burden score (CBS)*: It is a scale ranging from 0 to 10 used to assess the extent of thrombus in the proximal anterior circulation. Acute ischemic stroke patients with high CBS within 3 h of onset have small final infarct volume and good 3-month outcome. A cutoff of >6 was identified for favorable outcome (sensitivity 73% and specificity 64.6%). Combined with ASPECTS on CTA, CBS predicts both functional outcome and mortality in patients treated with IV thrombolysis [162, 176].
3. *Thrombus length:* SWI, sensitive to deoxyhemoglobin and hemosiderin, enables the visualization of thrombus (with the signal intensity related to the amount of red blood cells) in ischemic stroke patients and the measurement of its length, i.e., distance between the proximal and distal ends of the thrombus. Thrombus length >20 mm in MCA seems to be associated with the absence of recanalization and poor outcome after IV thrombolysis. The length of thrombus in MCA can be measured also on CTP and at the best cutoff values of 11.3 mm and 9.9 mm predicts recanalization and unfavorable outcome, respectively [162, 176].
4. *Thrombus attenuation increase from NCCT to CTA*: It is related to the permeability of the clot which is associated with lower fraction of red blood cell count and more fibrin/platelet conglomerations. These changes have been found to correlate with improved functional outcomes in patients receiving IV thrombolysis or thrombectomy [162].

9.6.1.3 Collaterome

Collateral circulation efficiency represents one of the important aspects underlying the pathophysiology of stroke [10]. For this reason, imaging of collateral circulation has become increasingly important in the field of precision medicine. Indeed, the imaging profile of collateral pattern, i.e., collaterome, represents another important and emerging field in stroke precision medicine useful for personalizing the prediction of treatment response and prognosis in patients with cerebrovascular diseases [181–183].

Collaterome refers to the innate compensatory ability of the brain and vasculature to contrast hypoperfusion when normal arterial inflow is compromised. Robust leptomeningeal collaterals on CTA or PWI in the acute phase of an ischemic stroke have been already proved to be a reliable marker of good outcome at 3 months and patients with poor collaterals are more likely to develop symptomatic intracerebral hemorrhage [181].

A wide range of cerebrovascular disorders from silent stroke to TIA, stroke, cerebral small vessel diseases, intra- and extracranial atherosclerotic diseases, or vascular cognitive impairment involve the damage from ischemia and the compensatory effects of collateral circulation patterns that vary from one individual to another. Mapping the collaterome does not simply imply the identification of specific anastomotic collection and, hence the potential brain vascular supply, but also the assessment of the potential brain plasticity to offset hypoperfusion and ischemic injury. Collaterome should be considered as a system biology like the neurovascular unit is, i.e., a system where multiple different mechanisms and cells interact to produce specific responses in the brain. While, as mentioned above, the evaluation of collateral circulation in terms of leptomeningeal or pial collaterals in acute stroke has been helpful in determining the degree of perfusion derived from collaterals and their impact on the response to acute treatments and clinical outcome, on the other side little is known about the actual dynamic parameters; genomic, proteomic, and metabolic correlates of this collateral, and reverse arterial blood flow. Precision medicine using topography imaging could help in systematically categorizing and developing an atlas of the patterns of collateral circulation for both acute and chronic cerebrovascular diseases in order to understand on an individual basis specificity of pathophysiological mechanisms, vascular adaptation, and therapeutic implications [181].

Determinants of collaterome can be genetic but there are also environmental determinants to neurovascular physiology, including hemodynamics, microvascular and venous phenomena, and correlates on routine imaging studies or triage pathways [181].

As of today, if on the one side from a clinical point of view collateral circulation status, as a modulator of hypoperfusion-induced ischemia, has been considered an important predictor of outcome, on the other side their assessment has been mostly qualitative so far. Indeed, for the acute stroke collateral vessel status has been grossly categorized as "poor" or "good" with MRA or CTA, and partial or complete with digital subtraction angiography (DSA), and the nature of the reverse arterial blood flow to a specific brain area is not routinely investigated. Similarly, in athero-sclerotic carotid disease and Moyamoya there is no standard assessment of distal collateral physiology and there is no study on collaterome in other chronic neuro-vascular conditions such as cerebral small vessel disease and vascular cognitive impairment/dementia, where hypoperfusion is involved in the underlying patho-physiology and etiopathogenesis. Finally, studies with serial blood flow imaging investigating the longitudinal changes in blood flow or collaterome over time are lacking. Even in connectomics, the science that has the objective to understand brain structure, function, and plasticity, the role of collaterals has been neglected. No systematic study on vascular networks spreading through the brain parenchyma, their variability across individuals, and their dynamic adaptation to brain perfusion changes in response to a wide range of cerebrovascular disorders has been performed.

As pointed out above, all types of cerebrovascular diseases can be considered as a *continuum* from the silent lesion to transient ischemic events or overt stroke, through the slow and sneaky progression of vascular lesion burden that is associated with mild cognitive impairment/dementia.

Mapping the collaterome even using routine serial blood flow imaging to study the temporal and evolution of hypoperfusion could provide a set of data serving as a basis for tailoring the management of patients with acute stroke and chronic cere-brovascular disorders. This is particularly true if it is taken into account that isch-emic damage, both acute and chronic, is a dynamic process with a fluctuating course that unfortunately cannot be studied only by imaging the parenchyma and assessing the degree of vessel stenosis at a single time point [181].

The clinical relevance of assessing collaterals has been further confirmed by the recently published successful trials on mechanical thrombectomy in large vessel occlusion-related stroke where the selection approaches using neuroimaging led to inclusion of patients with more robust collaterals [184, 185]. Subsequent post hoc analyses, such as that on the MR CLEAN CTA data, revealed the importance of accurate grading of collateral status in determining clinical outcomes [186]. However, in these cases a delayed intervention could have a different impact on patient outcome despite the presence of good collateral status.

Similarly, for chronic vascular conditions such as intracranial atherosclerotic dis-eases where the focus is on the stenosis degree, collateral status was found to be an important determinant of clinical outcomes [187]. The collateral status may explain why the pattern characterized by downstream collateral perfusion delays measured on CT or MRI as Tmax can reflect the ischemic penumbra that could progress to infarction while in patients with intracranial atherosclerosis the same pattern could not evolve to infarction because the associated cerebral blood volume (CBV) in these regions is adequate to guarantee a mechanism of compensation for the delayed perfusion. In these last cases, Tmax lesions may also become chronic and asymp-tomatic [181].

These findings have not been translated into clinical trials mainly for feasibility reasons related to the difficulties in rapidly and reliably assessing collateral circulation in clinical practice even within the ideal setting of a trial. Therefore, mapping the collaterome, the use of noninvasive techniques such as multimodal MRI and CT, including MRA and arterial spin-labeled MRI (ASL) and CTA, and the development of automated software to speed the imaging reading could implement future algorithms that incorporate this important pathophysiological aspect of cerebrovascular diseases. Post-processing with perfusion angiography can already associate anatomical characteristics of the collaterals with corresponding perfusion and give quantitative and more reliable information for outcome prediction [188]. It would be clinically relevant to phenotype for precision medicine conditions that are apparently homogeneous such as a proximal MCA occlusion, while they can be actually characterized by different responses to treatment and clinical outcomes due to diverse and variable patterns of hypoperfusion and collaterals serving the downstream vasculature and territory, within the different brain areas across individuals and in the same individual over time. Currently, these differences are neglected and the management of these patients with proximal MCA occlusion is the same [181].

Collaterals have the same importance in large subcortical strokes, lacunar strokes, or other vascular disorders related to small vessel diseases such as leukoaraiosis/white matter hyperintensity. In chronic neurovascular conditions, symptoms may become overt later and after changes in collateral status in terms of collateral recruitment, arteriogenesis, and brain perfusion have already occurred. It is biologically plausible that even minor changes in collateral status may transform a chronic and silent cerebrovascular condition in an acute clinical manifestation. For example, this can happen with an asymptomatic carotid stenosis. Unfortunately, imaging of brain and vessels is usually obtained after symptom onset [181].

Collateromics through the collection of meta-data/big data from routine imaging available from a large population and their systematic analysis could provide the opportunity to implement our prevention strategies, to better match cases with the most appropriate treatment and, hence, to improve both the short- and long-term outcome of cerebrovascular diseases, and to identify novel therapeutic targets for collateral circulation augmentation. Furthermore, the use of precision medicine with the mapping of the collateral perfusion patterns could help (1) to address some unanswered questions on the impact of aging, sex difference, and number and type of comorbidities on the burden and outcome of cerebrovascular conditions; (2) to provide the potential to identify even more specific individual therapeutic windows for acute treatments; (3) to clarify the relationship between systemic blood pressure and CBF and the role of hypoperfusion in atrial fibrillation and vascular dementia; and (4) to better understand the basis of arteriogenesis and the relationship with the BBB alterations. Specific methodological approaches can allow a real-time collaterome determination that in acute stroke can guide the endovascular treatment for example in terms of the number of procedural steps in revascularization or in intracranial atherosclerosis to determine whether particular treatments such as angioplasty or medical therapies are tailored to a specific individual [181].

9.6.2 Neuroimaging in Intracerebral Hemorrhage

Among the available myriad of imaging modalities, it is important for patients with intracerebral hemorrhage to understand the framework for choosing a rational imaging plan and the most adequate marker for a better individualized outcome prediction [189].

1. *Hematoma volume, hematoma growth, intraventricular hemorrhage*: On NCCT or MRI, volumes are measured using bedside manual methods (e.g., ABC/2 formula) or automated software. All these markers represent independent predictors of clinical outcome and mortality.
2. *Age of hematoma volume on CT*: Measured by evaluating the density of the lesions measured in Hounsfield units (i.e., according to the value of X-ray attenuation corrected for the attenuation coefficient of water) from the early stage with the presence of fluid levels (over the first 48 h) (also associated with the presence of coagulopathies [i.e., abnormal prothrombin time and partial thromboplastin time], higher hemorrhage volumes, and frequent in thrombolysis-related ICH) and presence of edema surrounding the lesion (over the first 72 h) to the later stages (3–20 days) with the shrinkage of the lesion, reduction of the cerebral edema, and pseudoabscess appearance (ringlike) as seen on contrast. On MRI, hematoma age depends on the stage of the blood degradation products (mainly the chemical state of iron molecules in hemoglobin as well as the state of the red blood cell membrane) given their different paramagnetic properties. Gradient echo (GE) imaging is as sensitive as NCCT and detects acute ICH with an excellent accuracy, while a complete MRI has a higher sensitivity for chronic hemorrhage. However, in case of minor bleeding, such as cerebral microbleeds (see below), GE may not be sufficient to distinguish between acute and chronic hemorrhage, so NCCT should be performed. Of note, it should be taken into account for prognostic implications that, compared to CT, MRI has a higher rate of detecting secondary cause of ICH, including vascular malformations (although better identified with DSA), tumors, cerebral vein thrombosis, and hemorrhagic transformation of cerebral infarctions [189].
3. *Spot sign on CTA*: It is an angiography CT imaging marker, indicating potential contrast extravasation, mostly detectable with 3 h from symptom onset, which predicts early intracerebral hematoma growth with a positive predictive value of 73%, a negative predictive value of 84%, sensitivity of 63%, and specificity of 90%. This marker is associated with poor prognosis, high rate of early clinical deterioration, and high mortality. However, the utility of detecting the spot sign on clinical decision-making and outcome improvement remains questionable. Therefore, further studies are needed to demonstrate the feasibility of CTA in the hyperacute phase and the reliability of spot sign in emergency setting for guiding the therapy with factor VII or other prothrombotic treatment to avoid hematoma expansion and, therefore, a worse outcome [189].
4. *Cerebral microbleeds (CMBs)*: They are chronic and silent small (smaller than 5–10 mm) dot-like lesions, not detectable on CT, having a hypointense appear-

ance on GE sequence. CMBs are considered markers of vascular pathology, including hyperintense vasculopathy and cerebral amyloid angiopathy (CAA), and have been reported to predict ICH in both patients with ICH and ischemic stroke. Furthermore, they can indicate bleeding-prone angiopathy and a high rate of hemorrhagic transformation in patients on anticoagulation, antithrombotic, or thrombolytic therapies. CMBs seem to be associated with small vessel disease-related ischemic stroke (lacunes). Lobar localization of CMBs and their association with ICH in the elderly patients make CMBs possible indicators of CAA. As chronic lesions, they provide a snapshot of the hemorrhages across the patient's life span [189].

5. *PET using compound capable of binding beta-amyloid*: For the identification of CAA and the prediction of ICH in patients with CAA [190].

6. *Fraction anisotropy alterations and corticospinal injury on diffusion tensor imaging (DTI)*: This advanced technique could provide information regarding the risk of damage to white matter tracts. Indeed, DTI has been found to be able to detect reduced levels of integrity and fiber counts and alterations in fractional anisotropy in white matter regions in patients with ICH in the acute phase indicative of potential worse outcome. However, it is not clear whether these alterations persist or increase in the long term. Of particular promise is the use of DTI tractography in the assessment of corticospinal tract injury after ICH along with the decrease of fractional anisotropy relative to the same area of ICH in the non-affected side, and of their association with functional recovery. These findings could be incorporated in precision medicine-based outcome models together with clinical scores in order to personalize prognosis determination. However, studies with large sample size and wider range of volumes and locations of ICH are needed for validating these findings as prognostic markers and not only in the acute phase of hemorrhage but also at later time points with longitudinal neuroimaging evaluations [190].

7. *Perihematomal hypoperfusion*: Detectable by MRI or SPECT, it suggests that aggressive measures to maintain perfusion and oxygenation to tissues could improve outcomes. Unfortunately, the outcome was not assessed in terms of the level of radiographic improvement. However, these data are yet to be fully validated, and significant debate on the ischemic versus metabolic nature of these findings persists [190].

9.6.3 Imaging of Functional Connectivity in Ischemic and Hemorrhagic Stroke

Resting-state functional MRI (rs-fMRI) is a task-independent functional neuroimaging approach based on the blood oxygenation level-dependent (BOLD) signal, which is the optimal choice to investigate functional networks and connectivity-based reorganization in stroke patients. Longitudinal studies after acute ischemic stroke demonstrated the value of rs-fMRI in capturing early changes in functional connectivity and in predicting motor outcome after stroke. Also, in ICH, with the use of functional connectivity measures it may be possible to develop sophisticated model of recovery/prognostication. The potential value of this imaging method in predicting clinical outcomes and mainly functional recovery in the acute/subacute phase of ischemic stroke or ICH needs to be investigated in future studies [176, 190].

9.6.4 Radiomics

Advances in computational technologies, particularly in machine learning, have placed neuroimaging, which contains important information on the pathophysiology of cerebrovascular diseases, in a central role for patient-centered management. Radiomics is emerging in this context as a computer-aided process (including image data acquisition, segmentation, feature extraction, exploratory analysis, and modeling) in which a large number of radiological features (e.g., shape, intensity, or texture) can be extracted from images in an objective and reproducible manner establishing a quantitative relationship between multimode data sources [191]. This is expected to address accurate prognosis prediction and therefore to improve treatment decision.

In the last few years, some progress has been made in the application of radiomics in both ischemic and hemorrhagic stroke for early outcome prediction and long-term prognosis evaluation.

In <u>ischemic stroke</u>, regarding the prediction of short-term outcome, the role of radiomics has been evaluated: (1) in the response to IV thrombolysis in terms of hemorrhagic transformation within 72 h and it was shown that the predictive ability of texture parameters was higher than that of visual evidence of post-contrast enhancement on T1-weighted MR images (AUC >0.75 vs. <0.6); (2) in the prediction of early recanalization of internal carotid artery and M1 segment of MCA occlusion by IV thrombolysis, for which the combination of radiomic features from non-contrast CT (NCCT), CTA, and radiomic changes (i.e., CTA-NCCT) was superior (AUC = 0.85) compared with the sole conventional thrombus imaging characteristics such as length, volume, or permeability [191].

Regarding the long-term prognosis determination, radiomics has also been applied for the quantification of the penumbra and core from both apparent diffusion coefficient and CBF maps in patients within 9 h from symptom onset. The radiomics nomogram could strongly predict favorable clinical outcomes at 7 days and 3 months with AUCs of 0.88 and 0.77, respectively. Therefore, radiomics seems to have the potential to select patients likely to benefit from systemic thrombolysis and/or endovascular treatment also beyond the therapeutic windows. Interestingly, texture features of MR images in the hippocampus and entorhinal cortex at 72 h after stroke onset were significantly different between patients with and without 6-month cognitive impairment. This suggests that radiomics could capture mild neuron loss in areas implicated in cognition at an early stage after stroke by measuring changes in image gray values and could have a role as an imaging marker for screening of long-term CI in patients with AIS [191].

In <u>hemorrhagic stroke</u>, as of prediction of early outcome like hematoma expansion, which is usually associated with neurological deterioration and poor prognosis, radiomics model was found to be superior to the radiological model that incorporates NCCT markers (AUC 0.9 vs. 0.8). Furthermore, radiomic signature has also been reported to be highly predictive of the early development of edema surrounding basal ganglia hematoma. Radiomics data on long-term prognosis are scarce [191].

Due to the potential variability of the radiomics workflow derived by the lack of standardization of neuroimaging protocols widely accepted in the stroke research community, reproducibility of this approach, comparability across studies, reliability, and precision should be improved by implementing a standardized general image processing workflow and by generating classifier models with high robustness and generalization through the use of large-scale data shared among different centers. By increasing its full potential of radiomics in the field of stroke, radiomics is expected to optimize secondary prevention strategies and facilitate the development of personalized precision medicine in post-stroke patients [191].

9.6.5 Conclusion on Neuroimaging

The development of imaging technologies has led to the individuation of all the above-indicated multiple prognostic markers in both ischemic and hemorrhagic stroke.

The findings of studies on neuroimaging in cerebrovascular diseases contradict the supposition that patients who appear clinically similar, fitting for example all inclusion criteria of a trial, are similar. Indeed, this assumption can be considered wrong and contribute to reaching non-correct conclusions on prognosis determination without more precise pathophysiological data, especially imaging data. Neuroimaging needs to be definitely considered not only in outcome predictive models but also in the epidemiology of cerebrovascular disorders that should not be limited to counting of event rates [192].

Therefore, the collection of neuroimaging data is critical for stroke precision medicine, from plain CT useful in the monitoring of the evolution of an ischemic stroke or expansion of an intracerebral hemorrhage to the most modern and advanced neuroimaging including post-processing techniques which can leverage routine CT or MRI to obtain a number of parameters that are characteristics of stroke. Furthermore, including neuroimaging characterization of cerebrovascular diseases of stroke in precision medicine increases the validity of genomic and other biomarker data [192].

Starting from large clinical trials, the collection of imaging data could allow to have those data to analyze in order to improve the selection of patients for future outcome studies. This could be obviously more feasible if noninvasive imaging methods using post-processing techniques are adopted, such as the fractional flow assessed by TOF-MRA or CTA that could be used in stroke secondary prevention trial to investigate, for example, the risk of recurrent stroke and therefore the outcome of patients with 40–69% carotid artery stenosis. Furthermore, in precision medicine, besides anatomical aspects also functional aspects should be considered for better assessing patient prognosis. Consistently, clinical studies or pharmacological trials could be designed differently around baseline pathophysiology of the cerebrovascular condition under investigation. Another aspect that contributes to stroke imaging precision medicine is the need to not only simply measure the abnormality but also the degree of abnormality [192].

Noninvasive neuroimaging data routinely collected could be stored and reanalyzed for specific aims in the future. An example of utility of reanalyzing imaging data of clinical trials, including those with negative results, comes from the WASID trial on intracranial atherosclerosis where subsequent analyses showed that collaterals assessed on conventional angiography were superior to the degree of arterial stenosis for predicting patient outcome and this was confirmed by the SAMMPRIS study [13].

This approach in clinical trials could lead to the creation of an imaging library that could serve as a collaborative multicenter repository data to analyze silent and/ or symptomatic lesion characterization within the multitude of stroke phenotypes and its impact on patient clinical outcome on an individual basis.

The mandate of neuroimaging is expanding with the ultimate goal of discovering novel tools or techniques that should be sensitive, specific, safe, rapid, affordable, and widely available which allows optimized and personalized patient management for the best possible outcome. Finally, it is expected that future studies would focus on the potential combination of image markers and try to establish a perfect neuroimaging paradigm for each of the main cerebrovascular disorders based on a precise outcome prediction [192].

9.7 Theranostic

Theranostic represents an emerging concept of precision medicine that aims to improve patient outcome by providing the right treatment for the right patient at the right time using all the information derived by the precision medicine approach. It is based on the availability of data that relate to a specific individual but also to a broader population. Results from RCTs may not properly take into account key variables such as pathophysiology or concomitant factors that impact long-term brain health, such as stroke etiology, chronic cerebrovascular conditions such as silent infarcts, or conditions related to small vessel disease such as white matter hyperintensities or cerebral microbleeds, longitudinal evaluation of brain resilience, and all the other multitude of variables that can affect the long-term outcome of stroke patients. In routine clinical practice, clinicians tend to switch therapies based on the conclusion that the previous therapy failed. However, it should be taken into account that compliance and pharmacogenomics may impact the effectiveness of secondary stroke prevention treatments. Furthermore, the definition of stroke etiology still remains crucial. For example, in the last years the use of implantable loop recorder has increased the chance to detect atrial fibrillation in stroke patients and this can improve the outcome by leading clinicians to start anti-coagulant treatment, but still the etiology of the index stroke could not be atrial fibrillation if the patient also presents a carotid stenosis for which anticoagulant therapies do not represent an adequate treatment strategy despite its role in preventing cardioembolic stroke.

Advances in technology could improve the theranostic approach in precision medicine. For example, theranostic nanoparticles that can be used to deliver into the body both imaging and therapeutic agents are an emerging technology that has gained interest in recent years for disease management and patient prognosis improvement [152]. Nanoparticles have been investigated in stroke animal models such as ceria nanoparticles and HSP72-vectorized immunoliposome with a potential role of protecting against ischemic stroke, and fibrin-targeted gold nanoparticles to direct imaging of cerebral thromboemboli on CT scan [193–195]. However, no theranostic drug has been approved yet by regulatory authorities for safety concerns.

The future realization of theranostics in stroke precision medicine depends on large-scale data and their integration.

9.8 Big Data and Data Integration

The general belief is that precision medicine is only molecular and/or imaging based, while other types of data have an important role in developing prognostic models such as epidemiological data that could be derived by large datasets, for example the administrative claims.

There is the need of big and longitudinal patient-specific data. Since the outcome of stroke patients is influenced by several variables in both the acute and the subsequent phases, an individual patient may have a unique course of the disease in both the earlier and later periods after stroke, for example he/she can be discharged after 1–2 days or may spend weeks in hospital [196].

The disease course and therefore the outcome of a patient with a neurovascular disorder are influenced by the eligibility to the acute reperfusion/recanalization treatments, by complications such as hemorrhagic transformation in patients with ischemic stroke and myocardial infarction, and by changes in the dynamics of collaterals, or cerebral edema, that require individualized approach.

A plethora of data, besides those included in the patient's medical record, such as imaging, laboratory, physiologic, and other diagnostic data, should be mined, used for linking the short- and long-term outcome, and managed through the use of informatics to help with their storage and analysis to better understand the complex relationship between variables and to guide the theranostic of stroke [196].

For precision medicine, it is crucial to predetermine data definition, collection, storage, and analysis, and to have all the infrastructure to realize that, in order to have large and high-quality dataset and, where applicable, new analytic methods.

The data collection is usually multicenter and therefore there should be efforts in reducing the variability in the availability of advanced techniques, for example neuroimaging and data interpretation. The concept is to shift from large not to narrow but to precise [4], so for example large studies on stroke evaluating outcomes in response to a specific treatment in the setting of precision could still enroll a broad patient population but at the same time they should clearly identify specific phenotypes and have the power to adequately investigate the outcomes in different subgroups of patients. Another example can be represented by clinical trials focused on the therapeutic effect of an endovascular device for stroke, where only select interventional variables may be collected while other data types are ignored, and this can impair the validity of the results for certain groups of patients with specific pathophysiological aspects of the disease. In fact, many of these data types are critical for generalizability and generation of real-world evidence that is recently raising interest in regulatory agencies [196].

A large amount of data, from clinical to laboratory of neuroimaging data, are collected every day for a number of patients with cerebrovascular diseases around the world in routine clinical practice. However, such data are not either considered at all or systematically organized in specific datasets or analyzed.

**Registries**, that usually have been secondary and ancillary to RCTs in importance, may represent the proper instrument to greatly leverage the role of phase IV studies (mostly utilized for post-marketing surveillance and for demonstrating generalizability and transferability of RCT results to clinical practice) and big data in stroke and advance precision medicine to assess the longitudinal or temporal course of a specific individual's neurovascular disorder and inform personalized clinical decision-making [5]. Nevertheless, with the progress in technology, informatics, and neuroimaging methods, and the introduction of endovascular treatment, with the consequent increase of neuroimaging acquisition (including angiography and perfusion imaging sequences), among the standard of care, there is the need to modernize and innovate registries into efficient and imaging-intensive resources that can add value to clinical activity and research on cerebrovascular diseases. In particular, registries reflecting clinical practice can be deployed to address those questions on specific clinical scenarios that have been left unanswered by clinical trials, for example on acute stroke, intracranial atherosclerosis, carotid disease, or vascular cognitive impairment, and therefore to investigate those subgroups of patients left out from RCTs [5].

Precision medicine represents the opportunity for systematically incorporating in stroke registries, even in those already existing, routine neuroimaging performed either at a single time point or serially/longitudinally, omics data, or cognitive/neuropsychology assessments to refine their informative properties. Furthermore, the inclusion of centralized imaging reading and assessment of standardized methods of clinical data collection would markedly enhance the value of the registries, as well as the use of a dynamic format that allows continuing updates (e.g., additional variables or later assessments) with the possibility to generate new data using novel post-processing imaging methods, new imaging signs, or omics assays on stored blood samples. The barriers to the development and implementation of this type of innovative registries would be accuracy of data, privacy concerns, workload, and cost. However, these shortcomings can be overcome with informatics, periodic data monitoring, and incentives. The great advantage is that the more complex the registry becomes the more the precision is refined and the better the neurovascular disorder course and prognosis of an individual patient may be ascertained [5].

Other approaches are under screening, such as that of the ***crowdsourcing***, an unusual approach in medicine that exploits the outstanding capacity of big data in the cloud that could better serve to study precision medicine [197]. Crowdsourcing allows individuals to voluntarily contribute to aggregate data on large populations while preserving anonymity and the right to have specific information on their own brain health. The cloud offers endless storage of data, the opportunity to use neuroimaging applications for post-processing and to avoid redundant repetition of neuroimaging for the same individual. The sharing of these large-size imaging data across a wide pool of experts could provide generalizability, allow specific analyses, and facilitate clinical practice and research on cerebrovascular diseases, with important prognostic implications. However, this type of approach is still in its embryonal state because undoubtedly there are limitations such as (1) acceptance to upload individual's brain imaging and clinical data to a repository; (2) issues on variability and quality of imaging data coming from different sources in terms of machine and standards of acquisition; (3) selection bias regarding the non-uploaded imaging data; (4) validity of nonclinical data; and (5) challenge to involve a sufficient number of experts to manage this large amount of data [197].

9.9   Artificial Intelligence and Machine Learning

Predictive analytics and machine learning represent the foundation of precision medicine. Recent advances in this field associated with the increase of available large amounts of data will transform stroke and neurovascular research and medicine, and the approach to patient management and treatment decisions, from general to tailored with the aim to improve clinical outcome on individual basis. It is true that there are several prognostic scoring systems that have been developed for outcome prediction; however machine learning algorithms have been proved to better describe the complex, variable, and unpredictable human physiology [198]. Conversely to the traditional predictive model that includes selected variable for individuating outcome predictors, machine learning techniques can incorporate a large number of variables that may have, even slight, impact on prediction [198]. In stroke machine learning, for example the deep neural network model has been used for prognosis determination particularly in acute stroke and, mainly, after endovascular treatment [199–201].

The deep neural network comprises layers of interconnected artificial neurons that could well represent the complexity of outcome in a stroke patient. An artificial neuron is designed based on the biological neuron itself and receives multiple inputs multiplied by weights and outputs the sum of the inputs. It can learn complex structures using a training dataset and use that knowledge to predict outcome. In fact, artificial neural networks are effective in capturing nonlinear relationships between dependent and independent variables and have the ability to detect all possible interactions between predictor variables which makes them suitable for complex diseases like stroke. In particular, the random forest algorithm consists of a multitude of decision trees comprising multiple true or false conditions using input variables. The sum of the decisions made by the decision trees is used for the final classification [199].

Despite this, the promises have not been translated into clinically meaningful results so far and in some cases improvement of predictability from traditional stroke outcome score is small, particularly considering the additional burden for entering many variables for the machine learning model. Furthermore, it should be taken into consideration that artificial intelligence-based models, for example those based on artificial neural network, cannot be generalized because it can happen that the training set is unbalanced and under/overrepresents certain characteristics of the data and this can lead to over- or underrepresentation of certain populations. Therefore, machine learning methods should be programmed and designed on large balanced datasets in order to capture linear and nonlinear relationships among variables [198].

With the implementation of electronic health record systems, automatic calculations are built into the system, and this can reduce the need for the models to be simple. Since machine learning can be self-taught with additional data, the results obtained with machine learning can be improved, for example by introducing methods to predict missing values and, hence, by including patients with missing variables. Finally, future integration of model into electronic medical records may enable early outcome prediction [199].

Nevertheless, it should be always taken in mind that artificial intelligence should be only a tool that can help and guide clinicians but it cannot be used as the only methods for prognosis prediction and cannot replace the experience, background, and clinical and ethical judgement of a physician.

9.10 Conclusion

Precision medicine will be a key area for future stroke research and treatment and therefore for improvement of patient management and outcome prediction. The continuing establishment of large dataset, the increase in the collection of omics data, and the development of advanced neuroimaging techniques have led the establishment of the basis for the realization of precision medicine in stroke for a tailored prognosis determination.

Indeed, despite guidelines being essential for supporting the clinicians' decision-making process, in some cases of our clinical activity they could not be helpful particularly because we daily face the challenges posed by the heterogeneity of cerebrovascular disease phenotypes and the complexity of individual cases. Therefore, while on the one hand the emphasis put onto "get with the guidelines" is more than correct, on the other side for some cases there is the need to go beyond the general standards suggested by the current guidelines which are overall applicable to a general population of patients with cerebrovascular diseases. This can occur, for example, in complex scenarios where there are variables such as advanced age, delayed time window from symptom onset, marked hypertension or hyperglycemia, large ischemic damage on plain CT scan, or all various combinations of these and other similar findings. In these cases, the clinicians have to offer whatever may lead to the best outcome possible in the setting of relatively uncommon circumstances [202]. It also happens that some of the variables considered in the stroke guidelines are usually removed by multivariate statistical models in the analysis on outcome prediction. There are tens of registries that collect the majority of the multitude and diversity of variables characterizing neurovascular disorders in most of their aspects. However, strong recommendations from guidelines come from RCTs where in most cases for feasibility reasons and study design, the complexity of cerebrovascular disease pathophysiology can be neglected. These trial shortcomings could just be overcome by precision medicine that with the help of multimodal neuroimaging and molecular data associated with clinical data can better stratify the individual cases by investigating the dynamics of the stroke course and defining the stroke phenotype and etiopathogenesis, and could allow to predict outcome and to adjust the decision for acute and secondary prevention treatment strategies accordingly [202].

However, as pointed out above, the implementation of this concept in clinical practice is still far from being a reality and healthcare disparities could limit the acceleration of the translation from the science of precision medicine into clinical practice around the world. Nevertheless, stroke patients already request personalized management of their disease conditions.

This goal could be achieved by putting together multidisciplinary teams including clinicians, experts of omics, imaging techniques, computational science, and biostatisticians with expertise in the development of novel statistical analysis methods to handle new variables and their weighing in outcome prediction models. Multicenter collaborative efforts should be put in place through the establishment of consortia and of adequate infrastructure for a standardized collection of data.

Revolution of digital health, particularly in the electronic health records, could help along with secure cloud-based resources, cloud computing, and metadata. Informatics serves not only for the storage of this big data but also for accurately and reliably analyzing them with subsequent interpretation of the results by pools of experts. Sustainability of these projects through research funds is of paramount importance. What is certain is that a philosophic and paradigm shift in the stroke community and a raise to a superior management level should occur because individualized treatments based on prognosis prediction models incorporating precision medicine-based variables represent the challenge for the future and the next frontier.

References

1. Norrving B, Barrick J, Davalos A, et al. Action plan for stroke in Europe 2018-2030. Eur Stroke J. 2018;3:309–36.
2. Goyal M, Menon BK, van Zwam WH, et al., HERMES Collaborators. Endovascular thrombectomy after large-vessel ischaemic stroke: a meta-analysis of individual patient data from five randomised trials. Lancet. 2016;387:1723–31.
3. Yang H-T, Shah RH, Tegay D, Onel K. Precision oncology: lessons learned and challenges for the future. Cancer Manag Res. 2019;11:7525–36.

4. Hinman JD, Rost NS, Leung TW, et al. Principles of precision medicine in stroke. J Neurol Neurosurg Psychiatry. 2017;88:54–61.
5. Liebeskind DS. Innovative interventional and imaging registries: precision medicine in cerebrovascular disorders. Interv Neurol. 2015;4:5–17.
6. Neuhaus AA, Couch Y, Hadley G, Buchan AM. Neuroprotection in stroke: the importance of collaboration and reproducibility. Brain. 2017;140:2079–92.
7. Juang F, Juang Y, Zhi H, et al. Artificial intelligence in healthcare: past present, and future. Stroke Vasc Neurol. 2017;2:230–43.
8. Krittanawong C, Zhang H, Wang Z, Aydar M. Artificial intelligence in precision cardiovascular medicine. J Am Coll Cardiol. 2017;21:2657–64.
9. Yang S-H, Lou M, Luo B, Jiang W-J, Liu R. Precision medicine for ischemic stroke, let's move beyond time is brain. Transl Stroke Res. 2018;9:93–5.
10. Liebeskind DS, Feldmann E. Data considerations in ischemic stroke trials. Neurol Res. 2014;36:423–6.
11. Feldmann E, Liebeskind DS. Developing precision stroke imaging. Front Neurol. 2014;5:29.
12. Whiteley W, Chong WL, Sengupta A, et al. Blood markers for the prognosis of ischemic stroke: a systematic review. Stroke. 2009;40(5):e380–9.
13. Montaner J, Ramiro L, Simats A, et al. Multilevel omics for the discovery of biomarkers and therapeutic targets for stroke. Nat Rev Neurol. 2020;16:247–64.
14. Falcone GJ, Malik R, Dichgans M, et al. Current concepts and clinical applications of stroke genetics. Lancet Neurol. 2014;13:405–18.
15. Cheng YC, Stanne TM, Giese A-K, et al. Genome-wide association analysis of young-onset stroke identifies a locus on chromosome 10q25 near HABP2. Stroke. 2016;47:307–16.
16. Cole JW, Xu H, Ryan K, et al. Genetics of the thrombomodulin–endothelial cell protein C receptor system and the risk of early-onset ischemic stroke. PLoS One. 2018;13:e0206554.
17. Dichgans M. Genetics of ischaemic stroke. Lancet Neurol. 2007;6:149–61.
18. Sharp FR, Jickling GC, Stamova B, et al. Molecular markers and mechanisms of stroke: RNA studies of blood in animals and humans. J Cereb Blood Flow Metab. 2011;31:1513–31.
19. Malik R, Chauhan G, Traylor M, et al. Multiancestry genome-wide association study of 520,000 subjects identifies 32 loci associated with stroke and stroke subtypes. Nat Genet. 2018;50:524–37.
20. Malik R, Rannikmäe K, Traylor M, et al. Genome-wide meta-analysis identifies 3 novel loci associated with stroke. Ann Neurol. 2018;84:934–9.
21. Woo D, Falcone GJ, Devan WJ, et al. Meta-analysis of genome-wide association studies identifies 1q22 as a susceptibility locus for intracerebral hemorrhage. Am J Hum Genet. 2014;94:511–21.
22. Debette S, Kamatan Y, Metso TM, et al. Common variation in PHACTR is associated with susceptibility to cervical artery dissection. Nat Genet. 2014;47:78–83.
23. Rannikmäe K, Davies G, Thomson PA, et al. Common variation in COL4A1/COL4A2 is associated with sporadic cerebral small vessel disease. Neurology. 2015;84:918–26.
24. Chauhan G, Arnold CR, Chu AY, et al. Identification of additional risk loci for stroke and small vessel disease: a meta-analysis of genome-wide association studies. Lancet Neurol. 2016;15:695–707.
25. Söderholm M, Pedersen A, Lorentzen E, et al., International Stroke Genetics Consortium, the NINDS-SiGN Consortium, and the Genetics of Ischaemic Stroke Functional Outcome (GISCOME) Network. Genome-wide association meta-analysis of functional outcome after ischemic stroke. Neurology. 2019;92:e1271–83.
26. Marini S, Devan WJ, Radamanesh F, et al. 17p12 influences hematoma volume and outcome in spontaneous intracerebral hemorrhage. Stroke. 2018;49:1618–25.
27. Pfeiffer D, Chen B, Schlicht K, et al. Genetic imbalance is associated with functional outcome after ischemic stroke. Stroke. 2019;50:298–304.
28. Schlunk F, Greenberg SM. The pathophysiology of intracerebral hemorrhage formation and expansion. Transl Stroke Res. 2015;6:257–63.

29. Biffi A, Anderson CD, Jagiella JM, et al. APOE genotype and extent of bleeding and outcome in lobar intracerebral haemorrhage: a genetic association study. Lancet Neurol. 2011;10:702–9.
30. Meschia JF. Pharmacogenetics and stroke. Stroke. 2009;40:3641–5.
31. Paré G, Eriksson N, Lehr T, et al. Genetic determinants of dabigatran plasma levels and their relation to bleeding. Circulation. 2013;127:1404–12.
32. del Rio-Espínola A, Fernández-Cadenas I, Giralt D, et al. A predictive clinical-genetic model of tissue plasminogen activator response in acute ischemic stroke. Ann Neurol. 2012;72:716–29.
33. Sealock R, Zhang H, Lucitti JL, et al. Congenic fine-mapping identifies a major causal locus for variation in the native collateral circulation and ischemic injury in brain and lower extremity. Circ Res. 2014;114:660–71.
34. Traylor M, Zhang CR, Adib-Samii P, et al. Genome-wide meta-analysis of cerebral white matter hyperintensities in patients with stroke. Neurology. 2016;86:146–53.
35. Paternoster L, Chen W, Sudlow CL. Genetic determinants of white matter hyperintensities on brain scans: a systematic assessment of 19 candidate gene polymorphisms in 46 studies in 19,000 subjects. Stroke. 2009;40:2020–6.
36. Traylor M, Tozer DJ, Croall ID, et al. Genetic variation in *PLEKHG1* is associated with white matter hyperintensities (n = 11,226). Neurology. 2019;92:e749–57.
37. Lyall DM, Cox SR, Lyall LM, et al. Association between APOE e4 and white matter hyperintensity volume, but not total brain volume or white matter integrity. Brain Imaging Behav. 2020;14:1468–76.
38. Adib-Samii P, Devan W, Traylor M, et al. Genetic architecture of white matter hyperintensities differs in hypertensive and nonhypertensive ischemic stroke. Stroke. 2015;46:348–53.
39. Nadareishvili Z, Kelley D, Simpkins AN, et al. Molecular signature of penumbra in acute ischemic stroke: a pilot transcriptomics study. Ann Clin Transl Neurol. 2019;6:817–20.
40. Soriano-Tárraga C, Mola-Caminal M, Giralt-Steinhauer E, et al. Biological age is better than chronological as predictor of 3-month outcome in ischemic stroke. Neurology. 2017;89:830–6.
41. Gallego-Fabrega C, Carrera C, Rebny J-L, et al. PPM1A methylation is associated with vascular recurrence in aspirin-treated patients. Stroke. 2016;47:1926–9.
42. Mishra A, Chauan G, Violleau M-H, et al. Association of variants in HTRA1 and NOTCH3 with MRI-defined extremes of cerebral small vessel disease in older subjects. Brain. 2019;142:1009–23.
43. Jickling GC, Xu H, Stamova B, et al. Signatures of cardioembolic and large-vessel ischemic stroke. Ann Neurol. 2010;68:681–92.
44. Jickling GC, Stamova B, Ander BP, et al. Profiles of lacunar and nonlacunar stroke. Ann Neurol. 2011;70:477–85.
45. Zhao H, Wang J, Gao L, et al. MiRNA-424 protects against permanent focal cerebral ischemia injury in mice involving suppressing microglia activation. Stroke. 2013;44:1706–13.
46. Stary CM, Xu L, Sun X, et al. MicroRNA-200c contributes to injury from transient focal cerebral ischemia by targeting Reelin. Stroke. 2015;46:551–6.
47. Jickling GC, Ander BP, Stamova B, Zhan X, Liu D, Rothstein L, et al. RNA in blood is altered prior to hemorrhagic transformation in ischemic stroke. Ann Neurol. 2013;74(2):232–40.
48. Kamtchum-Tatuene J, Jickling GC. Blood biomarkers for stroke diagnosis and management. NeuroMolecular Med. 2019;21:344–68.
49. Dykstra-Aiello C, Jickling GC, Ander BP, et al. Altered expression of long noncoding RNAs in blood after ischemic stroke and proximity to putative stroke risk loci. Stroke. 2016;47:2896–903.
50. Deng Q-W, Li S, Wang H, et al. Differential long noncoding RNA expressions in peripheral blood mononuclear cells for detection of acute ischemic stroke. Clin Sci. 2018;132:159701501614.
51. Wang W, Gao F, Zhao Z, et al. Integrated analysis of lncRNA-mRNA co-expression profiles in patients with Moyamoya disease. Sci Rep. 2017;7:42421.

52. Holdt LM, Teupser D. Long noncoding RNA ANRIL: Lnc-ing genetic variation at the chromosome 9p21 locus to molecular mechanisms of atherosclerosis. Front Cardiovasc Med. 2018;5:45.
53. Wang J, Ruan J, Zhu M, et al. Predictive value of long noncoding RNA ZFAS1 in patients with ischemic stroke. Clin Exp Hypertens. 2018;41:615–21.
54. Xu H, Tang Y, Liu D-Z, et al. Gene expression in peripheral blood differs after cardioembolic compared with large-vessel atherosclerotic stroke: biomarkers for the etiology of ischemic stroke. J Cereb Blood Flow Metab. 2008;28:1320–8.
55. Jickling GC, Stamova B, Ander BP, et al. Prediction of cardioembolic, arterial, and lacunar causes of cryptogenic stroke by gene expression and infarct location. Stroke. 2012;43:2036–41.
56. Jickling GC, Ander BP, Shroff N, et al. Leukocyte response is regulated by microRNA let7i in patients with acute ischemic stroke. Neurology. 2016;87:2198–205.
57. Gilles ME, Slack FJ. Let-7 microRNA as a potential therapeutic target with implications for immunotherapy. Expert Opin Ther Targets. 2018;22:929–39.
58. Tiedt S, Prestel M, Malik R, et al. RNA-seq identifies circulating MIR-125a-5p, MIR-125b-5p, and MIR-143-3p as potential biomarkers for acute ischemic stroke. Circ Res. 2017;121:970–80.
59. Eyileten C, Wicil Z, De Rosa S, et al. MicroRNAs as diagnostic and prognostic biomarkers in ischemic stroke—a comprehensive review and bioinformatic analysis. Cell. 2018;7:249.
60. Jickling GC, Ander BP, Zhan X, et al. MicroRNA expression in peripheral blood cells following acute ischemic stroke and their predicted gene targets. PLoS One. 2014;9:e99283.
61. Cuadrado E, Rosell A, Colomé N, et al. The proteome of human brain after ischemic stroke. J Neuropathol Exp Neurol. 2010;69:1105–15.
62. Ulm L, Ohlraun S, Harms H, et al. STRoke Adverse outcome is associated With NoSocomial Infections (STRAWINSKI): procalcitonin ultrasensitive-guided antibacterial therapy in severe ischaemic stroke patients—rationale and protocol for a randomized controlled trial. Int J Stroke. 2013;8:598–603.
63. Katan M, Fluri F, Morgenthaler NG, et al. Copeptin: a novel, independent prognostic marker in patients with ischemic stroke. Ann Neurol. 2009;66(6):799–808.
64. De Marchis GM, Katan M, Weck A, et al. Copeptin adds prognostic information after ischemic stroke: results from the CoRisk study. Neurology. 2013;80(14):1278–86.
65. Bustamante A, Garcia-Berrocoso T, Llombart V, et al. Neuroendocrine hormones as prognostic biomarkers in the setting of acute stroke: overcoming the major hurdles. Expert Rev Neurother. 2014;14(12):1391–403.
66. Xu Q, Tian Y, Peng H, et al. Copeptin as a biomarker for prediction of prognosis of acute ischemic stroke and transient ischemic attack: a meta-analysis. Hypertens Res. 2017;40(5):465–71.
67. Greisenegger S, Segal HC, Burgess AI, et al. Copeptin and long-term risk of recurrent vascular events after transient ischemic attack and ischemic stroke: population-based study. Stroke. 2015;46(11):3117–23.
68. Katan M, Nigro N, Fluri F, et al. Stress hormones predict cerebrovascular re-events after transient ischemic attacks. Neurology. 2011;76(6):563–6.
69. De Marchis GM, Weck A, Audebert H, et al. Copeptin for the prediction of recurrent cerebrovascular events after transient ischemic attack: results from the CoRisk study. Stroke. 2014;45(10):2918–23.
70. Senn R, Elkind MSV, Montaner J, Christ-Crain M, Katan M. Potential role of blood biomarkers in the management of nontraumatic intracerebral hemorrhage. Cerebrovasc Dis. 2014;38:395–409.
71. Zweifel C, Katan M, Schuetz P, et al. Copeptin is associated with mortality and outcome in patients with acute intracerebral hemorrhage. BMC Neurol. 2010;10:34.
72. Katan M, Elkind MSV. The potential role of blood biomarkers in patients with ischemic stroke: an expert opinion. Clin Transl Neurosci. 2018:1–7. https://doi.org/10.1177/2514183X18768050.

73. Montaner J, Molina CA, Monasterio J, et al. Matrix metalloproteinase-9 pretreatment level predicts intracranial hemorrhagic complications after thrombolysis in human stroke. Circulation. 2003;107(4):598–603.
74. Castellanos M, Sobrino T, Millan M, et al. Serum cellular fibronectin and matrix metalloproteinase-9 as screening biomarkers for the prediction of parenchymal hematoma after thrombolytic therapy in acute ischemic stroke: a multicenter confirmatory study. Stroke. 2007;38(6):1855–9.
75. Castellanos M, Leira R, Serena J, et al. Plasma metalloproteinase-9 concentration predicts hemorrhagic transformation in acute ischemic stroke. Stroke. 2003;34(1):40–6.
76. Wang L, Wei C, Deng L, et al. The accuracy of serum matrix metalloproteinase-9 for predicting hemorrhagic transformation after acute ischemic stroke: a systematic review and meta-analysis. J Stroke Cerebrovasc Dis. 2018;27:1653–65.
77. Montaner J, Alvarez-Sabin J, Molina C, et al. Matrix metalloproteinase expression after human cardioembolic stroke: temporal profile and relation to neurological impairment. Stroke. 2001;32:1759–66.
78. Serena J, Blanco M, Castellanos M. The prediction of malignant cerebral infarction by molecular brain barrier disruption markers. Stroke. 2005;36:1921–6.
79. Montaner J, Rovira A, Molina CA, et al. Plasmatic level of neuroinflammatory markers predict the extent of diffusion-weighted image lesions in hyperacute stroke. J Cereb Blood Flow Metab. 2003;23:1403–7.
80. Barr TL, Latour LL, Lee KY, et al. Blood-brain barrier disruption in humans is independently associated with increased matrix metalloproteinase-9. Stroke. 2010;41(3):123–8.
81. Silva Y, Leira R, Tejada J, Lainez JM, Castillo J, Davalos A. Molecular signatures of vascular injury are associated with early growth of intracerebral hemorrhage. Stroke. 2005;36:86–91.
82. Nash DL, Bellolio MF, Stead LG. S100B as a marker of acute brain ischemia: a systematic review. Neurocrit Care. 2008;8(2):301–7.
83. Foerch C, Otto B, Singer OC, et al. Serum S100B predicts a malignant course of infarction in patients with acute middle cerebral artery occlusion. Stroke. 2004;35(9):2160–4.
84. Brea D, Sobrino T, Blanco M, Cristobo I, et al. Temporal profile and clinical significance of serum neuron-specific enolase and S100 in ischemic and hemorrhagic stroke. Clin Chem Lab Med. 2009;47(12):1513–8.
85. Martin AJ, Price CI. A systematic review and meta-analysis of molecular biomarkers associated with early neurological deterioration following acute stroke. Cerebrovasc Dis. 2018;46:230–41.
86. Lorenzano S, Rost NS, Khan M, et al. Early molecular oxidative stress biomarkers of ischemic penumbra in acute stroke. Neurology. 2019;93:e1288–98.
87. Lorenzano S, Rost NS, Khan M, et al. Oxidative stress biomarkers of brain damage: hyperacute plasma F2-isoprostane predicts infarct growth in stroke. Stroke. 2018;49:630–7.
88. The Emerging Risk Factors Collaboration. C-reactive protein concentration and risk of coronary heart disease, stroke, and mortality: an individual participant meta-analysis. Lancet. 2010;375:132–40.
89. Elkind MSV, Luna JM, Moon YP, et al. High sensitivity C-reactive protein predicts mortality but not stroke: the Northern Manhattan Study. Neurology. 2009;73:1300–7.
90. Woodward M, Lowe GD, Campbell DJ, et al. Associations of inflammatory and hemostatic variables with the risk of recurrent stroke. Stroke. 2005;36:2143–7.
91. Welsh P, Lowe GD, Chalmers J, et al. Associations of proinflammatory cytokines with the risk of recurrent stroke. Stroke. 2008;39(8):2226–30.
92. Elkind MS, Tai W, Coates K, et al. High-sensitivity C-reactive protein, lipoprotein-associated phospholipase A2, and outcome after ischemic stroke. Arch Intern Med. 2006;166(19):2073–80.
93. Fang HY, Ko WJ, Lin CY. Inducible heat shock protein 70, interleukin-18, and tumor necrosis factor alpha correlate with outcomes in spontaneous intracerebral hemorrhage. J Clin Neurosci. 2007;14:435–41.

94. Castillo J, Davalos A, Alvarez-Sabin J, et al. Molecular signatures of brain injury after intracerebral hemorrhage. Neurology. 2002;58:624–9.

95. Wang KW, Cho CL, Chen HJ, et al. Molecular biomarker of inflammatory response is associated with rebleeding in spontaneous intracerebral hemorrhage. Eur Neurol. 2011;66:322–7.

96. Fang HY, Ko WJ, Lin CY. Plasma interleukin 11 levels correlate with outcome of spontaneous intracerebral hemorrhage. Surg Neurol. 2005;64:511–7, discussion 517–8.

97. Zhou Y, Xiong KL, Lin S, et al. Elevation of high-mobility group protein box-1 in serum correlates with severity of acute intracerebral hemorrhage. Mediators Inflamm. 2010. pii: 142458. https://doi.org/10.1155/2010/142458. Epub 2010 Sept 29.

98. Elkind MS, Tai W, Coates K, et al. Lipoprotein-associated phospholipase A2 activity and risk of recurrent stroke. Cerebrovasc Dis. 2009;27(1):42–50.

99. Han L, Zhong C, Bu X, et al. Prognostic value of lipoprotein-associated phospholipase A2 mass for all-cause mortality and vascular events within one year after acute ischemic stroke. Atherosclerosis. 2017;266:1–7.

100. Bustamante A, Nin MM, Garcìa-Berrocoso, et al. Usefulness of ADAMTS13 to predict response to recanalization therapies in acute ischemic stroke. Neurology. 2018;90:e995–e1004.

101. Sobrino T, Arias S, Perez-Mato M, et al. CD34+ progenitor cells likely are involved in the good functional recovery after intracerebral hemorrhage in humans. J Neurosci Res. 2011;89:979–85.

102. Sobrino T, Arias S, Rodriguez-Gonzalez R, et al. High serum levels of growth factors are associated with good outcome in intracerebral hemorrhage. J Cereb Blood Flow Metab. 2009;29:1968–74.

103. Castellanos M, Castillo J, García MM, et al. Inflammation-mediated damage in progressing lacunar infarctions: a potential therapeutic target. Stroke. 2002;33:982–7.

104. Azurmendi L, Degos V, Tiberti N, et al. Measuring serum amyloid a for infection prediction in aneurysmal subarachnoid hemorrhage. J Proteome Res. 2015;14:3948–56.

105. Yuan D, Liu C, Hu B. Dysfunction of membrane trafficking leads to ischemia–reperfusion injury after transient cerebral ischemia. Transl Stroke Res. 2018;9:215–22.

106. Herrmann M, Vos P, Wunderlich MT, de Bruijn CH, Lamers KJ. Release of glial tissue-specific proteins after acute stroke: a comparative analysis of serum concentrations of protein S-100B and glial fibrillary acidic protein. Stroke. 2000;31:2670–7.

107. Hoffmann S, Harms H, Ulm L, et al. Stroke-induced immunodepression and dysphagia independently predict stroke-associated pneumonia—the PREDICT study. J Cereb Blood Flow Metab. 2017;37:3671–82.

108. Perez de la Ossa N, Sobrino T, Silva Y, et al. Iron-related brain damage in patients with intracerebral hemorrhage. Stroke. 2010;41:810–3.

109. Leira R, Davalos A, Silva Y, et al. Early neurologic deterioration in intracerebral hemorrhage: predictors and associated factors. Neurology. 2004;63:461–7.

110. Marti-Fabregas J, Borrell M, Silva Y, et al. Hemostatic proteins and their association with hematoma growth in patients with acute intracerebral hemorrhage. Stroke. 2010;41:2976–8.

111. Castellanos M, Leira R, Serena J, et al. Plasma cellular-fibronectin concentration predicts hemorrhagic transformation after thrombolytic therapy in acute ischemic stroke. Stroke. 2004;35:1671–6.

112. Castellanos M, Sobrino T, Millán M, et al. Serum cellular fibronectin and matrix metalloproteinase-9 as screening biomarkers for the prediction of parenchymal hematoma after thrombolytic therapy in acute ischemic stroke: a multicenter confirmatory study. Stroke. 2007;38:1855–9.

113. Ribo M, et al. Admission fibrinolytic profile is associated with symptomatic hemorrhagic transformation in stroke patients treated with tissue plasminogen activator. Stroke. 2004;35:2123–7.

114. Marti-Fabregas J, Borrell M, Cocho D, et al. Hemostatic markers of recanalization in patients with ischemic stroke treated with rt-PA. Neurology. 2005;65:366–70.

115. Lee SH, Kim BJ, Bae HJ, Lee JS, Lee J, Park BJ, Yoon BW. Effects of glucose level on early and long-term mortality after intracerebral haemorrhage: the Acute Brain Bleeding Analysis Study. Diabetologia. 2010;53:429–34.

116. Rodriguez-Luna D, Rubiera M, Ribo M, et al. Serum low-density lipoprotein cholesterol level predicts hematoma growth and clinical outcome after acute intracerebral hemorrhage. Stroke. 2011;42:2447–52.

117. García-Berrocoso T, Penhalba A, Boada C, et al. From brain to blood: new biomarkers for ischemic stroke prognosis. J Proteome. 2013;94:138–48.

118. García-Berrocoso T, Llombart V, Colàs-Campàs L, et al. Single cell immuno-laser microdissection coupled to label-free proteomics to reveal the proteotypes of human brain cells after ischemia. Mol Cell Proteomics. 2018;17:175–89.

119. Simats A, Garcì-Berrocoso T, Ramiro L, et al. Characterization of the rat cerebrospinal fluid proteome following acute cerebral ischemia using an aptamer-based proteomic technology. Sci Rep. 2018;8:7899.

120. Hernandez-Guillamon M, Garcia-Bonilla L, Solé M, et al. Plasma VAP-1/SSAO activity predicts intracranial hemorrhages and adverse neurological outcome after tissue plasminogen activator treatment in stroke. Stroke. 2010;41:1528–35.

121. Llombart V, Antolin-Fontes A, Bustamante A, et al. B-type natriuretic peptides help in cardioembolic stroke diagnosis: pooled data meta-analysis. Stroke. 2015;46:1187–95.

122. Bai J, Sun H, Xie L, Zhu Y, Feng Y. Detection of cardioembolic stroke with B-type natriuretic peptide or N-terminal pro-BNP: a comparative diagnostic meta-analysis. Int J Neurosci. 2018;128:1100–8.

123. Santamarina E, Penalba A, Garcì-Berrocoso T, et al. Biomarker level improves the diagnosis of embolic source in ischemic stroke of unknown origin. J Neurol. 2012;259:2538–45.

124. Longstreth WT Jr, Kronmal RA, Thompson JL, et al. Amino terminal pro-B-type natriuretic peptide, secondary stroke prevention, and choice of antithrombotic therapy. Stroke. 2013;44(3):714–9.

125. Kamel H, Longstreth W, Tirschwell DL, et al. The atrial cardiopathy and antithrombotic drugs in prevention after cryptogenic stroke randomized trial: rationale and methods. Int J Stroke. 2019;14:207–14.

126. James ML, Blessing R, Phillips-Bute BG, Bennett E, Laskowitz DT. S100B and brain natriuretic peptide predict functional neurological outcome after intracerebral haemorrhage. Biomarkers. 2009;14:388–94.

127. Cascino I, Fiucci G, Papoff G, Ruberti G. Three functional soluble forms of the human apoptosis-inducing Fas molecule are produced by alternative splicing. J Immunol. 1995;154:2706–13.

128. Delgado P, Cuadrado E, Rosell A, et al. Fas system activation in perihematomal areas after spontaneous intracerebral hemorrhage. Stroke. 2008;39:1730–4.

129. Hu L, Dong MX, Zhao H, Xu GH, Qin XY. Fibulin-5: a novel biomarker for evaluating severity and predicting prognosis in patients with acute intracerebral haemorrhage. Eur J Neurol. 2016;23(7):1195–201.

130. Whiteley W, Wardlaw J, Dennis M, et al. The use of blood biomarkers to predict poor outcome after acute transient ischemic attack or ischemic stroke. Stroke. 2012;43:86–91.

131. Rodriguez-Yanez M, Sobrino T, Arias S, Vazquez-Herrero F, Brea D, Blanco M, et al. Early biomarkers of clinical diffusion mismatch in acute ischemic stroke. Stroke. 2011;42(10):2813–8.

132. Dayon L, Turck N, Garcì-Berrocoso T, et al. Brain extracellular fluid protein changes in acute stroke patients. J Proteome Res. 2011;10:1043–51.

133. Lescuyer P, Allard L, Zimmermann-Ivo CG, et al. Identification of post-mortem cerebrospinal fluid proteins as potential biomarkers of ischemia and neurodegeneration. Proteomics. 2004;4:2234–41.

134. Dayon L, Hainard A, Licker V, et al. Relative quantification of proteins in human cerebrospinal fluids by MS/MS using 6-plex isobaric tags. Anal Chem. 2018;8:2921–31.

135. Katan M, Morgenthaler N, Widmer I, et al. Copeptin, a stable peptide derived from the vasopressin precursor, correlates with the individual stress level. Neuro Endocrinol Lett. 2008;29(3):341–6.

136. Ulm L, Hoffman S, Nabavi D, et al. The randomized controlled STRAWINSKI trial: procalcitonin-guided antibiotic therapy after stroke. Front Neurol. 2017;8:153.

137. Elkind MS, Luna JM, McClure LA, et al. C-reactive protein as a prognostic marker after lacunar stroke: levels of inflammatory markers in the treatment of stroke study. Stroke. 2014;45(3):707–16.

138. Sheth SA, Verma A, Liebeskind DS, et al. Endothelial cell collection from ipsilateral middle cerebral artery in acute ischemic stroke. In: International stroke conference, Houston, TX, 2016.

139. Sviri GE, Soustiel JF, Zaaroor M. Alteration in brain natriuretic peptide (BNP) plasma concentration following severe traumatic brain injury. Acta Neurochir (Wein). 2006;148:529–33.

140. Hernandez-Guillamon M, Sole M, Delgado P, et al. VAP-1/SSAO plasma activity and brain expression in human hemorrhagic stroke. Cerebrovasc Dis. 2012;33:55–63.

141. Kim SH, Smith CJ, Van Eldik LJ. Importance of MAPK pathways for microglial pro-inflammatory cytokine IL-1 beta production. Neurobiol Aging. 2004;25:431–9.

142. Ponath G, Schettler C, Kaestner F, et al. Autocrine S100B effects on astrocytes are mediated via RAGE. J Neuroimmunol. 2007;184:214–22.

143. Hu YY, Dong XQ, Yu WH, Zhang ZY. Change in plasma S100B level after acute spontaneous basal ganglia hemorrhage. Shock. 2010;33:134–40.

144. Stegemann C, Pechlaner R, Willeit P, et al. Lipidomics profiling and risk of cardiovascular disease in the prospective population-based Bruneck study. Circulation. 2014;129:1821–31.

145. Sun D, Tiedt S, Yu B, et al. A prospective study of serum metabolites and risk of ischemic stroke. Neurology. 2019;92:e1890–8.

146. Choi JY, Kim J-S, Kim JH, et al. High free fatty acid level is associated with recurrent stroke in cardioembolic stroke patients. Neurology. 2014;82:1142–8.

147. Nelson SE, Ament Z, Wolcott Z, Gerszten RE, Kimberly WT. Succinate links atrial dysfunction and cardioembolic stroke. Neurology. 2019;92:e802–10.

148. Marklund M, Wu JHY, Imamura F, et al., Cohorts for Heart and Aging Research in Genomic Epidemiology (CHARGE) Fatty Acids and Outcomes Research Consortium (FORCE). Biomarkers of dietary omega-6 fatty acids and incident cardiovascular disease and mortality. Circulation. 2019;139:2422–36.

149. Frank PG, Woodman SE, Park DS, Lisanti MP. Caveolin, caveolae, and endothelial cell function. Arterioscler Thromb Vasc Biol. 2003;23:1161–8.

150. Bang OY, Chung JW, Kim SJ, et al. Caveolin-1, ring finger protein 213, and endothelial function in Moyamoya disease. Int J Stroke. 2016;11:999–1008.

151. Sonveaux P, Martinive P, DeWever J, et al. Caveolin-1 expression is critical for vascular endothelial growth factor-induced ischemic hindlimb collateralization and nitric oxide-mediated angiogenesis. Circ Res. 2004;95:154–61.

152. Bang OY. Advances in biomarker for stroke patients: from marker to regulator. Prec Fut Med. 2017;1:32–42.

153. Urra A, Cervera A, Obach V, et al. Monocytes are major players in the prognosis and risk of infection after acute stroke. Stroke. 2009;40:1262–8.

154. Nadareishvili ZG, Li H, Wright V, Maric D, Warach S, et al. Elevated pro-inflammatory CD4+CD28- lymphocytes and stroke recurrence and death. Neurology. 2004;63:1446–51.

155. Bogoslovsky T, Chaudhry A, Latour L, et al. Endothelial progenitor cells correlate with lesion volume and growth in acute stroke. Neurology. 2010;75:2059–62.

156. Raffield LM, Tu AT, Szeto MD, et al. Coagulation factor VIII: relationship to cardiovascular disease risk and whole genome sequence and epigenome-wide analysis in African Americans. J Thromb Haemost. 2020;18:1335–47.

157. Hartwig FP, Davies NM, Hemani G, Davey SG. Two-sample Mendelian randomization: avoiding the downsides of a powerful, widely applicable but potentially fallible technique. Int J Epidemiol. 2016;45:1717–26.

158. Larsson SC, Traylor M, Markus HS. Homocysteine and small vessel stroke: a Mendelian randomization analysis. Ann Neurol. 2019;85:495–501.
159. Georgakis MK, Gill D, Rannikmae K, et al. Genetically determined levels of circulating cytokines and risk of stroke. Circulation. 2019;139:256–68.
160. Georgakis MK, Malik R, Bjorkbacka H, et al. Circulating monocyte chemoattractant protein-1 and risk of stroke: meta-analysis of population-based studies involving 17 180 individuals. Circ Res. 2019;125:773–82.
161. Sun L, Clarke R, Bennett D, et al. Causal associations of blood lipids with risk of ischemic stroke and intracerebral hemorrhage in Chinese adults. Nat Med. 2019;25:569–74.
162. Fitzgerald S, Mereuta OM, Doyle KM, et al. Correlation of imaging and histopathology of thrombi in acute ischemic stroke with etiology and outcome. J Neurointerv Surg. 2017;9:529–34.
163. Bivard A, Levi C, Krishnamurthy V, et al. Perfusion computed tomography to assist decision making for stroke thrombolysis. Brain. 2015;138:1919–31.
164. Gonzalez RG. Imaging-guided acute ischemic stroke therapy: from "time is brain" to "physiology is brain". AJNR Am J Neuroradiol. 2006;27:728–35.
165. Adams HP Jr, Bendixen BH, Kappelle LJ, et al. Classification of subtype of acute ischemic stroke. Definitions for use in a multicenter clinical trial. TOAST. Trial of ORG 10172 in Acute Stroke Treatment. Stroke. 1993;24:35–41.
166. Parsons MW, Spratt N, Bivard A, et al. A randomised trial of tenecteplase versus alteplase for acute ischaemic stroke. N Engl J Med. 2012;366:1099–107.
167. Huang XY, Cheripelli BK, Lloyd SM, et al. Alteplase versus tenecteplase for thrombolysis after ischaemic stroke (ATTEST): a phase 2, randomised, open-label, blinded endpoint study. Lancet Neurol. 2015;14:368–76.
168. Saver JL, Goyal M, Bonafe A, et al. Stent-retriever thrombectomy after intravenous t-PA vs. t-PA alone in stroke. N Engl J Med. 2015;372:2285–95.
169. Campbell BC, Mitchell PJ, Kleinig TJ, et al. Endovascular therapy for ischemic stroke with perfusion-imaging selection. N Engl J Med. 2015;372:1009–18.
170. Berkhemer OA, Fransen PS, Beumer D, et al. A randomized trial of intraarterial treatment for acute ischemic stroke. N Engl J Med. 2015;372:11–20.
171. Jovin TG, Chamorro A, Cobo E, et al. Thrombectomy within 8 hours after symptom onset in ischemic stroke. N Engl J Med. 2015;372:2296–306.
172. Nogueira RG, Jadhav AP, Haussen DC, et al. Thrombectomy 6 to 24 hours after stroke with a mismatch between deficit and infarct. N Engl J Med. 2018;378:11–21.
173. Albers GW, Marks MP, Kemp S, et al. DEFUSE 3 Investigators. Thrombectomy for stroke at 6 to 16 hours with selection by perfusion imaging. N Engl J Med. 2018;378:708–71.
174. Thomalla G, Simonsen CZ, Boutitie F, et al., WAKE-UP Investigators. MRI-guided thrombolysis for stroke with unknown time of onset. N Engl J Med. 2018;379:611–22.
175. Rocha M, Jovin TG. Fast versus slow progressors of infarct growth in large vessel occlusion stroke: clinical and research implications. Stroke. 2017;48:2621–7.
176. Zhou Y, Zhang S, Lou M. Imaging markers in acute phase of stroke: implications for prognosis. Brain Hemorrhages. 2020;1:19–23.
177. Mundiyanapurath S, Diatschuk S, Loebel S, et al. Outcome of patients with proximal vessel occlusion of the anterior circulation and DWI-PWI mismatch is time-dependent. Eur J Radiol. 2017;91:82–7.
178. Dani KA, Thomas RGR, Chappell FM, et al. Systematic review of perfusion imaging with computed tomography and magnetic resonance in acute ischemic stroke: heterogeneity of acquisition and postprocessing parameters a translational medicine research collaboration multicentre acute stroke imaging study. Stroke. 2012;43:563–6.
179. Feldmann E, Liebesking DS. Developing precision stroke imaging. Front Neurol. 2014;5:29.
180. Dani KA, Warach S. Metabolic imaging of ischemic stroke: the present and future. Am J Neuroradiol. 2014;35:S37.
181. Liebeskind DS. Mapping the collaterome for precision cerebrovascular health: theranostics in the continuum of stroke and dementia. J Cereb Blood Flow Metab. 2018;38:1449–60

182. Liebeskind DS, Feldman E. Imaging of cerebrovascular disorders: precision medicine and the collaterome. Ann N Y Acad Sci. 2016;1366:40–8.
183. Liebeskind DS, Woolf GW, Shuaib A, Collaterals 2016 Consortium. Collaterals 2016: translating the collaterome around the globe. Int J Stroke. 2017;12:338–42.
184. Leng X, Fang H, Leung TW, et al. Impact of collaterals on the efficacy and safety of endovascular treatment in acute ischaemic stroke: a systematic review and meta-analysis. J Neurol Neurosurg Psychiatry. 2016;87:537–44.
185. Leng X, Fang H, Leung TW, et al. Impact of collateral status on successful revascularization in endovascular treatment: a systematic review and meta-analysis. Cerebrovasc Dis. 2015;41:27–34.
186. Berkhemer OA, Jansen IG, Beumer D, et al. Collateral status on baseline computed tomographic angiography and intra-arterial treatment effect in patients with proximal anterior circulation stroke. Stroke. 2016;47:768–76.
187. Liebeskind DS, Cotsonis GA, Saver JL, et al. Collaterals dramatically alter stroke risk in intracranial atherosclerosis. Ann Neurol. 2011;69:963–74.
188. Scalzo F, Liebeskind DS. Perfusion angiography in acute ischemic stroke. Comput Math Methods Med. 2016;2016:2478324.
189. Macellari F, Paciaroni M, Agnelli G, Caso V. Neuroimaging in intracerebral hemorrhage. Stroke. 2014;45:903–8.
190. McDowell MM, Kellner CP, Barton SM, et al. The role of advanced neuroimaging in intracerebral hemorrhage. Neurosurg Focus. 2013;34:E2.
191. Chen Q, Xia T, Zhang M, et al. Radiomics in stroke neuroimaging: techniques, applications, and challenges. Aging Dis. 2021;12:143–54.
192. Liebeskind SD, Malhotra K, Hinman JD. Imaging as the Nidus of precision cerebrovascular health: a million brains initiative. JAMA Neurol. 2017;74:257–8.
193. Kim CK, Kim T, Choi IY, Soh M, Kim D, Kim YJ, et al. Ceria nanoparticles that can protect against ischemic stroke. Angew Chem Int Ed Engl. 2012;51:11039–43.
194. Agulla J, Brea D, Campos F, Sobrino T, Argibay B, Al-Soufi W, et al. In vivo theranostics at the peri-infarct region in cerebral ischemia. Theranostics. 2013;4:90–105.
195. Kim JY, Ryu JH, Schellingerhout D, Sun IC, Lee SK, Jeon S, et al. Direct imaging of cerebral thromboemboli using computed tomography and fibrin-targeted gold nanoparticles. Theranostics. 2015;5:1098–114.
196. Liebeskind SD. Big data for a big problem: precision medicine of stroke in neurocritical care. Crit Care Med. 2018;46:1189–91.
197. Liebeskind SD. Crowdsourcing precision cerebrovascular health: imaging and cloud seeding A Million Brains Initiative™. Front Med. 2016;3:62.
198. Saber H, Somai M, Rajah GB, Scalzo F, Liebeskind DS. Predictive analytics and machine learning in stroke and neurovascular medicine. Neurol Res. 2019;41:681–90.
199. Heo J, Yoon JG, Park H, Kin YD, Nam HS, Heo JH. Machine learning-based model for prediction of outcomes in acute stroke. Stroke. 2019;40:1263–5.
200. van Os HJA, Ramos LA, Hilbert A, et al. Predicting outcome of endovascular treatment for acute ischemic stroke: potential value of machine learning algorithms. Front Neurol. 2018;9:784.
201. Cuadrado-Godia E, Dwivedi P, Sharma S, Ois Santiago A, Roquer Gonzalez J, Balcells M, et al. Cerebral small vessel disease: a review focusing on pathophysiology, biomarkers, and machine learning strategies. J Stroke. 2018;20:302–20. https://doi.org/10.5853/jos.2017.02922.
202. Liebeskind SD. Editorial commentary: beyond the guidelines to expertise in precision stroke medicine. Trends Cardiovasc Med. 2017;27:67–8.

Artificial Intelligence Applications in Stroke

10

Arlindo L. Oliveira

10.1 Introduction

Artificial intelligence (AI) techniques, namely those that are based in machine learning (ML), can be used effectively in order to improve the diagnostic and treatment of stroke. Machine learning techniques can leverage the significant amounts of data obtained by clinicians in order to provide insights on the seriousness of stroke incidents, improve the quality of the diagnosis, and predict patient outcomes. Machine learning techniques make it possible to use data to create models that can be used to support decisions in the different phases of stroke diagnostic and treatment. The application of machine learning is widely viewed as a key research priority, as academic institutions, companies, and clinicians strive to improve the treatment of stroke.

Until recently, the data that could be used to support decisions in this area was mainly the clinical data obtained during admission and stay of patients at the hospital. This data can be very informative and, duly analyzed, can be used to effectively make diagnosis and predictions about the future evolution of stroke patients. However, in the last few years, the emergence of deep learning techniques that can effectively process image data enabled machine learning-based systems to use other sources of information, in particular imaging data obtained using computed tomography (CT), with or without contrast, and magnetic resonance imaging (MRI). Furthermore, the increased availability of patient genetic data creates the possibility of integrating clinical, imaging, and genetic data in order to improve the prediction ability of the models. The number of applications of artificial intelligence and machine learning in the area of stroke is, therefore, increasing rapidly, from early detection of ischemia on CT images to the determination of key metrics on

A. L. Oliveira (✉)
INESC-ID/Instituto Superior Técnico, Lisbon, Portugal
e-mail: arlindo.oliveira@tecnico.ulisboa.pt

© Springer Nature Switzerland AG 2021
A. C. Fonseca, J. M. Ferro (eds.), *Precision Medicine in Stroke*,
https://doi.org/10.1007/978-3-030-70761-3_10

perfusion or blood flow in specific areas of the brain. Improving decision support systems with the use of machine learning techniques will be an important objective in the years to come.

10.2 Using Machine Learning to Infer Predictive Models

The key technology behind the most recent advances in artificial intelligence is machine learning, a designation that stands for a vast set of techniques that aim at inferring general rules from specific examples.

In its simpler form, inductive learning infers a general rule from a set of labeled instances, called the training set. Each instance is defined by a set of attributes (or variables) and their respective values. To provide a concrete example, one may build a table with patient information at the time of admission, which includes the age and gender of the patient, the existence of past stroke events, the delay between stroke onset and hospital arrival, and the NIH Stroke Score (NIHSS). In this example, one wishes to infer, from the available data, the expected final outcome, 3 months after the stroke incident, in the modified Rankin Scale (mRS). The relevant data could be organized into something that would resemble Table 10.1, where the specific values for each attribute, for each patient, are listed in the corresponding column, one row per patient.

The organization of data in tabular form is familiar to many readers and is extensively used to keep track of many types of patient information. It turns out that the existence of data in tabular format makes possible the direct application of machine learning techniques to the problem of inferring the outcome (the target label, listed in the last column of Table 10.1) from the independent patient attributes, listed in columns 2–6 of that table. The patient ID is simply an identifier of the patient and has no predictive value. In many cases, it is used to preserve the anonymity of the patients, by making sure that the correspondence between the patient ID and the real identification of the patients is kept reserved.

Over many decades machine learning researchers have developed hundreds, if not thousands, of methods and algorithms that can be used to infer the target label from the independent attributes, a problem known as supervised learning. If the label is discrete, as is the case in this table, the problem is called a classification problem. If the label is continuous (typically a real number) the problem is called a

Table 10.1 Example of table with instances of stroke incidents

Patient ID	Age	Gender	Past events	Delay (h)	NIHSS	mRS
001	57	Male	No	3.5	12	2
002	65	Male	Yes	4.0	27	5
003	71	Female	No	1.5	14	3
004	58	Female	No	3.5	20	2
005	66	Male	Yes	6.0	27	5
006	68	Male	No	1.0	25	4

regression problem. In this chapter, we focus mainly on classification problems, but many of the techniques developed for classification problems can also be used in regression problems, although sometimes they require some modifications.

This problem is known as supervised learning because a supervisor (or teacher) provides the value of the labels in the training set, the dataset that can be used to train the machine learning system. If labels are not available, the problem is known as unsupervised learning. In that case, the objective is usually to aggregate the instances into classes that share a significant similarity, a problem known as clustering, but other objectives are also possible, such as the identification of outliers or the cleaning of data. In this chapter, we focus on the problem of supervised learning, since the availability of labels for a subset of the instances (the training set) usually enables the algorithms to perform more interesting predictions.

Supervised machine learning algorithms infer a model from the data available in the training set. Such a model can take many different forms. It can be a mathematical formula, a set of rules, the parameters of a network, and several other forms. In practice, the model enables the user to apply a fixed set of computations to the attributes of an instance in order to obtain the value of the target label. One significant issue in machine learning is overfitting. Overfitting occurs when the model performs well in the available data (training set) but does not perform equally well on future data (test set). Since the objective of creating the model is to use it to predict future instances, avoiding overfitting is essential when machine learning techniques are used.

Machine learning algorithms can be classified into one of the four categories: symbolic, statistical, similarity based, and connectionist. These categories are not mutually exclusive, and one method may share features of more than one category. It is also possible to partition the methods in a different and more or less numerous set of categories. Pedro Domingos, for instance, considered an additional category, genetically inspired machine learning algorithms, obtaining a five-category taxonomy [1]. In the sequence, I will provide a brief introduction to each of these families of machine learning algorithms.

10.2.1 Symbolic Methods

Symbolic methods derive symbolic rules that can be used to derive the target labels of unseen instances. One may imagine, for instance, a symbolic rule of the type *"if age > 60 and NIHSS > 24 then mRS = 5,"* which would enable us to predict that persons older than 60 that obtain an NIHSS larger than 24 will be expected to have a final modified Rankin Scale of 5. Such a rule is just an example, of course. In a realistic case, a set of such rules would enable clinicians to derive the predicted Rankin Scale for any incoming patient. Symbolic methods have a significant advantage: the classification they perform can be, in many cases, intelligible to a human, and the inferred rules can be analyzed and checked for consistency.

Although there are many methods that use a symbolic approach, one of them is particularly popular and effective: decision trees. A decision tree inference algorithm, such as ID3 [2], C4.5 [3], or CART [4], processes the tabular data and derives a decision tree that closely matches the target labels in the training set. Decision tree inference algorithms aim at deriving compact trees, which are more likely to have high predictive values for unseen instances. Such trees not only match closely the target labels in the training set, but can also be used to effectively predict these labels in new instances, never seen before. For instance, the decision tree in Fig. 10.1 correctly labels all the instances in Table 10.1, and can be used to infer the outcomes of patients who are not in that table.

By inspection, it is fairly easy to understand the set of rules that correspond to the tree in Fig. 10.1. For instance, the tree predicts that patients with an NIHSS larger than 24 who have been admitted to the hospital more than 3 h after the stroke incident are expected to have a final mRS of 5. This tree should not be viewed as an accurate classifier for this particular problem, as it is being used solely to illustrate the approach. In practice, trees are inferred from much larger datasets and are usually significantly more complex [5]. Other symbolic models, such as decision lists [6], have also been proposed since they exhibit, over other approaches, the advantage of being more easily understandable. One popular and effective approach, random forests, is based on the creation of a population of decision trees that "vote" on the predicted outcome. The most popular outcome (the one that gets more votes from the trees) is selected as the predicted outcome. In reality, decision forests can also be viewed as a statistical method, since it is sampling from a distribution of trees that models the phenomenon under study.

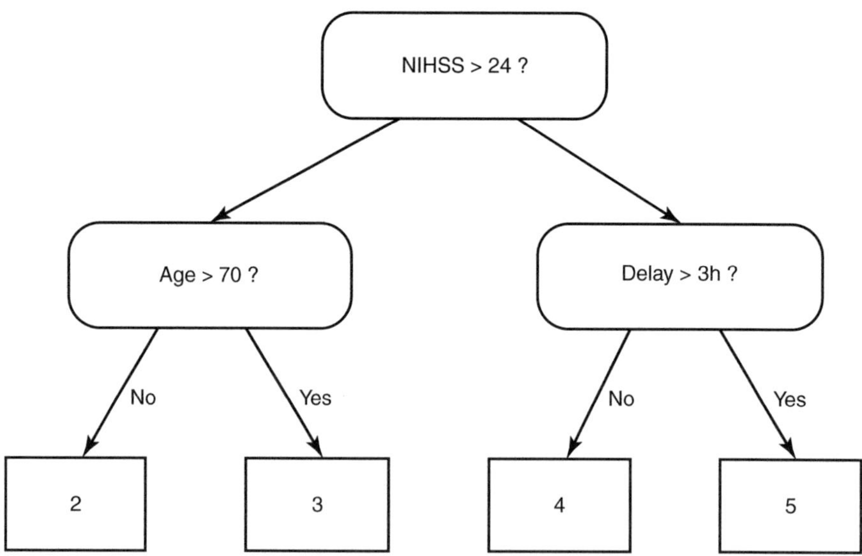

Fig. 10.1 Decision tree for the instances in Table 10.1

10.2.2 Statistical Methods

Statistical methods aim at inferring relevant probabilistic relations between the independent attributes and the target label, in order to predict the most likely value of the target label from the values of the attributes. More formally, statistical methods estimate the joint probability distributions (either implicitly or explicitly) of the input/output attributes and use this joint distribution to infer the most likely value of the target output. One of the most relevant and well-known statistical methods is regression, a simple technique that is, however, very relevant in many practical settings. In its simplest form, single linear regression finds a linear relation between an independent continuous variable and a dependent continuous variable, by looking for a set of parameters that minimize the sum of the squares of the differences between the model and the observed values of the independent variable. Multiple linear regression finds a relation between a set of continuous variables and a single independent variable. In some cases, one expects a nonlinear relationship between the independent variables and the dependent variable. In these cases, polynomial regression can be used, a technique that derives the coefficients of a polynomial relating the input and output variables.

Single or multiple, linear or polynomial, regression is not applicable in classification problems, where the independent variable is discrete, as is the example in Table 10.1. In these cases, logistic regression should be used. Logistic regression is directly applicable when the independent variable, the target class label, is binary. As in linear regression, the coefficients derived by the mathematical optimization algorithm provide an indication of the relevance of a given input variable in the determination of the class label. Multinomial logistic regression is used when there are more than two possible values for the target label.

Regularization can be used to improve the performance of regression methods. When there are many input variables, standard regression (linear or logistic) tends to weight many, or even all, input variables, leading in many cases to the phenomenon of overfitting, introduced above. Overfitting can be controlled in regression if one forces a significant fraction of the coefficients to become zero, forcing the regression function to depend only on a small subset of the input variables. The mathematical formulation of regularized regression adds a term to the sum of the squares of the errors that penalizes the existence of many coefficients different from zero. Depending on the form of the penalty, this formulation may lead to ridge regression, Lasso regression, or other possibilities. Regression-based methods have been extensively used in the prediction of stroke outcomes [7, 8], with good results.

Another important statistical method is based on the direct application of Bayes' theorem, which relates the probability of a given value of the target label with the probability of observing a specific value in the independent attributes, for each value of the target. Although a direct application of Bayes' theorem is usually not doable, since it involves the estimation of the joint probability distribution of the input variables for each possible class, a simplified method, called naive Bayes, can be applied and can be very effective, in practice [9].

10.2.3 Similarity-Based Methods

A third category of methods used to infer a classification method from a set of labeled instances is similarity-based methods. The fundamental idea behind similarity-based methods is to classify a new instance in the same class as the most similar instance or instances in the training set. For example, given the instances in Table 10.1, if one is asked to determine the most likely outcome for a new male patient, with 57 years and no prior incidents, admitted 3 hours after the stroke incident and classified with an NIHSS of 12, it would be reasonable to estimate that the mRS outcome would be 2, since this case is very similar to the patient that corresponds to the first instance in the table. This classification method is called the nearest-neighbor algorithm, and is reasonably effective in some specific conditions. When the algorithm considers a fixed number of nearest neighbors (k) and decides the class by looking at the most common class among these neighbors, it is called the k-nearest neighbor algorithm.

In general, the application of similarity-based methods requires the definition of a metric of similarity (a distance) between two instances that takes into account the nature of the different input attributes. For instance, in our example, a difference of 1 year in age is probably less significant than a difference of 1 h in the admission delay. Furthermore, both categorical and continuous attributes have to contribute to this metric in such a way that the distances between instances make sense. Defining such a similarity metric can be challenging, but there are algorithms that perform this task automatically, adjusting the scales of the different dimensions.

Although the basic idea behind similarity-based methods is very simple, very sophisticated approaches based on this idea have been developed, and some of them involve very sophisticated mathematical machinery. One method that can be classified in the family of similarity-based methods (although it can also be viewed as a modified form of regression) is support vector (SVM) classification. Support vector classification (or support vector machines) can be used in a wide range of circumstances, although it is based on the simple idea of finding a hyperplane in input space that separates the two classes under analysis. Modified versions of the algorithm can work with more than two classes. Since a hyperplane can only separate the instances of two classes in very particular cases, when the classes are linearly separable, one would think that SVMs have a very narrow range of applicability. However, that is not so, because SVM algorithms perform a transformation on the original space into a high-dimensional space using what is known as the kernel trick [10, 11], enabling SVM classifiers to work even in cases where the stroke data is not linearly separable [12].

10.2.4 Connectionist Methods

The original idea behind connectionist methods was inspired in the behavior of the human brain, which performs very sophisticated computations using millions of simple computational units (biological neurons) interconnected in complex, and mostly unknown, patterns. Biological neurons are complex cells, which perform computations by integrating incoming information, generated by upstream neurons and received in the dendritic trees. When the neuron excitation is sufficient to generate a signal at the output, the neuron generates a pulse or a train of electric pulses that are transmitted through the axon to other neurons downstream. The actual behavior of individual neurons is very complex, and can only be modeled by considering the actual physical characteristics of the neuron and the electrical parameters of the neuron membrane, among many other factors. However, the idea that supports connectionist methods, also known as artificial neural networks (ANN), or simply neural networks (NN), is to use a very simplified model of the behavior of neurons, illustrated in Fig. 10.2. In this simplified model, an artificial neuron simply computes a weighted sum of the inputs it receives and generates, at the output, a nonlinear function of this weighted sum. In this example, the nonlinear function is simply the Heaviside step function (equal to 1 if the input is positive, 0 otherwise), but other functions are extensively used, such as the sigmoid/logistic, the hyperbolic tangent, or the rectified linear unit.

A simple artificial neuron, like the one depicted in Fig. 10.2, does not perform a very useful computation. The true computational power of artificial neural networks derives from the fact that artificial neurons can be connected, in networks, in order to perform complex tasks, mimicking, in this way, the behavior of brains. Networks of artificial neurons, called multilayer perceptrons (MLPs), depicted in Fig. 10.3 can indeed perform very complex tasks, if the connection weights between the artificial neurons are set to the appropriate values.

The idea of using artificial neurons to process information is more than 60 years old [13] but this approach is only useful if appropriate algorithms to set the weights are available. Indeed, one of the winters of artificial intelligence was caused mainly by the realization that a single artificial neuron is not particularly useful and that

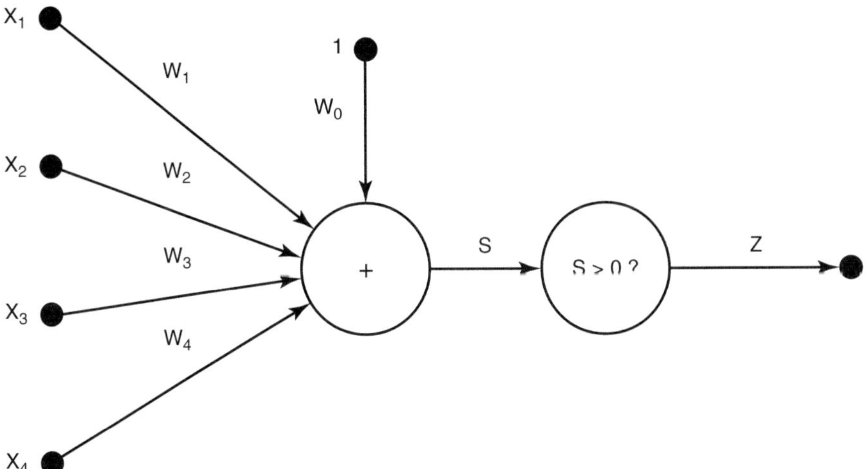

Fig. 10.2 Simplified mathematical model of a neuron

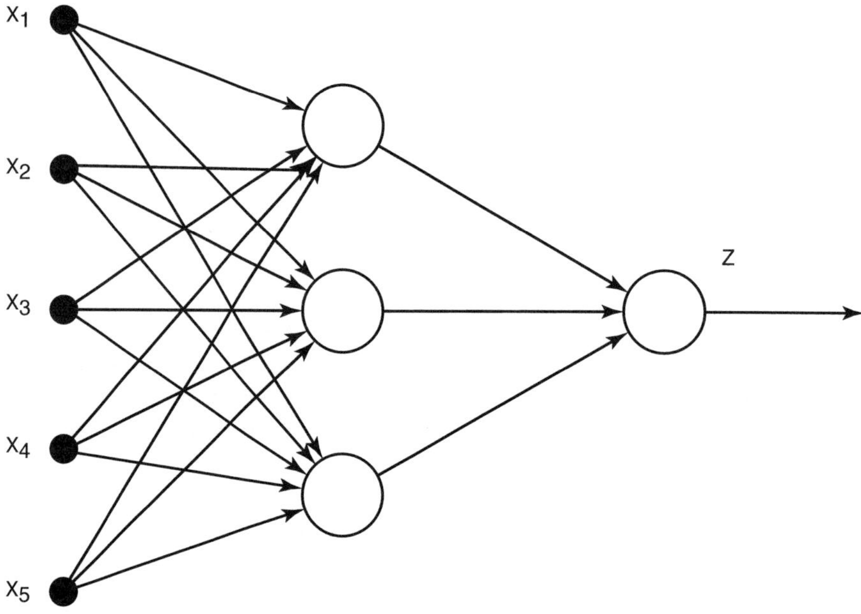

Fig. 10.3 Multilayer perceptron

finding the right value for the interconnection weights in a network is a very difficult computational problem [14]. However, the (re)discovery of the backpropagation [15] enabled researchers to apply artificial neural networks to a wide variety of problems. Backpropagation is a mathematical optimization method that derives the weights on an artificial neural network by computing the derivative of the error function with respect to each of the weights in the network. The error function can take several forms, but in general has a minimum when the network output is equal to the desired output, for all instances. One popular error function is the sum of the squares of the difference between the target output and the network output.

The set of derivatives of the error function with respect to each network weight is called, in mathematical terms, the gradient, and can be computed using standard mathematical operations, in particular the chain rule. Once computed, the gradient can be used to minimize the error at the output of the network, by performing a (typically very long) series of small changes in the weights, a process known as gradient descent. Gradient descent methods, which include backpropagation and conjugate gradient algorithms, among others, find the combination of weights that minimize the output error of the network. Such a configuration of weights can then be used to compute the network output for any combination of variables in the inputs.

For ANNs to be useful, the weights in the network have to be set in such a way as to make the network map the input variables to the desired output value. Using our running example, variables X_1–X_5 could be the attributes in columns 2–6 of Table 10.1 and the output Z would be the target label, the mRS value. When the weights are set to the right values, the network will compute the correct mRS value from the value of the input variables, the age, gender, past events, elapsed time, and NIHSS value of the admitted patient. Variables that are categorical have to be encoded as an integer, in order to be processed by the network units.

In this particularly straightforward problem of inferring the mRS from these five clinical and personal attributes, ANNs have a performance that is, probably, comparable to other methods we already discussed [8]. However, the power of artificial neural networks is that they can be applied to perform computations using high-dimensional data, such as images or sounds, which no other known machine learning method can cope with. Deep learning methods use artificial neural networks with many levels (in some cases, hundreds of levels) and hundreds of thousands of artificial neurons to perform image classification tasks that we were unable to perform, until only a few years ago.

10.3 Deep Learning for Image Processing

The problem of obtaining diagnosis from medical images is not different, in its essence, from the basic problem we have been discussing, that of inferring the target labels from a set of labeled instances. An image could in principle be described by a set of independent attributes, leading to a formulation not very different from the one that is exemplified in Table 10.1. Consider, for example, a grayscale, one-megapixel image obtained using any standard imaging technique. Such an image could be described by 1 million attributes, one attribute for each pixel in the image. The equivalent of Table 10.1 for such a task would consist of a table with 1 million columns, each column corresponding to the value of a pixel. Each entry in the table would be a number between 0 (for a black pixel) and 1 (for a white pixel), and intermediate values corresponding to intermediate levels of gray. For a color image, of the same dimension, the table would have 3 million attributes, since each pixel is described by three continuous values, for each of the three-color channels.

In principle, one could learn a classification rule from a table with 1 million columns (or 3 million columns, for color images) by using any of the techniques described in the previous section: decision trees, logistic regression, naive Bayes, nearest-neighbor, or support vector machines. In practice, such an approach does not work, because no single pixel provides any significant information about the target class. The relevant information is hidden in complex patterns that involve thousands or tens of thousands of pixels, patterns that are easily recognized by human experts but that are opaque to these basic machine learning methods. For that reason, the application of machine learning techniques to the classification of medical images was neither practical nor relevant, until a few years ago. Image processing algorithms were used to enhance the images, by manipulating contrast and by applying other image transformations, but stand-alone systems that could process and classify medical images were not common, if they existed at all. However, in the last decade, a significant number of developments took place, which enabled machine learning techniques to process and classify high-dimensional data, such as medical images or 3D medical images, obtained using magnetic resonance imaging or computed tomography.

The key development was the ability to apply convolutional neural networks to the processing of high-dimensional image data. Convolutional neural networks are multilayer perceptrons with a particular architecture where the first layers perform convolution operations on the image. Figure 10.4 shows an example of a convolutional neural network, with two convolutional layers and one fully connected layer at the output. Each convolutional layer applies a filter to the image, specified by a kernel, which is used to "scan" the image, applying the same filter over and over again as it is swept over the rows and columns of the image. In the simplified network in Fig. 10.4, only one kernel is used, leading to a single channel as an output of the first convolutional layer. In practice, several kernels are used in each layer, leading to a number of channels in each convolutional layer. The last layer (or layers) is usually a fully connected layer, enabling the output units (there is only one in this simplified case) to compute the desired output by combining the outputs of the neurons in the last convolutional layer. The kernel parameters (which are the input weights of the neurons in the convolutional layers) as well as all the other network weights are computed using gradient descent, as in standard neural networks. Other types of operations, such as pooling (selecting the largest value in a range), are also commonly used in convolutional neural networks.

In the last decade convolutional neural networks became the architecture best suited for many kinds of image processing tasks, among many other applications. Although convolutional neural networks have been proposed decades ago [16, 17] they became the solution of choice only more recently, with the availability of large datasets that can be used to train the networks, and the appearance of faster computers that speed up the computation of the solution using gradient descent methods, in many cases using graphic processing units (GPUs) developed for gaming

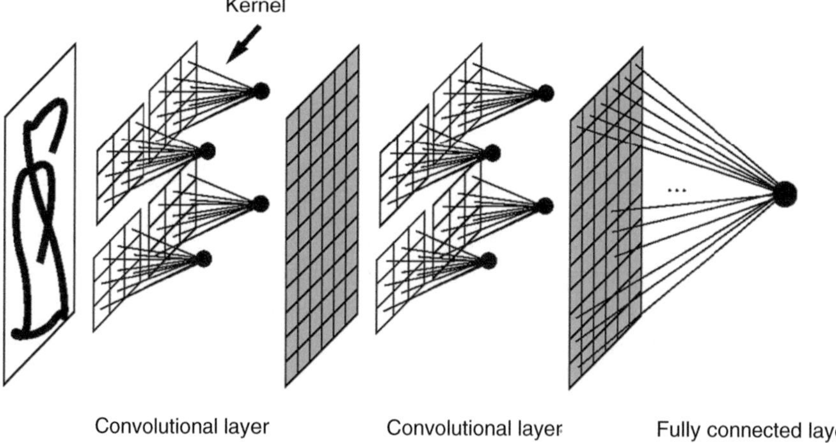

Fig. 10.4 Convolutional neural network

applications. After the first evidence that convolutional neural networks outperform any competing approaches in image recognition and labeling problems [18] many architectures with ever-increasing complexity [19–21] have been proposed and used in many different problems. These architectures have in common the fact that they included hundreds of thousands or even millions of artificial neurons, organized in very deep networks that exhibit many layers (in some cases, hundreds of layers).

10.4   Applications of Machine Learning in Stroke

Given the inherent flexibility of machine learning methods, and its ability to process many different types of data, it is no surprise that the number of applications in the area of stroke has exploded in the last few years. Applications include outcome prediction from clinical and/or imaging data, segmentation of lesions, and assessment of treatment effectiveness, among others.

The basic idea of outcome prediction is to infer the most likely outcome from clinical data available. Although a number of scores have been proposed to that effect [22], machine learning methods hold the promise of increasing the accuracy by being able to use more effectively all the available data. A number of authors developed methods to predict outcomes from clinical information, using support vector machines [12]; random forests, support vector machines, logistic regression, and decision trees [7]; decision trees [5]; neural networks, random forests, and logistic regression [8]; and support vector machines, random forests, and neural networks [23].

A number of high-profile public competitions to develop the most accurate methods to process MRI stroke data were held between 2015 and 2017. The 2015 edition of the ISLES (Ischemic Stroke Lesion Segmentation) challenge [24] proposed two tasks to the participants, subacute ischemic stroke lesion segmentation and acute stroke outcome/penumbra estimation. The 2016 edition consisted of two tasks: lesion outcome prediction and clinical outcome prediction, while the 2017 edition asked the participants to predict the lesion outcome [25]. In all cases, the available training data was multispectral MRI scans of acute stroke patients. Many other authors proposed to apply deep neural networks to process different types of stroke imaging data [26–29].

Given the increased availability of clinical and imaging data, and the ever-increasing effectiveness of machine learning methods, one should expect significant developments in the application of machine learning technologies to the task of outcome prediction from available information.

References

1. Domingos P. The master algorithm. London: Allen Lane; 2015.
2. Quinlan JR. Induction of decision trees. Mach Learn. 1986;1(1):81–106.
3. Quinlan JR. C4.5—programs for machine learning. San Mateo: Morgan Kaufmann; 1993.

4. Breiman L, Friedman J, Stone CJ, Olshen RA. Classification and regression trees. Boca Raton, FL: CRC Press; 1984.
5. Saraee MH, Keane J. Using T3, an improved decision tree classifier, for mining stroke-related medical data. Methods Inf Med. 2007;46(5):523–9.
6. Letham B, Rudin C, McCormick TH, Madigan D. Interpretable classifiers using rules and Bayesian analysis: Building a better stroke prediction model. Ann Appl Stat. 2015;9(3):1350–71.
7. Monteiro M, Fonseca AC, Freitas AT, Pinho E, Melo T, Francisco AP, Ferro JM, Oliveira AL. Using machine learning to improve the prediction of functional outcome in ischemic stroke patients. IEEE/ACM Trans Comput Biol Bioinform. 2018;15(6):1953–9.
8. Heo JN, Yoon JG, Park H, Kim YD, Nam HS, Heo JH. Machine learning-based model for prediction of outcomes in acute stroke. Stroke. 2019;50(5):1263–5.
9. Domingos P, Pazzani M. On the optimality of the simple Bayesian classifier under zero-one loss. Mach Learn. 1997;29(2–3):103–30.
10. Cortes C, Vapnik V. Support-vector networks. Mach Learn. 1995;20(3):273–97.
11. Scholkopf B, Smola AJ. Learning with kernels: support vector machines, regularization, optimization, and beyond, Adaptive computation and machine learning series. Cambridge, MA: MIT Press; 2018.
12. Jeena RS, Kumar S. Stroke prediction using SVM. In: 2016 International conference on control, instrumentation, communication and computational technologies (ICCICCT 2016). Piscataway, NJ: IEEE; 2017. p. 600–2.
13. Rosenblatt F. The perceptron: a probabilistic model for information storage and organization in the brain. Psychol Rev. 1958;65(6):386–408.
14. Minsky M, Papert S. Perceptrons. Cambridge: MIT Press; 1969.
15. Rumelhart DE, Hinton GE, Williams RJ. Learning representations by back-propagating errors. Nature. 1986;5(6088):533–6.
16. Fukushima K, Miyake S. Neocognitron: a self-organizing neural network model for a mechanism of visual pattern recognition. In: Competition and cooperation in neural nets. Berlin: Springer; 1982. p. 267–85.
17. LeCun Y, Boser B, Denker JS, Henderson D, Howard RE, Hubbard W, et al. Backpropagation applied to handwritten ZIP code recognition. Neural Comput. 1989;1(4):541–51.
18. Krizhevsky A, Sutskever I, Hinton GE. Imagenet classification with deep convolutional neural networks. In: Advances in neural information processing systems, 2012. p. 1097–105.
19. He K, Zhang X, Ren S, Sun J. Deep residual learning for image recognition. In: Proceedings of the IEEE computer society conference on computer vision and pattern recognition, Dec 2016. p. 770–8.
20. Szegedy C, Vanhoucke V, Ioffe S, Shlens J, Wojna Z. Rethinking the inception architecture for computer vision, 2015
21. Huang G, Liu Z, Van Der Maaten L, Weinberger KQ. Densely connected convolutional networks. In: Proceedings of the 30th IEEE conference on computer vision and pattern recognition (CVPR 2017), Jan 2017. p. 2261–9.
22. Drozdowska BA, Singh S, Quinn TJ. Thinking about the future: a review of prognostic scales used in acute stroke. Front Neurol. 2019;10:274.
23. Lin C-H, Hsu K-C, Johnson KR, Fann YC, Tsai C-H, Sun Y, et al. Evaluation of machine learning methods to stroke outcome prediction using a nationwide disease registry. Comput Methods Programs Biomed. 2020;190:105381.
24. Maier O, Menze BH, von der Gablentz J, Häni L, Heinrich MP, Liebrand M, et al. ISLES 2015—a public evaluation benchmark for ischemic stroke lesion segmentation from multispectral MRI. Med Image Anal. 2017;35:250–69.
25. Winzeck S, Hakim A, McKinley R, Pinto JA, Alves V, Silva C, et al. ISLES 2016 and 2017-benchmarking ischemic stroke lesion outcome prediction based on multispectral MRI. Front Neurol. 2018;9:679.

26. Kamal H, Lopez V, Sheth SA. Machine learning in acute ischemic stroke neuroimaging. Front Neurol. 2018;9:7–12.
27. Sheth SA, Lopez-Rivera V, Barman A, Grotta JC, Yoo AJ, Lee S, et al. Machine learning-enabled automated determination of acute ischemic core from computed tomography angiography. Stroke. 2019;50(11):3093–100.
28. Nielsen A, Hansen MB, Tietze A, Mouridsen K. Prediction of tissue outcome and assessment of treatment effect in acute ischemic stroke using deep learning. Stroke. 2018;49(6):1394–401.
29. Chauhan S, Vig L, De Grazia MDF, Corbetta M, Ahmad S, Zorzi M. A comparison of shallow and deep learning methods for predicting cognitive performance of stroke patients from MRI lesion images. Front Neuroinform. 2019;13:53.

Registry-Based Stroke Research

11

Niaz Ahmed and Tiago Prazeres Moreira

11.1 Introduction

Clinical research can be generally divided into interventional and observational studies. The most common interventional study is the randomized controlled trial (RCT) in which certain interventions such as a new drug, surgical method or device are tested on participants. The RCT can be single or double blinded and has strict inclusion and exclusion criteria. Randomization usually balances potential confounding factors between active and control arms. High-quality RCT is the gold standard for clinical research and basis for national and international guidelines. However, a RCT also has its limitations. For example, when a too strict experimental condition is applied and patients are highly selected in a RCT, the results may not be easily translated into routine clinical practice and may be difficult to implement in a broader patient population. Consequently, clinicians often treat patients based on knowledge derived from a minority of highly selected patients. In this scenario, the conclusions from RCTs may not be generalizable to 'real-world' patients. On the other hand, registry-based observational studies with big data may provide some insights into future direction of clinical trials and fill the gap when RCTs seem impossible to perform or are sometimes unethical [1–4].

11.2 Registry-Based Studies

In clinical studies, big data refers to the information collected using electronic databases such as a clinical or administrative registry. A Registry is a place where official names and/or items are kept forming an official list or register. A patient registry

N. Ahmed · T. Prazeres Moreira (✉)
Department of Neurology, Karolinska University Hospital-Solna, Stockholm, Sweden

Department of Clinical Neuroscience, Karolinska Institutet, Stockholm, Sweden
e-mail: niaz.ahmed@sll.se; tiago.prazeres.moreira@ki.se

© Springer Nature Switzerland AG 2021
A. C. Fonseca, J. M. Ferro (eds.), *Precision Medicine in Stroke*,
https://doi.org/10.1007/978-3-030-70761-3_11

is an organized system to collect data that uses observational study methods. Patient registries often collects demographic, risk factors, treatments, outcomes and other clinical data to evaluate specified characteristics, management, follow-up, benchmarking or outcomes for a defined population of a particular disease, condition, or exposure. The registry serves a predetermined scientific, clinical or policy purpose(s). Patient registries are usually created by researchers, research institutions, academic clinical institutions or multidisciplinary clinical teams. Registries may be funded by statal, private or other sources for the purpose of quality assessment or observational data collection that can be used for a specific research purpose. Registries may be organized and operated in a variety of forms and formats. Researcher-generated patient registries currently exist for a wide range of acute, chronic, or rare conditions. Pharmaceutical companies may create or sponsor registries for post-marketing studies and to identify rare complications.

11.3 Types of Studies Generated from a Registry

Risk factor evaluation, effectiveness of intervention, prediction model, epidemiological study (e.g. incidence and prevalence), implementation and efficacy of healthcare policy are some examples of a registry-based study. Effectiveness of intervention requires high-quality data and advanced statistical analysis to control for confounding factors. Multivariable models, stratification and propensity score analyses are useful tools for such kind of analysis [4].

11.4 Data Processing

This consists of data management and statistical analysis. Data management is the most time-consuming process and correctly performed data management is essential for a sound statistical analysis and valid results. Data management can include several steps or approaches such as (I) data cleaning, e.g. remove erroneous, impossible values (e.g. weight = 1000 kg, age 300 years) and convert various units into one if various unit measures are collected for a variable (e.g. blood glucose from mmol to mg/dL or vice versa; (II) generating new variables, for example, when transforming the continuous variable systolic blood pressure (SBP) into categorical variable (e.g. high SBP >140 mmHg, vs. normal SBP <140 mmHg); (III) transforming ordinal variables (e.g. mild stroke, moderate stroke, severe stroke and very severe stroke) into numerical variable, or vice versa; and (IV) combining data sets, e.g. if data sources are different then they should preferably be combined into one data set for the purpose of statistical analysis [4]. A correct method of statistical analysis is also crucial to draw a conclusion. A statistical analysis plan should be developed preferably with the help of a statistician. It is wise to consult a statistician before finalising the statistical analysis plan rather than consulting the statistician after the analysis has been performed.

11.5 Strengths and Limitations of Registry-Based Studies

Registry-based studies have both strengths and limitations compared to randomized studies.

11.5.1 Strengths

As registry data come from daily routine clinical practice without strict inclusion and exclusion criteria, therefore keeping its real clinical practice features, a registry can generate large amounts of data in a relatively short time frame. Registries provide a relatively inexpensive and quick option for big data collection from large populations and geographically diverse areas. Registries may also provide data over a long time period if needed and, provided that funding is available, make it possible to detect rare complications. As a registry should record all consecutive patients with a certain disease, it follows that more risk factors and subpopulations that are often excluded in RCTs get registered and analysed. A Phase IV study is an example of a registry-based study that is often carried out after an intervention has been shown to be efficacious in a Phase III trial. The registry can be used to describe a disease and outcome patterns over time and might follow changes in clinical care timely if it runs sufficiently long. After registration or implementation of guidelines of a new drug, surgical method or device, international registry data allows for comparisons between regions, countries, continents, and populations, thus reflecting the so-called 'real-world' data. Registries may shed light on risk factors for disease outcomes and enable hypothesis generation in less understood disease processes.

11.5.2 Limitations

Registry studies are, by definition, observational and in most cases retrospective and therefore cannot establish causality. In an observational study, the investigator does not act upon study participants, but instead observes natural relationships between factors and outcomes. Registries can only provide evidence of associations in support of potential cause-effect relationships and be used for generating hypotheses. On the contrary, a RCT can establish causality if done properly. The main risk to correct inference with registry studies is bias, which can impact the internal or external validity of the study. Identification of and control for bias are critical for registry-based studies. A careful examination for potential sources of bias should guide study design, analysis and interpretation of registry-based studies. This is particularly important for studies using already collected data from a registry. Data necessary for a specific study may not have been collected, the baseline characteristics may not be well balanced between the groups, and the conclusion may not be generalizable if restricted to a certain geographic population. The ability to conduct sound research using a registry is also highly dependent upon the quality of the data collected [3].

11.6   Internal vs. External Validity

Registry studies need to balance for internal validity and external validity. Internal validity is the degree to which a study is free from systematic error and measures what it was intended to. Precision is the degree to which a study is free from random error [5].

Internal validity thus refers to the degree of confidence that the causal association being tested is trustworthy and not influenced by other factors or variables. It means how well we are measuring the strength of association in the study population. The researcher needs to ask whether their conclusion accurately describes what actually ensued in the study.

External validity refers to the extent to which results from a study can be applied or generalized to other situations, groups or events. It means to what extent we can generalize the results obtained in the study population to a larger population of interest or how well do our results obtained in this specific cohort translate to 'real-world' patients.

11.7   Bias

Bias is a systematic error introduced through the measurement mechanism itself (e.g. diagnostic testing or questionnaire errors), as opposed to random error or statistical uncertainty of the measurement. To understand bias, it is helpful to keep in mind the difference between the overall research question and the specific study being undertaken. Bias can also be conceptualized as a systematic difference between the research question and the specific study that may lead to incorrect results. Bias associated with selective treatment may play an important role and should be considered in study design. One key issue is how to conceive research ideas that can be addressed with the database. The researcher may have a good research idea, but it may be difficult to carry out the research if the database does not have the necessary variables and the quality of the data is not sufficiently high. One approach could be the modification of the research idea. Another way could be to conceive a research idea based on available data. For this purpose, the researchers need to have a good overview of the collected data in the registry and be aware of its limitations. Prospective data collection with variables needed to test a certain research question may solve the issue of data not being available in the existing data set.

11.7.1 Categories of Bias

Bias has generally been divided into three broad categories: selection bias information bias and confounding.

11.7.1.1 Selection Bias

Selection bias occurs when the sample of subjects in the study is not representative of the population from which they were drawn, e.g. study participants have a different association between exposure and outcome than non-participants. Inclusion and exclusion criteria are the most common methods to control for selection bias, though in a registry-based study the investigator has little control over selection bias as it relates to a registry population. This can also occur if a large number of participants are lost to follow-up. When differing results are obtained between studies, it is important to ask whether differing answers are 'real' or are due to different characteristics of the subjects being evaluated. Non-response and study drop-out can also result in selection bias.

The effect of random error decreases with a larger size of the study population while systematic error in principle does not change [6, 7]. So, a large data set with systematic error will give invalid conclusions compared to a small data set without any systematic error. The precision increases and confidence intervals become narrower when the size of the study increases but systematic errors remain the same. So, researchers should make the utmost effort to minimize systematic bias in a registry study, which may not be possible if the study is done in an existing database.

11.7.1.2 Information Bias

Information bias refers to distortions in the exposure and outcome data measures. Measurement error and missing data are the most commonly encountered sources of information bias in registry studies. Information bias can have a substantial impact on the integrity of registry data if the quality of the collected data is poor or the proportion of missing data is high. Measurement error is the difference between the measured value of a variable and the true value. Misclassification is the most common form of measurement error and refers to the incorrect assignment of exposure or outcome status. As an example, obesity and overweight are sometimes misclassified according to body mass index; hypertension cut-off values have also changed in recent guidelines and differ between Europe and the United States. Pre-stroke disability as defined by the modified Rankin scale can also be misclassified as a score of 1 instead of 2 and so forth. Non-differential (random) misclassification occurs when the probability of misclassification is independent of exposure or outcome status. Generally, non-differential misclassification attenuates the observed exposure-disease relationship; in other words, it may mask an association where one truly exists. In contrast, differential misclassification occurs when the probability of misclassification is related to the exposure or the outcome. It can either artificially magnify or diminish the apparent association between an exposure and an outcome. Information bias may potentially also occur in the assessment of outcomes [8]. Evaluation is normally not blinded in registry studies as the exposure is known. This may lead to expectations from the medical professionals, from patients or from relatives when evaluating outcomes. This could affect clinical outcome measurement and lead to misclassification [7]. As for misclassification, it is important to consider whether missing data is differential or non-differential. In other words, is the probability of missing data related to either exposure or outcome? Exploration of the pattern of missing data is an important preliminary step in data analysis.

11.8 Confounding

Confounding is due to extrinsic factors that are associated with both the exposure and the outcome and not in the causal pathway for the association being investigated. Confounding can occur because of measured or unmeasured factors. If confounding factors are not measured or not completely accounted for in the analysis, they can change the observed association between the predictor and the outcome, resulting in inaccurate results.

Confounding can be a particular problem in the analyses of existing data, since the investigator has no control over what data have been collected and bound by the available data [9]. Unmeasured confounding factors cannot be controlled by statistical methods and may affect the outcome.

Confounding by indication is a special case to consider in studies evaluating outcomes associated with specific therapies. For example, patients receiving a certain therapy in a registry study had a greater risk of death compared to those not receiving the therapy, in direct contrast to the results of randomized clinical trials demonstrating strong benefits of this treatment. The patients who received the treatment in the registry study were shown to be the sickest and therefore at greatest risk of dying.

11.9 Local, National, and International Stroke Registries

Currently, there are several national but few international stroke registries serving different purposes and with different types of funding. In 2015, there were 28 national stroke registries active in 26 countries as identified by a systematic review of the literature [10]. Naturally, each country has its own priorities for which type of data is to be recorded for quality or research purposes. This creates many variables in each registry that have different definitions, measurement units or follow-up criteria making international comparisons troublesome, but help guiding each country's own health policies. However, an example of a national registry with international reach is the Get With The Guidelines (GTWG) Stroke Registry. The GTWG was started in 2001 by the American Heart Association in the United States and is a well-known hospital-based programme designed to improve care and outcomes of stroke patients by promoting the use and adherence to scientific treatment guidelines. The registry has more than 5 million included patients and provides clinical tools and resources for health professionals as well as patient education resources. Importantly, the GTWG Registry has a national and local recognition programme for hospital team performance [11]. The GTWG Registry has produced research publications of high impact for stroke treatment such as estimating risks of intracranial haemorrhage among patients with acute ischaemic stroke receiving warfarin and treated with intravenous thrombolysis (IVT) [12]. As one of the longest-running national stroke registries, the RIKSSTROKE in Sweden is another example of a stroke registry providing scientific publications in international journals [13]. Founded in 1994 and sponsored by the Ministry of Health and regional councils, it is used by 72 hospitals nationwide. Similarly, local but long running single-center registries such as the ASTRAL stroke registry of Lausanne, in the swiss canton of Vaud, can also be more detailed and stricter in the number of variables and provide systematic follow-up, allowing for high-quality research output [14]. A more recent systematic review of stroke registries in the world by a Japanese group of investigators identified 38 non-Japanese and 13 Japanese stroke registries, with a predominance of Europe over Africa and Asia. An expected finding of this review was the fact that the number of registered patients was higher in the registries with an opt-out clause or without required consent compared to those requiring consent [15]. The SITS Registry, the largest international stroke database, which uses opt-out or written informed consent in agreement with each country's legislation and ethical approval, is discussed below.

11.10 The SITS Registry

The SITS Registry, Safe Implementations of Treatments in Stroke-International Stroke Treatment Registry (SITS-ISTR), is a prospective, Internet-based, academic-driven, non-profit, multinational stroke register and international collaboration established in 1996 (https://www.sitsinternational.org). The SITS Registry was created to monitor safe implementation of intravenous (IV) thrombolysis with alteplase in acute ischaemic stroke. In 2002 the SITS Registry was given a broader international role and the European Medicines Agency (then EMEA, currently EMA) requested that all patients treated with intravenous thrombolysis should be registered in SITS for a period of 3 years [16]. Registration in SITS became a condition for approval of treatment with IVT in the European Union. The EMA also endorsed SITS as the registry for follow-up on thrombolysis treatment in acute ischaemic stroke. SITS has since then developed its services to enable follow-up of other evidence-based treatments in acute stroke such as thrombectomy, as well as secondary prevention. As per 2020, about 1680 stroke centres from more than 80 countries on 5 continents have participated in the SITS Registry and over 287,000 patient files are included, with more than 80 scientific reports published in international peer-reviewed journals based on data from SITS Registry.

In the last decade SITS has expanded and currently includes nine different data entry forms (IVT—standard, minimum; endovascular thrombectomy (EVT)—standard, minimum; general stroke registry—standard, minimum; intracerebral haemorrhage; atrial fibrillation; and a quality registry). Currently in deployment are cerebral venous thrombosis, decompressive hemicraniectomy, and spinal ischaemia data entry protocols.

<table>
<tr>
<td>

The SITS Scientific committee (SC) consists of World leading stroke experts. The SCs role is overseeing the scientific activities of SITS, review and approve the SITS studies, project proposals and manuscript before submission to peer reviewed journals.

</td>
<td>

The SITS International Coordination team assists the global SITS activities, maintains the database and supports international, national and local coordinators.

</td>
</tr>
<tr>
<td>

SITS International Regional Coordinators are leading stroke experts in the certain international geographic regions such as South America, Middle East and North Africa (MENA)

</td>
<td>

SITS National, associate National and Regional Coordinators are leading stroke experts in the country, and are responsible for assuring that the national rules and regulations are followed and to support the centres within the country

</td>
</tr>
</table>

<table>
<tr>
<td>

The SITS centre/ Local coordinator is the head of the Stroke unit in the centre and is responsible for following local rules and regulations and for assuring that the data entered in the SITS registry is accurate and completed

</td>
</tr>
</table>

<table>
<tr>
<td>

The SITS centre/ Local user is the person (s) who actually entered data in the registry. SITS centre user could a physician, research nurse or other administrative personals

</td>
</tr>
</table>

Fig. 11.1 Structure of the SITS Registry network

Figure 11.1 shows the structure of the SITS Registry.

11.11 Impact of SITS Data on Stroke Treatment

SITS Registry-based studies contributed to the license for IV alteplase within 3 h in Europe [16] and extension of the treatment time window >3 h [17, 18]. The SITS Registry also contributed to asserting the safety of off-label IV thrombolysis in a number of studies such as in the elderly (>80 years) [19–21], patients with a combination of diabetes mellitus and previous stroke [22], patients with stroke within 3 months [23], patients with severe (NIHSS scores 15–25) and very severe (NIHSS scores >25) acute ischaemic stroke [24], patients on vitamin K antagonist (e.g. warfarin) treatment with INR ≤ 1.7 [25], and more recently patients on dual-antiplatelet therapy [26] low-dose low-molecular-weight heparins [27] and with pre-stroke disability [28]. Risk prediction of intracerebral haemorrhage following treatment with

IVT [29] and safety and outcomes of IVT in young patients [30] are other examples of SITS contributions.

Studies based on SITS data have been referred to in the American Stroke Association guidelines [31]. SITS has proved useful as a tool to monitor guideline adherence. Retrospective database analysis showed that when European Stroke Organisation guidelines for intravenous thrombolysis were updated in 2008/2009 to include patients aged >80 years and to extend the treatment time window from 3 to 4.5 h, there was widespread and prompt adherence of stroke physicians to these new recommendations and no longer adherence to the unchanged pharmaceutical label for these previous contraindications. This prompt change was more pronounced in high-volume IV thrombolysis centres (especially treating > 100 patients over 2 years) than in centres treating less than 50 patients over a 2-year period. Experience with large IVT patient cohorts is thus a factor to consider when exploring guideline adherence, requiring large data sets for analysis [32].

The geographical presence of the SITS Registry through its regional networks is also believed to have encouraged stroke awareness and raised the interest of physicians in contributing to patient recruitment for scientific studies. Indeed, studies from the Middle East and North Africa [33, 34], South America [35], and Eastern Europe [36, 37] regions were often followed by an increase of patient recruitment in these regions (https://www.sitsinternational.org/sits-report-2019/).

11.12 Benefits of Participation in the SITS Registry

One of the major roles of SITS is to address scientific questions which are unanswered by RCTs. SITS can complement data from RCTs by performing an observational study where an RCT would be unfeasibly complex in design. Clinical practice data collected from individual clinics and countries can contribute to research results or raise new questions that impact clinical practice.

There are also benefits for the individual centre such as access to the data analysis toolkit, and active utilization of the knowledge gained to improve outcomes and quality of stroke care. Each centre can compare and analyse performance with national and international data, and benchmark centre performance results against others locally, regionally, or nationally using the SITS online, real-time report tool.

SITS is also a partner of the ESO-Angels and Angels Awards Programme and the American Stroke Association Stroke certification programme.

11.13 Limitations of the SITS Registry

The SITS Registry inherits all limitations of registry-based studies as discussed in the published articles based on SITS data sets [16, 18]. Data is reported by local investigators and there is no regular source data monitoring after the SITS-MOST study. So, there is no absolute certainty that data recorded in the registry is correct and consecutive according to the data entry form. Consequently, the potential for systematic bias must be taken into account. However, in 2011–2012, the Karolinska

Trial Alliance performed an independent monitoring of some selected Swedish centres and verified that data entered in the registry from these centres were accurate. Furthermore, the SITS Registry has a logical automatic validation system that prevents the entry of erroneous or impossible data in the registry, to some extent. Indeed, results from observational studies of intravenous thrombolysis and endovascular treatment from the SITS database have so far been comparable to those of RCTs, which is reassuring.

Patients recorded in the SITS Registry are a selected group compared to the general stroke population, which may limit generalizability. In most cases, patients included in studies had received reperfusion therapy. Patients receiving reperfusion therapy have more often severe neurological deficits. Patients who received reperfusion therapy may also have less concomitant disease than patients with similar stroke severity that did not receive such therapy. If a patient is missing from follow-up, the degree of activity in searching for the patient is up to the local investigator and probably varies between persons, populations and hospitals. Losses to follow-up at 3 months in the SITS Registry-based studies are about 20% which could be due to selection or random bias and weakens conclusions of these studies.

11.14 Management of a Large Data Set Derived from a Registry for Analysis

If we consider the SITS Registry data set as big data, it is crucial to consider certain issues for handling such a big data set. When the entire data set is downloaded it contains more than 280,000 cases and more than 400 raw variables. Researchers must go through the entire data set to understand it first. This may take a while if one is not familiar to the data set. This also applies for any data set. The next decision is how to clean data and what variables to keep for the purpose of the analysis. Data cleaning is a very important step for analysis. Sometimes a variable may contain several sub-variables, which is not so uncommon in the SITS Registry. Researchers need to agree on which data is erroneous and which are outliers but still valid. A data management protocol or handbook is necessary to serve this purpose. The person who performs the statistical analysis needs to understand the data and have the knowledge on where to look for inconsistency. Has any mistake occurred during data transport from one programme to another? Descriptive data is very helpful to identify any potential source of error. For example, if previous analysis of a certain variable gives a proportion of 30% and the current data gives a proportion of 50% then the researcher needs to carefully review the variable. What has happened? Was it an error in the data or has the clinical practice changed due to other reasons?

11.15 Who Can Get Access to SITS Database?

An active SITS user may submit a scientific project proposal based on the SITS Registry data to the SITS Scientific Committee (SC). The SITS SC reviews the project proposal and defines if the quality of the project is relevant and the quality of the project is high enough to use the SITS international data. If approved by the SITS SC, necessary data is provided to the investigator to run the project. National data can be used by the National Coordinator and any centre within the country without any need for approval from the SITS SC.

11.16 Novel Challenges in Registry-Based Research

In order to sustain or increase enrolment of larger patient populations, registries need to adapt to novel healthcare information technology semantics in order to increase interoperability between electronic health records (EHRs) and structure of the registry database. Many registries now extract data directly from EHRs and reduce manual input as well as sources of entry error. One such development is the use of open-source EHR language (openEHR) applied to guidelines, the so-called guideline definition language (GDL). The use of openEHR GDL technology applied to a stroke registry can be useful in checking guideline adherence. In a recent experiment we were able to try this technology in the SITS Registry; however, several manual steps were still required since the SITS Registry does not operate on openEHR [38]. Interoperability is thus becoming a key issue for the development and sustainability of large clinical registries with implications for planning, design, and analysis of databases.

Another recent development in the last decade is patient-centred outcomes research (PCOR) [39–41]. These are outcomes that should be valuable, meaningful and preferable for the patients and their families and should guide better decision-making by the physicians and the patients. This concept has had some influence on the creation of patient registries, in which the patient can report outcome measures directly or including sections dedicated to the patient-reported outcomes in existing registries, thus reshaping registry design. Registries may also consider adding a patient representative to the advisory board. However, there are still several unresolved ethical and regulatory issues such as to which extent patients need to be protected in these new responsibility roles, and to which extent one needs to ensure that they are acquainted with new technology for data input as well as ensure data privacy protection. The SITS coordination team is developing a subsection of PCOR questions in the cerebral venous thrombosis protocol which will be asked to the patient by the physician but can in the future be inserted via a mobile phone-based application directly by the patient or relatives themselves.

11.17 Conclusions

In contrast to RCTs, registry-based observational studies cannot establish causality; they can only provide evidence of associations in support of potential cause-effect relationships. Study design is critical when utilizing registry data. Bias is the most important threat to the validity of any registry study. Bias will differ for each scientific question and for each registry. Interpretation of results should be made within the context of the population under study. Data management protocol to clean a large data set and a pre-specified statistical analysis plan is essential before performing any analysis.

References

1. Gail MH, Altman DG, Cadarette SM, et al. Design choices for observational studies of the effect of exposure on disease incidence. BMJ Open. 2019;9:e031031. https://doi.org/10.1136/bmjopen-2019-031031.
2. Workman TA. Engaging patients in information sharing and data collection: the role of patient-powered registries and research networks. Rockville, MD: Agency for Healthcare Research and Quality (US); 2013.
3. Zhang Z. Big data and clinical research: perspective from a clinician. J Thorac Dis. 2014;6:1659–64. https://doi.org/10.3978/j.issn.2072-1439.2014.12.12.
4. Gliklich REDN, Leavy MB. Registries for evaluating patient outcomes: a user's guide. Rockville, MD: Agency for Healthcare Research and Quality (US); 2014.
5. Porta M. A dictionary of epidemiology. 5th ed. New York: Oxford University Press; 2008.
6. Vetter TR, Mascha EJ. Bias, confounding, and interaction: lions and tigers, and bears, oh my! Anesth Analg. 2017;125:1042–8. https://doi.org/10.1213/ANE.0000000000002332.
7. Rothman K. Epidemiology: an introduction. 2nd ed. New York: Oxford University Press; 2012.
8. Carlson MD, Morrison RS. Study design, precision, and validity in observational studies. J Palliat Med. 2009;12:77–82. https://doi.org/10.1089/jpm.2008.9690.
9. Norgaard M, Ehrenstein V, Vandenbroucke JP. Confounding in observational studies based on large health care databases: problems and potential solutions—a primer for the clinician. Clin Epidemiol. 2017;9:185–93. https://doi.org/10.2147/CLEP.S129879.
10. Cadilhac DA, Kim J, Lannin NA, et al. National stroke registries for monitoring and improving the quality of hospital care: a systematic review. Int J Stroke. 2016;11:28–40. https://doi.org/10.1177/1747493015607523.
11. American Heart Association. Get with the Guidelines®—stroke overview. 2020. https://www.heart.org/en/professional/quality-improvement/get-with-the-guidelines/get-with-the-guidelines-stroke/get-with-the-guidelines-stroke-overview. Accessed 30 Nov 2020.
12. Xian Y, Liang L, Smith EE, et al. Risks of intracranial hemorrhage among patients with acute ischemic stroke receiving warfarin and treated with intravenous tissue plasminogen activator. JAMA. 2012;307:2600–8. https://doi.org/10.1001/jama.2012.6756.
13. Asplund K, Hulter Asberg K, Norrving B, et al. Riks-stroke—a Swedish national quality register for stroke care. Cerebrovasc Dis. 2003;15(Suppl 1):5–7. https://doi.org/10.1159/000068203.
14. Michel P, Odier C, Rutgers M, et al. The Acute STroke Registry and Analysis of Lausanne (ASTRAL): design and baseline analysis of an ischemic stroke registry including acute multimodal imaging. Stroke. 2010;41:2491–8. https://doi.org/10.1161/STROKEAHA.110.596189.
15. Sato S, Sonoda K, Yoshimura S, Miyazaki Y, Matsuo R, Miura K, Imanaka Y, Isobe M, Saito Y, Kohro T, Nishimura K, Yasuda S, Ogawa H, Kitazono T, Iihara K, Minematsu K. Stroke registries in the world: a systematic review. Jpn J Stroke. 2018;40:331–42. https://doi.org/10.3995/jstroke.10587.

16. Wahlgren N, Ahmed N, Davalos A, et al. Thrombolysis with alteplase for acute isch-aemic stroke in the Safe Implementation of Thrombolysis in Stroke-Monitoring Study (SITS-MOST): an observational study. Lancet. 2007;369:275–82. https://doi.org/10.1016/S0140-6736(07)60149-4.
17. Ahmed N, Wahlgren N, Grond M, et al. Implementation and outcome of thrombolysis with alteplase 3-4.5 h after an acute stroke: an updated analysis from SITS-ISTR. Lancet Neurol. 2010;9:866–74. https://doi.org/10.1016/S1474-4422(10)70165-4.
18. Wahlgren N, Ahmed N, Eriksson N, et al. Multivariable analysis of outcome predictors and adjustment of main outcome results to baseline data profile in randomized controlled trials: Safe Implementation of Thrombolysis in Stroke-MOnitoring STudy (SITS-MOST). Stroke. 2008;39:3316–22. https://doi.org/10.1161/STROKEAHA.107.510768.
19. Ford GA, Ahmed N, Azevedo E, et al. Intravenous alteplase for stroke in those older than 80 years old. Stroke. 2010;41:2568–74. https://doi.org/10.1161/STROKEAHA.110.581884.
20. Mishra NK, Ahmed N, Andersen G, et al. Thrombolysis in very elderly people: controlled comparison of SITS International Stroke Thrombolysis Registry and Virtual International Stroke Trials Archive. BMJ. 2010;341:c6046. https://doi.org/10.1136/bmj.c6046.
21. Ahmed N, Lees KR, Ringleb PA, et al. Outcome after stroke thrombolysis in patients >80 years treated within 3 hours vs. >3–4.5 hours. Neurology. 2017;89:1561–8. https://doi.org/10.1212/WNL.0000000000004499.
22. Mishra NK, Davis SM, Kaste M, et al. Comparison of outcomes following thrombolytic ther-apy among patients with prior stroke and diabetes in the Virtual International Stroke Trials Archive (VISTA). Diabetes Care. 2010;33:2531–7. https://doi.org/10.2337/dc10-1125.
23. Karlinski M, Kobayashi A, Czlonkowska A, et al. Intravenous thrombolysis for stroke recurring within 3 months from the previous event. Stroke. 2015;46:3184–9. https://doi.org/10.1161/STROKEAHA.115.010420.
24. Mazya MV, Lees KR, Collas D, et al. IV thrombolysis in very severe and severe ischemic stroke: results from the SITS-ISTR registry. Neurology. 2015;85:2098–106. https://doi.org/10.1212/WNL.0000000000002199.
25. Mazya MV, Lees KR, Markus R, et al. Safety of intravenous thrombolysis for ischemic stroke in patients treated with warfarin. Ann Neurol. 2013;74:266–74. https://doi.org/10.1002/ana.23924.
26. Tsivgoulis G, Katsanos AH, Mavridis D, et al. Intravenous thrombolysis for ischemic stroke patients on dual antiplatelets. Ann Neurol. 2018;84:89–97. https://doi.org/10.1002/ana.25269.
27. Cooray C, Mazya M, Mikulik R, et al. Safety and outcome of intravenous thrombolysis in stroke patients on prophylactic doses of low molecular weight heparins at stroke onset. Stroke. 2019;50:1149–55. https://doi.org/10.1161/STROKEAHA.118.024575.
28. Cooray C, Karlinski M, Kobayashi A, et al. Safety and early outcomes after intravenous throm-bolysis in acute ischemic stroke patients with prestroke disability. Int J Stroke. 2020; https://doi.org/10.1177/1747493020954605.
29. Mazya M, Egido JA, Ford GA, et al. Predicting the risk of symptomatic intracerebral hemor-rhage in ischemic stroke treated with intravenous alteplase: safe implementation of treatments in stroke (SITS) symptomatic intracerebral hemorrhage risk score. Stroke. 2012;43:1524–31. https://doi.org/10.1161/STROKEAHA.111.644815.
30. Toni D, Ahmed N, Anzini A, et al. Intravenous thrombolysis in young stroke patients: results from the SITS-ISTR. Neurology. 2012;78:880–7. https://doi.org/10.1212/WNL.0b013e31824d966b.
31. Powers WJ, Rabinstein AA, Ackerson T, et al. 2018 guidelines for the early management of patients with acute ischemic stroke: a guideline for healthcare professionals from the American Heart Association/American Stroke Association. Stroke. 2018;49:e46–e110. https://doi.org/10.1161/STR.0000000000000158.
32. Anani N, Mazya MV, Bill O, et al. Changes in European label and guideline adherence after updated recommendations for stroke thrombolysis: results from the safe implementation of treatments in stroke registry. Circ Cardiovasc Qual Outcomes. 2015;8:S155–62. https://doi.org/10.1161/CIRCOUTCOMES.115.002097.

33. Al-Rukn S, Mazya M, Akhtar N, et al. Stroke in the Middle East and North Africa: a 2-year prospective observational study of intravenous thrombolysis treatment in the region. Results from the SITS-MENA registry. Int J Stroke. 2019; https://doi.org/10.1177/1747493019874729.

34. Rukn SA, Mazya MV, Hentati F, et al. Stroke in the Middle East and North Africa: a 2-year prospective observational study of stroke characteristics in the region—results from the safe implementation of treatments in stroke (SITS)—Middle East and North Africa (MENA). Int J Stroke. 2019;14:715–22. https://doi.org/10.1177/1747493019830331.

35. Alonso de Lecinana M, Mazya MV, Kostulas N, et al. Stroke care and application of thrombolysis in Ibero-America: report from the SITS-SIECV Ibero-American Stroke Register. Stroke. 2019;50:2507–12. https://doi.org/10.1161/STROKEAHA.119.025668.

36. Tsivgoulis G, Katsanos AH, Kadlecova P, et al. Intravenous thrombolysis for ischemic stroke in the golden hour: propensity-matched analysis from the SITS-EAST registry. J Neurol. 2017;264:912–20. https://doi.org/10.1007/s00415-017-8461-8.

37. Korv J, Vibo R, Kadlecova P, et al. Benefit of thrombolysis for stroke is maintained around the clock: results from the SITS-EAST registry. Eur J Neurol. 2014;21:112–7. https://doi.org/10.1111/ene.12257.

38. Anani N, Mazya MV, Chen R, et al. Applying openEHR's Guideline Definition Language to the SITS international stroke treatment registry: a European retrospective observational study. BMC Med Inform Decis Mak. 2017;17:7. https://doi.org/10.1186/s12911-016-0401-5.

39. Xian Y, O'Brien EC, Fonarow GC, et al. Patient-centered research into outcomes stroke patients prefer and effectiveness research: implementing the patient-driven research paradigm to aid decision making in stroke care. Am Heart J. 2015;170:36–45, 45.e1–11. https://doi.org/10.1016/j.ahj.2015.04.008.

40. Ellis LE, Kass NE. Patient engagement in patient-centered outcomes research: challenges, facilitators and actions to strengthen the field. J Comp Eff Res. 2017;6:363–73. https://doi.org/10.2217/cer-2016-0075.

41. Rathert C, Wyrwich MD, Boren SA. Patient-centered care and outcomes: a systematic review of the literature. Med Care Res Rev. 2013;70:351–79. https://doi.org/10.1177/1077558712465774.

From Bedside to Bench: Methods in Precision Medicine

12

Filipe Cortes-Figueiredo, Vanessa A. Morais, and Helena Pinheiro

12.1 Introduction

The escalating amounts of data in biomedical research have recently arisen as a harbinger of a new approach to medicine—*precision medicine*. Precision medicine aims to consider individual characteristics when diagnosing, treating, and managing the prognosis of a patient by concentrating health interventions (preventive or therapeutic) on those who will benefit from them. Thus, unnecessary side effects may be avoided and the allocation of health resources might be made more efficiently [1, 2].

A key determinant in aiding the advent of precision medicine has been *biomarkers*, which are characteristics that are objectively measured and assessed as indicators of either normal biological processes, pathogenic processes, or pharmacologic responses to therapeutic interventions. Thus, biomarkers may serve numerous functions, namely detecting higher susceptibility/risk to a specific medical condition or

Illustrations by Helena Pinheiro.

F. Cortes-Figueiredo
VMorais Lab—Mitochondria Biology & Neurodegeneration, Instituto de Medicina Molecular João Lobo Antunes, Faculdade de Medicina, Universidade de Lisboa, Lisbon, Portugal

NeuroCure Clinical Research Center, Charité—Universitätsmedizin Berlin, Berlin, Germany
e-mail: filipe.figueiredo@medicina.ulisboa.pt

V. A. Morais (✉)
VMorais Lab—Mitochondria Biology & Neurodegeneration, Instituto de Medicina Molecular João Lobo Antunes, Faculdade de Medicina, Universidade de Lisboa, Lisbon, Portugal
e-mail: vmorais@medicina.ulisboa.pt

H. Pinheiro
EGomes Lab—Cell Architecture, Instituto de Medicina Molecular João Lobo Antunes, Faculdade de Medicina, Universidade de Lisboa, Lisbon, Portugal
e-mail: hpinheiro@medicina.ulisboa.pt

© Springer Nature Switzerland AG 2021
A. C. Fonseca, J. M. Ferro (eds.), *Precision Medicine in Stroke*,
https://doi.org/10.1007/978-3-030-70761-3_12

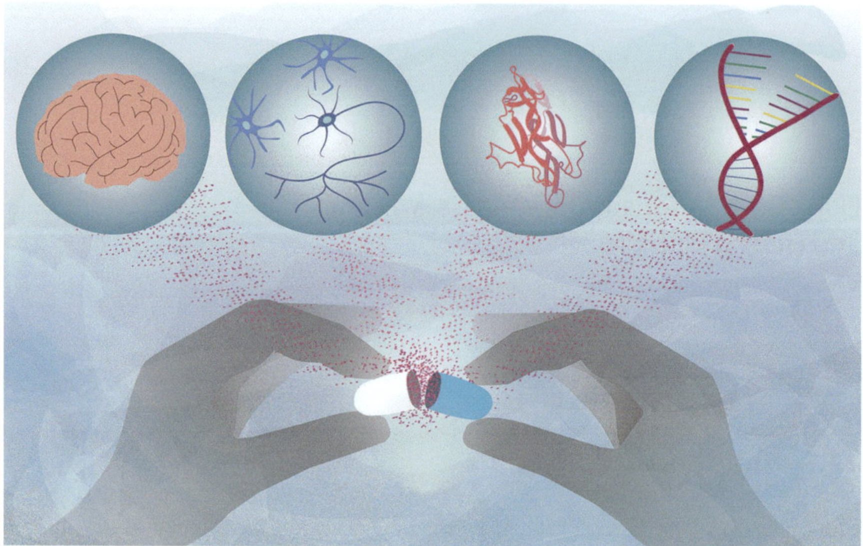

Fig. 12.1 Precision medicine makes use of multiple techniques in a diverse set of biological samples, ranging from organs (macroscopy) to tissues, cells, and molecules (microscopy and nanoscopy)

disease, diagnosing it, monitoring it longitudinally, and anticipating its prognosis. Similarly, biomarkers are pivotal in drug development, as they provide important insights in predicting favorable or unfavorable responses to therapies, assessing pharmacodynamics and safety concerns, and monitoring clinical responses [3, 4].

This chapter aims to peek behind the curtain of laboratorial methodology commonly used in biomedical research and laboratorial clinical settings aimed at identifying known disease biomarkers, as well as uncovering new ones. Precision medicine benefits from a multitude of *in vivo* biological samples (urine, blood, tissue biopsies), where we can go from a macroscopic approach, by analyzing whole organs, to a microscopic/nanoscopic approach, ranging among tissues, cells, and molecules (Fig. 12.1).

12.2 Organs, Tissues, Cells

Apart from autopsies and gross examination of surgical resections, which may assess organs macroscopically, studies in anatomic pathology focus on histologic practices, *i.e.*, the study of tissues and their two interacting components: cells and extracellular matrix. Histologic research is mostly performed *ex vivo*, following a complex process that aims to preserve the cellular architecture observed in the body while avoiding sample deterioration. Afterwards, thin translucent sections of these tissues are cut, allowing microscopic observation [5, 6].

Microscopy is broadly divided into *light microscopy* (*LM*) and *electron microscopy* (*EM*), depending on what interacts with tissue components: light for the former and beams of electrons for the latter. On the one hand, LM encompasses a vast variety of options: *bright-field microscopy*, *fluorescence microscopy*, *phase-contrast microscopy*, *confocal microscopy*, and *polarizing microscopy*. The type of LM will, in very plain terms, mostly depend on the choice of (1) wavelength range and divergence for light source, (2) filter, (3) condenser, and (4) lens system, among others. On the other hand, the beam of electrons in EM has a much shorter wavelength than light, which increases resolution 1000-fold, albeit in shades of black, gray, and white. There are two main types of EM: *transmission electron microscopy* (*TEM*), which provides a sectional view of the sample in shades of gray depending on electro-density (the darker, the denser), and *scanning electron microscopy* (*SEM*), which provides a 3D-like image of the surface of the sample, after a coat of metal ions is applied on the sample [6].

Since tissues and cells are colorless (excluding naturally occurring pigments), one must use a variety of tools to morphologically distinguish different cell types and microscopic components within the samples of interest (Fig. 12.2). This is achieved by [6, 7]:

- *Staining*—Dyes are used more or less selectively, depending on electrostatic linkages with ionizable radicals of macromolecules and acidic or basic compounds. Illustratively, hematoxylin-eosin (H&E), very commonly used, is composed by hematoxylin, a basic dye that binds to basophilic components such as DNA, RNA, and glycosaminoglycans, and eosin, an acidic dye that interacts with acidophilic components such as mitochondria, secretory granules, and collagen.
- *Autoradiography*—Radioactively labeled metabolites are provided to living cells in order to be incorporated into macromolecules of interest. After sample processing and sectioning, radioactivity is detected by silver bromide crystals and microscopic slides (LM or TEM) are developed photographically.
- *Enzyme histochemistry or cytochemistry*—The minimally processed tissue sections are subjected to an enzyme of interest (phosphatases, dehydrogenases, peroxidase) after the sections have already been exposed to their specific substrate. Afterwards, a marker compound that detects the enzymatic reaction is added and

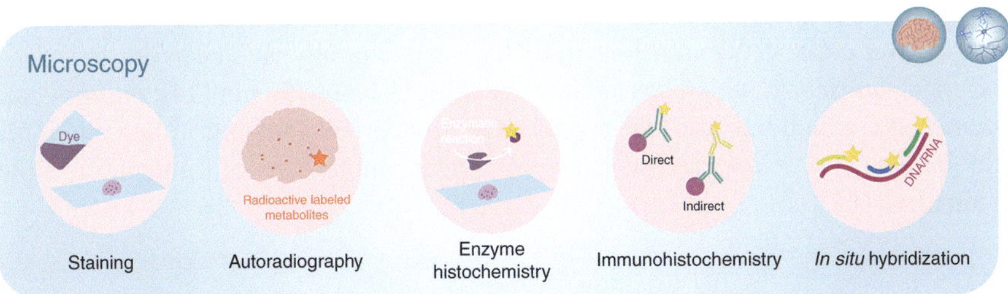

Fig. 12.2 Different techniques allow colorless cells to become visible under a microscope

its precipitation is detected by LM or EM, thus pointing out the sites of reaction in the cell.

- *Immunohistochemistry*—Antibodies are used to specifically target an antigen of interest, mostly proteins with high molecular weight [8–10], and are able to label them either directly through a tagged antibody (*direct immunohistochemistry*) or indirectly through a tagged secondary antibody that targets an untagged primary antibody, which, in turn, targets the antigen of interest (*indirect immunohisto-chemistry*). These tagged antibodies may be combined with different labels: fluorescent compounds for fluorescence microscopy, enzymes for enzyme histochemistry, and gold for TEM, thereby making use of established approaches to both LM and EM microscopy.
- *In situ hybridization (ISH)*—A single-stranded DNA- or RNA-tagged probe is used to bind specific complementary strands of interest (genes, viruses, among others). Probes may be tagged with radioactive nucleotides (autoradiography is used), with a compound, such as digoxigenin which interacts with peroxidase-labeled antibodies against digoxigenin (immunocytochemistry is used), or with a fluorochrome (fluorescence microscopy is used). ISH with a fluorescent probe is called fluorescent ISH (FISH).

The use of antibodies and fluorescence has revolutionized histologic research, but it has also ushered in a new era for cell biology, where microscopy may be complemented by indirect detection of specific cellular markers. Two main examples are *flow cytometry* and *mass cytometry*. Flow cytometry, commonly used in immunology and hematology, allows for the identification of cells or their intracellular components depending on the detection of fluorescent antibodies or dyes after excitation by a beam of lasers. As cells are in a laminar flow and each antibody or dye will have a different emission spectrum detected by different filters, it is possible to collect the many different spectra emitted per cell and, indirectly, assess various cellular components at once [11]. Similarly, mass cytometry uses antibodies but these are tagged with rare heavy metal isotopes. As cells in a single-cell suspension are nebulized and their heavy metal reporter ions are released, the time-of-flight (TOF) of each one, which depends on the mass of each atom, is detected by an atomic mass cytometer, allowing the decoding of the exact composition of metal atoms on each cell. Since emission spectra in flow cytometry have significant overlap, mass cytometry is able to analyze more parameters per cell at once [12, 13].

Currently, new efforts are being made towards expanding these technologies. Taking fluorescence microscopy as an example, which is commonly employed in imaging live cells, new extensions to its basic functioning have been created: *fluorescence nanoscopy*, which has attained resolutions below 50 nm [14]; *multiphoton microscopy*, which has allowed noninvasive *in vivo* cell imaging in humans [15]; and *imaging flow cytometry*, which has provided fluorescent cell imaging to flow cytometry [16].

> $\mathbf{Q}$ **Focus on Stroke**
>
> The *neutrophil-to-lymphocyte ratio* (*NLR*) might be used as a clinical marker of inflammation, by establishing a ratio between the balance of neutrophils, cells in the innate immune system associated with the phagocytosis of bacteria and direct tissue lesion, and lymphocytes, which orchestrate a directed and more adequate response in the adaptive immune system [17]. NLR has been linked to an increased risk to multiple cardiovascular diseases, including stroke [18], and it has also been shown to have a predictive role in assessing the risk of hemorrhagic transformation in ischemic strokes [19]. Far from the traditional methods of using hemocytometers and manual cell counting, currently most white blood cell (WBC) counts are performed automatically with a large variety of techniques, including *flow cytometry* and *cytochemistry* [20–24].

12.3 Proteins

Proteins are the largest contributor to a cell's dry mass and are the most complex macromolecules in the body. On the one hand, they are key pieces in cellular architecture, providing a "cellular skeleton", and, on the other hand, they are the main elements in the complex biochemical interactions that constitute life [25–27].

Proteins are translated from mRNA in a ribosome, forming a polypeptide chain of various amino acids. They then assume their structure, which is key for the protein's functions within the cell, through a sequence of increasingly complex post-translational modifications, such as folding, covalent modifications (*e.g.*, methylation, acetylation, phosphorylation, lipidation, and glycosylation), cleavage, and assembly into multi-subunit proteins [28, 29].

12.3.1 Protein Purification

Prior to any analysis with a focus on a specific protein or set of proteins, it is necessary to find ways of purifying our proteins of interest out of a cell homogenate with thousands of other proteins and macromolecules.

Firstly, different cell components might be separated by centrifugation: *differential centrifugation*, where varying levels of centrifugal force allow the separation of particles based on their sedimentation rates, or *density gradient centrifugation*, where a solution with a density gradient is able to separate another solution after a centrifugal force is applied, based on either the particles' size and mass (*rate zonal centrifugation*) or their density (*isopycnic centrifugation*) [30, 31]. Another approach is *selective precipitation*, where protein differential solubility is explored by altering the pH/salt balance or by adding precipitating agents such as ethanol, acetone, and polyethylene glycol, among many others [32]. *Immunoprecipitation* uses antibodies to precipitate a specific protein of interest [33].

12.3.2 Protein Separation

Chromatography offers a very versatile approach of separating a mixture of different proteins into its different constituents. Regardless of its various versions, chromatography relies on a *stationary phase* and a *mobile phase*, which do not mix and compete for the components in the mixture, depending on differing properties determined by the method chosen. The mobile phase serves as a medium of moving the proteins across the stationary phase, where they will move at varying speeds as they interact with both phases (Fig. 12.3) [27, 34]:

- *Column chromatography*—A vertical container made out of glass, plastic, or stainless steel (the column) is filled with a stationary phase (inorganic materials, synthetic organic polymers, or polysaccharides). The protein mixture is placed

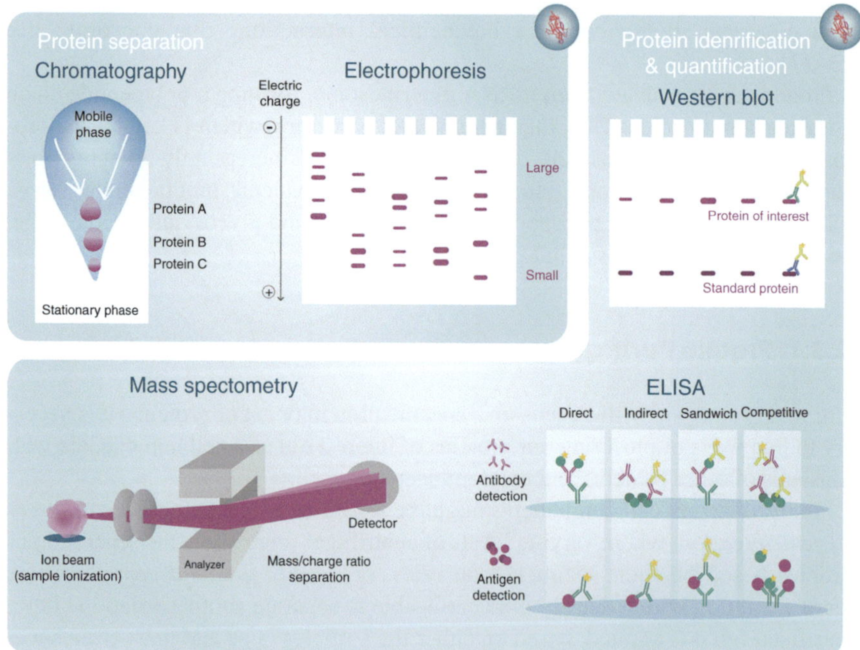

Fig. 12.3 Proteins are crucial macromolecules in cell biology which may be separated, identified, and quantified through a variety of techniques

atop the column and a mobile phase moves the proteins along the stationary phase at different speeds according to their adsorption or dispersion properties.

- *High-performance (high-pressure) liquid chromatography (HPLC)*—This variation of standard column chromatography uses much smaller beads as the stationary phase, usually silicon based, and stainless steel columns able to withstand much higher pressures of mobile phases passing through, which significantly increases the scalability and speed of the separation process.
- *Size-exclusion (gel-filtration) chromatography*—The column is filled by porous beads (the stationary phase) that will filter the proteins differently according to their molecular size. As the mobile phase moves the proteins along, the proteins small enough to go through the pores will travel faster than the ones excluded from them, which are forced to move around the beads. The most common stationary phases are dextran-based and agarose gels.
- *Ion-exchange chromatography*—The proteins will move along the stationary phase depending on the electrostatic interaction they have with it: stationary phases with positive groups, called *anion exchangers*, will make more negatively charged proteins move slower, retaining them, while stationary phases with negative groups, called *cation exchangers*, will do the exact opposite.
- *Hydrophobic interaction chromatography*—The stationary phase components are coated with hydrophobic groups that will retain proteins with a similar hydrophobic surface, while nonadherent proteins move freely with the mobile phase, usually of high ionic strength.
- *Affinity chromatography*—In contrast to the other nonspecific chromatography methods, this method is based on selective properties between the stationary phase, embedded with ligands for our protein of interest, and the protein we are interested in retaining. A few examples of common interactions are between antigen and antibody, enzyme and substrate, and hormone and receptor, among others.

Chromatography methods can also be a mix of several approaches such as high-performance affinity chromatography (HPAC), combining HPCL and affinity chromatography, which is commonly used in biomedical research [35, 36].

Gel electrophoresis is another method that separates proteins by applying an electric field to a solution of proteins in a semipermeable gel (*e.g.*, polyacrylamide, agarose) at different currents according to their net charge (Fig. 12.3). When the proteins are kept in their native structure, this is called a *native gel electrophoresis*. However, as protein structure might greatly impact their migration, proteins are subjected to sodium dodecyl sulfate (SDS), an anionic detergent; 2-mercaptoethanol, a reducing agent; and heat, which denature the protein and disassemble multimeric proteins, while increasing the protein's negative charge proportionally to its molecular weight. Thus, in *polyacrylamide gel electrophoresis (SDS-PAGE)* proteins will migrate according to their molecular weight in the polyacrylamide matrix. Proteins can be visualized with a dye such as Coomassie Blue [27, 34].

Isoelectric focusing (IEF) is another method that uses an electrical field to separate proteins according to their isoelectric point (pI), *i.e.*, when the net charge of the protein (sum of negative and positive charges at the amino acid chain regions) is null. To achieve this, a pH gradient is created within a polyacrylamide matrix using ionic buffers and an electric field that will allow proteins to migrate to a point where their pI is null [27, 34].

If one combines both methods by running an IEF first, followed by a SDS-PAGE, proteins with very similar molecular weights will be first separated by their pI and afterwards by their size. This technique is known as *two-dimensional gel electrophoresis (2DGel)* and it is very useful in analyzing complex protein mixtures [27, 34].

12.3.3 Protein Identification and Quantification

Mass spectrometry (MS) is a high-throughput technology that is able to detect and, in particular setups, also quantify an enormous variety of macromolecules, including proteins. This highly versatile technique has been responsible for the "-omics" revolution in molecular cell biology, giving rise to the fields of proteomics [37], lipidomics [38], and metabolomics [39]. Despite the many variants of *MS*, its functioning revolves around the following (Fig. 12.3) [27, 34, 37, 40]:

- Following protein purification and separation, proteins are digested into smaller peptides and undergo *molecular ionization* that fragments and charges the molecules. This creates a gaseous phase of intact ions.
- Afterwards, the ionized molecules are separated according to either their *mass-to-charge (m/z) ratio* or *TOF* in a *mass analyzer*, through magnetic, electric, or electromagnetic fields.
- Finally, the separated ionized molecules reach a *detector* that plots the results in a *mass spectrum*, with the *m/z ratio* plotted against signal intensity. This allows both the identification of various amino acids per the mass spectra and their quantification per the signal intensity.

There are three main MS-based protocols in biomedical research [34, 41]:

1. *Liquid chromatography-mass spectrometry (LC-MS)*, which uses liquid chromatography to separate proteins prior to MS analysis and *electrospray ionization* for molecular ionization of peptides, through the electron-charged dispersion of a liquid mixed with volatile components.
2. *Matrix-assisted laser desorption/ionization-time-of-flight mass spectrometry (MALDI-TOF)*, which uses MALDI for molecular ionization, through a laser beam that excites a liquid matrix that absorbs light and serves as a source of protons to the preprocessed peptides.
3. *Tandem mass spectrometry (MS/MS)*, which uses two or more MS steps performed sequentially (*e.g.*, two mass spectrometers connected to each other, two mass analyzers in the same instrument), through a first step that separates peptides according to their mass and a second step that isolates a peptide of interest and further dissects it into its mass spectra.

Another common method of protein quantification is *enzyme-linked immunosorbent assay (ELISA)*, which combines antibodies directed towards proteins of interest and linked to an enzyme. A substrate is then added to produce a change in color, luminescence, or fluorescence which is objectively assessed with a spectrophotometer or fluorometer, thus quantifying our proteins of interest proportionally to signal intensity. Depending on what is controlled in the experiment, it is possible to quantify either the antigens or the antibodies: by providing known antigens we may quantify antibodies and by providing antibodies for a specific antigen we may quantify the antigen. This technique is widely used in laboratorial research and has different variations (Fig. 12.3) [34, 42, 43]:

- *Direct ELISA* - It derives from the *direct* link between an enzyme-linked antibody and a specific antigen.
- *Indirect ELISA* - It derives from the link between a *secondary antibody*, which is enzyme-linked, directed towards *primary antibodies*, which, in turn, are linked to an antigen.
- *Sandwich ELISA* - It derives from the link between three antibodies: a *capture antibody* directed towards an antigen, the *primary antibody* linked to the captured antigen, and the *secondary antibody*, which is enzyme-linked and will react with the substrate. This is the most sensitive form of all ELISA approaches.
- *Competitive ELISA* - It derives from the competition between an enzyme-linked antibody or an enzyme-linked antigen and the antigen-antibody interaction we are interested in quantifying. In contrast to the other methods, the signal coming from the enzymatic reaction will be inversely proportional to the protein we are interested in studying, since higher signal intensity will correspond to the enzyme-linked protein (an antigen or an antibody) and not the antigen-antibody interaction we are interested in quantifying.

Western blot is a method commonly used for the *relative* quantification of proteins, *i.e.*, the levels of our protein of interest will be relative to another known standard protein. A Western blot starts with a gel electrophoresis (details provided in Sect. 12.3.2) followed by a transfer to a porous membrane (made of nitrocellulose or polyvinylidene difluoride) through an electrical current. After *electrotransfer*, the detection of specific proteins is done through antibodies: the membrane is *blocked* first to prevent nonspecific antibody binding; afterwards *primary antibodies* against our proteins of interest are added and incubated, followed by the addition of a *secondary antibody* targeting the host IgG of the primary antibodies previously added, which will be either radiolabeled or enzyme linked (Fig. 12.3). Proteins are then quantified by colorimetric, chemiluminescent, radioactive, or fluorescent detection [34, 44].

Due to its limited scalability, more high-throughput versions of Western blots have been developed [34, 45, 46]:

- *Reverse-phase protein lysate microarrays* (RPA)—it uses a microarray with a nitrocellulose slide to detect proteins of interest by immunochemistry, without, however, separating the peptides by molecular size.
- *Micro-Western arrays* (MWA)—which further expands on the technology of RPA and adds the possibility of separating the peptides by molecular size.

12.3.4 Protein Sequence and Structure

Prior to the advent of MS-based technology, protein sequencing was achieved through the *Edman method*, which is able to determine the amino acid composition and order of a polypeptide from its N-terminus. In it, proteins are first denatured to a polypeptide chain and phenyl isothiocyanate, the *Edman reagent*, is added. Upon addition of an anhydrous acid that breaks the peptide bond between the N-terminus amino acid and second amino acid, the first amino acid is released. Afterwards, the released amino acids are extracted sequentially, being further separated by HPLC [27, 34].

Proteins, however, are much more than a sequence of amino acids, the *primary structure* of a protein. Through covalent and noncovalent bonds (*e.g.*, hydrogen bonds, electrostatic attractions, van der Waals attractions, and hydrophobic clustering force) protein *conformation* determines the role it will execute in the cell. In addition to the primary structure of a protein, there is also the *secondary structure* (α-helices and β-sheets), the *tertiary structure* (the three-dimensional organization of a polypeptide chain), and the quaternary structure (a protein composed of various polypeptide chains). A few tools may be used to decipher these levels of protein structure: *circular dichroism (CD)*, *nuclear magnetic resonance (NMR) spectroscopy*, *X-ray crystallography*, and EM [26, 34].

> $\mathcal{Q}$ **Focus on Stroke**
>
> The *B-type natriuretic peptide (BNP)* is synthesized by cardiomyocytes in the heart ventricles in response to mechanical stretch, leading to a reduction in blood pressure and circulating volume, thus reducing cardiac preload and afterload. During its processing, both BNP and an inactive N-terminal proBNP (NT-proBNP) are released in equal amounts [47]. BNP and NT-proBNP have been linked to an increased risk of ischemic stroke, particularly cardioembolic strokes, as well as, for stroke patients, worse functional outcomes and higher mortality [48–52]. BNP was initially entitled *brain natriuretic peptide* because it was identified in the porcine brain in 1988, through precipitation, chromatography, and sequencing with the Edman method [53]. Currently, however, various *immunoassay techniques* (which are based on the principles of immunochemistry) are used instead [48, 49, 51].

12.4 Nucleic Acids

Human cells hold their genome, the entire set of genetic instructions, in ~3 billion base pairs (bps) of double-stranded *deoxyribonucleic acid (DNA)* molecules, densely packed in 46 chromosomes. *Genes* are transcribed into single-stranded *ribonucleic acid (RNA)*, a much more unstable but extremely versatile macromolecule that controls *gene expression* in a plethora of ways [26, 54]:

- *Messenger RNAs (mRNAs)* - Coding RNAs that might be translated into proteins.

- *Ribosomal RNAs* (*rRNAs*) - Basic elements of ribosomes and responsible for protein translation.
- *Transfer RNAs* (*tRNAs*) - Responsible for bridging amino acids and RNA translation into polypeptide chains.
- *Small nuclear RNAs* (*snRNAs*) - Responsible for alternative splicing of mRNAs, producing various protein isoforms.
- *microRNAs* (*miRNAs*) *and small interfering RNAs* (*siRNAs*) - Responsible for inhibiting gene expression at the RNA level.

12.4.1 Nucleic Acid Extraction

Both DNA and RNA extractions involve cell lysis with a detergent, protein digestion with proteases, centrifugation, and precipitation. While DNA extraction is very straightforward with a large variety of different kits due to its stability, extracting RNA involves careful handling of the samples due to ubiquitous enzymes that degrade RNA—*RNase* [7, 55, 56].

12.4.2 Nucleic Acid Visualization and Quantification

Akin to the Western blot for protein quantification (details provided in Sect. 12.3.3), *Southern* and *Northern blots* are used to visualize DNA and RNA, respectively. A gel electrophoresis separates fragments according to size, as nucleic acids are negatively charged. The gel is then transferred to a membrane or paper and a complementary labeled probe is added, thus revealing the location of the fragments of interest through hybridization (details provided in IHS, in Sect. 12.2). For Southern blot, DNA is digested with *restriction enzymes* that cut it into fragments prior to gel electrophoresis and must be denatured prior to membrane transferring to become single stranded. By using restriction enzymes that cut at specific locations, it is possible to *genotype* different samples that differ at *restriction sites*. For Northern blot, this technique may be used for relative quantification of gene expression, since the presence of more transcripts of interest will produce a band with increased signal [57, 58].

An absolute quantification of DNA and, indirectly, of RNA through cDNA, obtained by reverse transcriptase, can be attained with *quantitative polymerase chain reaction (qPCR)*. This approach is based on the biological method for DNA replication, where a thermostable DNA polymerase, two short oligonucleotide probes called primers designed to flank the gene or region we are interested in amplifying, and free nucleotides exponentially replicate DNA molecules through a cycle of denaturation of the double-stranded molecules, annealing of the primers, and elongation of the polynucleotides. Afterwards, the products of each cycle will serve as templates for the following cycles. By adding fluorescent dyes or probes that interact with the PCR products, it is possible to quantify the *in vitro* DNA production and, thereby, the initial concentration of DNA. This can be done both relatively, regarding a gene we view as our baseline, and absolutely, by performing a standard curve with serial dilutions and using it as a reference. *Genotyping* is also possible by analyzing the *melt curves* of fluorescent probes, since different genotypes will have different affinities to the same probes [7, 59].

Another approach to relative quantification of gene expression or genotyping is *DNA microarrays*. DNA microarrays are plated with numerous probes for specific genes or single-nucleotide polymorphisms (SNPs) of interest. Then, a labeled DNA/cDNA is added, usually using fluorochromes, and hybridization to the sequences of interest is recorded by fluorescence intensity. Thus, genes with higher fluorescence have more copies in our cDNA and SNPs with recorded fluorescence are present in our DNA samples. Usually, however, a comparison between a control and a sample of interest is performed. In this case, samples are labeled with different fluorochromes and the pattern of fluorescence is used to determine the number of differentially expressed genes and differing SNPs [7, 60].

Genome-wide analysis studies (GWAS) mostly use DNA microarrays to interrogate SNP differences in patients and controls and between different populations [61]. Shortly after the initial draft of the human genome was published [62], the search for different haplotypes in the human population, *i.e.*, a collection of SNPs that tend to be inherited together, launched the International HapMap Project [63] aiming to collect, organize, and make freely available the SNPs of multiple human ancestries. After the first study in 2002 [64], GWAS grew exponentially, uncovering 71,673 variant-trait associations from 3567 publications in 2018 [65].

12.4.3 Nucleic Acid Sequencing

Despite the 2004 publication of the Human Genome Project's final version of the human genome [66], the reference genome has been subjected to a variety of reviews, with its latest release in 2017 [67]. Similarly, sequencing methods have suffered a revolution since its origins with *Sanger sequencing* (Fig. 12.4).

Sanger sequencing uses *dideoxyribonucleoside triphosphates (ddNTPs)*, which, contrary to normal nucleotides, lack the 3′ hydroxyl group and block the elongation of a DNA strand being actively replicated. Following PCR amplification with a specific primer, exact copies of our DNA molecule of interest are divided into four tubes, each one with one of the ddNTPs and the remaining three nucleotides, plus a DNA polymerase. As we amplify the DNA molecules through PCR, we obtain fragments of different sizes that terminate at the ddNTP of each tube. Afterwards, by loading each tube and performing a gel electrophoresis, one is able to reconstruct the original DNA fragment sequence. Since this gel electrophoresis is very labor-intensive, the method was adapted to an automated capillary gel electrophoresis with fluorescently labeled ddNTPs, where each ddNTP has a different color (Fig. 12.4) [26].

Massively parallel sequencing (MPS) or *next-generation sequencing (NGS)* offers a completely different approach to Sanger sequencing by producing numerous *reads* that can be aligned to a consensus sequence bioinformatically. Despite significant differences between various platforms, the process overall starts by *library preparation* with DNA fragmentation and adapter ligation. Afterwards, each

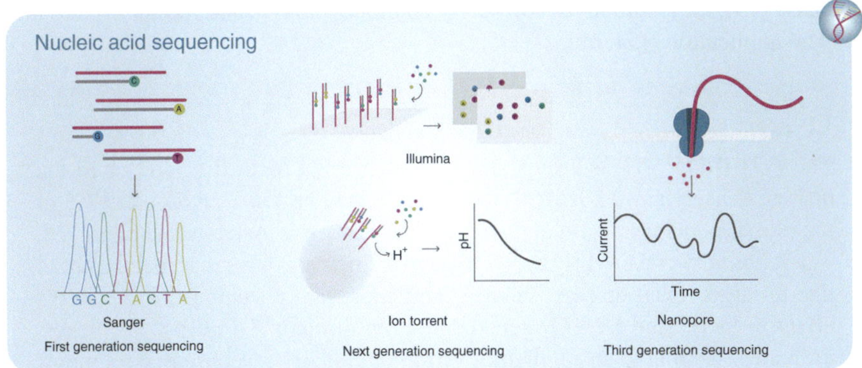

Fig. 12.4 Nucleic acid sequencing has suffered a revolution since its origins in Sanger sequencing with the advent of next-generation and third-generation sequencing approaches

DNA fragment with its unique adapter is amplified in a solid support that allows copies of the same oligonucleotide to be sequenced in *clusters*. Numerous clusters are then sequenced in parallel. The most common approaches are the following (Fig. 12.4) [26, 68, 69]:

- *Illumina sequencing*—The reaction is performed on a microarray, through sequencing-by-synthesis. It uses nucleotides labeled with different fluorochromes that block DNA elongation, similarly to ddNTPs in Sanger sequencing. However, the tags can be removed enzymatically and a further tagged nucleotide may be added afterwards. Thus, DNA sequences are determined by reading the sequence of different fluorescent colors.
- *Ion torrent sequencing*—The reaction is performed on DNA-covered beads spread throughout multiple wells, through semiconductor sequencing. Each bead is covered with the same DNA fragment after PCR enrichment. As the well is filled with a specific nucleotide, a voltage-sensitive semiconductor chip detects changes in pH, since a proton is released when a nucleotide is incorporated. If the pH changes, the nucleotide filling the well is registered as having been incorporated and the sequence is successively determined.

A completely alternative sequencing approach to the aforementioned NGS approaches is the *nanopore sequencing*, sometimes classified as a *third-generation sequencing technology*. Nanopore sequencing is able to sequence a single-DNA molecule through a stationary DNA polymerase, by measuring the time nucleotides with different removable fluorescent dyes reside on the polymerase. Nucleotides who linger the most before losing their dye are the ones incorporated by the polymerase (Fig. 12.4). Despite achieving reads with up to ~10,000 bps, error rate is significantly increased in this method [68, 70, 71].

NGS technologies have revolutionized the field of genomics, allowing the sequencing of whole genomes and exomes (the coding regions only), and launching the fields of transcriptomics (RNA-seq) and epigenomics (methylation sequencing), as well as the 1000 Genomes Project, which aims to collect a diverse set of whole genomes and make them public [7, 69, 70, 72–74]. As NGS prices continue to decrease [75], these initiatives will surely continue to thrive and further expand into clinical applications [54, 69].

> Q **Focus on Stroke**
> The *rs2107595 SNP* is a regulatory region variant located at 7p21.1 in the histone deacetylase 9 (*HDAC9*) locus which may be found in around 17% of the global population with an increased prevalence in Asian populations [76, 77]. It has very consistently been linked to an increased risk in ischemic stroke due to large vessel disease [78–81]. This most likely stems from the SNP's effect in increasing *HDAC9* gene expression through E2F3/Rb1 complexes, ultimately leading to an augmented pro-inflammatory response that promotes carotid plaque and carotid intima-media thickness (IMT) [82–84]. The rs2107595 SNP was found through a combination of *DNA microarrays*, *qPCR*, and *MALDI-TOF* [78–80].
>
> The *miR-106b-5p microRNA* is expressed from 7q22.1 and has been found to be upregulated in patients with ischemic stroke [85–87]. Data from experimental models suggests that this might be caused by an enhancement in glutamate-induced apoptosis and increased oxidative stress [88]. The miR-106b-5p was found through *DNA microarrays* and *qPCR* [85, 86].

12.5 Conclusion

This chapter summarizes the main methods used in biomedical research, with a primary focus on the ones applicable to medicine. Although methods were presented in a somewhat simplified fashion, in reality, many of the techniques are far more complex. Nonetheless, the promise of *precision medicine* and the discovery of novel biomarkers are dependent on reliable and robust scientific methods in biomedical research. Having a strong and broad knowledge of the available techniques in histology and cell and molecular biology fields is important not only for current scientific progress, but also for future endeavors in science, ultimately leading to scientific breakthroughs.

Regarding stroke per se, at present, the distinction of stroke mimics from transient ischemic attacks (*TIA*), ischemic strokes, and hemorrhagic strokes is made by combining a patient's medical and family history with clinical examination by an experienced neurologist and brain imaging. Similarly, the choice of treatment, etiology assessment, and prognosis prediction are based on the accrued clinical data, symptom severity, and time elapsed since the first symptoms [89–93]. Due to the complexity of this process, novel biomarkers that would be able to objectively and quickly ascertain stroke risk, subtype, etiology, and/or prognosis would be highly valuable in the clinical setting. Currently, however, single biomarkers, although promising, have failed to provide an effective solution to this problem [94–97]. Thus, panels of multiple biomarkers are actively being explored in clinical trials [98–100].

References

1. National Research Council. Toward precision medicine: building a knowledge network for biomedical research and a new taxonomy of disease. Washington, DC: The National Academies Press; 2011.
2. Haendel MA, Chute CG, Robinson PN. Classification, ontology, and precision medicine. N Engl J Med. 2018;379:1452–62.
3. Biomarkers Definitions Working Group. Biomarkers and surrogate endpoints: preferred definitions and conceptual framework. Clin Pharmacol Ther. 2001;69:89–95.
4. Califf RM. Biomarker definitions and their applications. Exp Biol Med (Maywood). 2018;243:213–21.
5. Funkhouser WK. Clinical practice: anatomic pathology. In: Reisner HM, editor. Pathology: a modern case study. 2nd ed. New York: McGraw-Hill Education; 2020.
6. Mescher AL. Histology & its methods of study. In: Junqueira's basic histology: text and atlas. 15th ed. McGraw-Hill Education: New York; 2018.
7. Gulley ML. Clinical practice: molecular pathology. In: Reisner HM, editor. Pathology: a modern case study. 2nd ed. New York: McGraw-Hill Education; 2020.
8. Mahanty S, Prigent A, Garraud O. Immunogenicity of infectious pathogens and vaccine antigens. BMC Immunol. 2015;16:31.
9. Sanchez-Trincado JL, Gomez-Perosanz M, Reche PA. Fundamentals and methods for T- and B-cell epitope prediction. J Immunol Res. 2017;2017:2680160.
10. Levinson W, Chin-Hong P, Joyce EA, Nussbaum J, Schwartz B. Overview of immunity. In: Review of medical microbiology & immunology: a guide to clinical infectious diseases. 16th ed. New York: McGraw-Hill; 2020.
11. Cossarizza A, Chang H-D, Radbruch A, Acs A, Adam D, Adam-Klages S, et al. Guidelines for the use of flow cytometry and cell sorting in immunological studies (second edition). Eur J Immunol. 2019;49:1457–973.
12. Spitzer MH, Nolan GP. Mass cytometry: single cells, many features. Cell. 2016;165:780–91.
13. Gadalla R, Noamani B, MacLeod BL, Dickson RJ, Guo M, Xu W, et al. Validation of CyTOF against flow cytometry for immunological studies and monitoring of human cancer clinical trials. Front Oncol. 2019;9:415.
14. Sahl SJ, Hell SW, Jakobs S. Fluorescence nanoscopy in cell biology. Nat Rev Mol Cell Biol. 2017;18:685–701.
15. Balu M, Mazhar A, Hayakawa CK, Mittal R, Krasieva TB, König K, et al. In vivo multiphoton NADH fluorescence reveals depth-dependent keratinocyte metabolism in human skin. Biophys J. 2013;104:258–67.
16. Zuba-Surma EK, Ratajczak MZ. Analytical capabilities of the ImageStream cytometer. Methods Cell Biol. 2011;102:207–30.
17. Haynes BF, Soderberg KA, Fauci AS. Introduction to the immune system. In: Jameson JL, Fauci AS, Kasper DL, Hauser SL, Longo DL, Loscalzo J, editors. Harrison's principles of internal Medicine. 20th ed. New York: McGraw-Hill Education; 2018.
18. Angkananard T, Anothaisintawee T, McEvoy M, Attia J, Thakkinstian A. Neutrophil lymphocyte ratio and cardiovascular disease risk: a systematic review and meta-analysis. Biomed Res Int. 2018;2018:2703518.
19. Zhang R, Wu X, Hu W, Zhao L, Zhao S, Zhang J, et al. Neutrophil-to-lymphocyte ratio predicts hemorrhagic transformation in ischemic stroke: a meta-analysis. Brain Behav. 2019;9:e01382.
20. Chabot-Richards DS, George TI. White blood cell counts: reference methodology. Clin Lab Med. 2015;35:11–24.
21. Kim J, Song T-J, Park JH, Lee HS, Nam CM, Nam HS, et al. Different prognostic value of white blood cell subtypes in patients with acute cerebral infarction. Atherosclerosis. 2012;222:464–7.

22. Saliba W, Barnett-Griness O, Elias M, Rennert G. Neutrophil to lymphocyte ratio and risk of a first episode of stroke in patients with atrial fibrillation: a cohort study. J Thromb Haemost. 2015;13:1971–9.

23. Guo Z, Yu S, Xiao L, Chen X, Ye R, Zheng P, et al. Dynamic change of neutrophil to lymphocyte ratio and hemorrhagic transformation after thrombolysis in stroke. J Neuroinflammation. 2016;13:199.

24. Suh B, Shin DW, Kwon H-M, Yun JM, Yang H-K, Ahn E, et al. Elevated neutrophil to lymphocyte ratio and ischemic stroke risk in generally healthy adults. PLoS One. 2017;12:e0183706.

25. Feijó Delgado F, Cermak N, Hecht VC, Son S, Li Y, Knudsen SM, et al. Intracellular water exchange for measuring the dry mass, water mass and changes in chemical composition of living cells. PLoS One. 2013;8:e67590.

26. Alberts B, Johnson A, Lewis J, Morgan D, Raff M, Roberts K, et al. Molecular Biology of the Cell. 6th ed. Garland Science, Taylor and Francis Group: New York; 2015.

27. Kennelly PJ, Rodwell VW. Proteins: determination of primary structure. In: Rodwell VW, Bender DA, Botham KM, Kennelly PJ, Weil PA, editors. Harper's Illustrated Biochemistry. 31st ed. New York: McGraw-Hill Education; 2018.

28. Kennelly PJ, Rodwell VW. Proteins: higher orders of structure. In: Rodwell VW, Bender DA, Botham KM, Kennelly PJ, Weil PA, editors. Harper's Illustrated Biochemistry. 31st ed. New York: McGraw-Hill Education; 2018.

29. Weil PA. Protein synthesis & the genetic code. In: Rodwell VW, Bender DA, Botham KM, Kennelly PJ, Weil PA, editors. Harper's Illustrated Biochemistry. 31st ed. New York: McGraw-Hill Education; 2018.

30. Brakke MK. Density gradient centrifugation: a new separation technique. J Am Chem Soc. 1951;73:1847–8.

31. Pertoft H. Fractionation of cells and subcellular particles with Percoll. J Biochem Biophys Methods. 2000;44:1–30.

32. Matulis D. Selective precipitation of proteins. Curr Protoc Protein Sci. 2016;83:4.5.1–4.5.37.

33. Bonifacino JS, Dell'Angelica EC, Springer TA. Immunoprecipitation. Curr Protoc Protein Sci. 2001;Chapter 9:Unit 9.8.

34. Büyükköroğlu G, Dora DD, Özdemir F, Hızel C. Chapter 15—Techniques for protein analysis. In: Barh D, Azevedo V, editors. Omics technologies and bio-engineering. London: Academic Press; 2018. p. 317–51.

35. Hage DS. Analysis of biological interactions by affinity chromatography: clinical and pharmaceutical applications. Clin Chem. 2017;63:1083–93.

36. Zhang C, Rodriguez E, Bi C, Zheng X, Suresh D, Suh K, et al. High performance affinity chromatography and related separation methods for the analysis of biological and pharmaceutical agents. Analyst. 2018;143:374–91.

37. Choudhary C, Mann M. Decoding signalling networks by mass spectrometry-based proteomics. Nat Rev Mol Cell Biol. 2010;11:427–39.

38. Züllig T, Trötzmüller M, Köfeler HC. Lipidomics from sample preparation to data analysis: a primer. Anal Bioanal Chem. 2020;412:2191–209.

39. Bujak R, Struck-Lewicka W, Markuszewski MJ, Kaliszan R. Metabolomics for laboratory diagnostics. J Pharm Biomed Anal. 2015;113:108–20.

40. Alsaleh M, Barbera TA, Andrews RH, Sithithaworn P, Khuntikeo N, Loilome W, et al. Mass spectrometry: a guide for the clinician. J Clin Exp Hepatol. 2019;9:597–606.

41. Pitt JJ. Principles and applications of liquid chromatography-mass spectrometry in clinical biochemistry. Clin Biochem Rev. 2009;30:19–34.

42. Levinson W, Chin-Hong P, Joyce EA, Nussbaum J, Schwartz B. Antigen–antibody reactions in the laboratory. In: Review of medical microbiology & immunology: a guide to clinical infectious diseases. 16th ed. New York: McGraw Hill; 2020.

43. Aydin S. A short history, principles, and types of ELISA, and our laboratory experience with peptide/protein analyses using ELISA. Peptides. 2015;72:4–15.

44. Mahmood T, Yang P-C. Western blot: technique, theory, and trouble shooting. N Am J Med Sci. 2012;4:429–34.

45. Spurrier B, Ramalingam S, Nishizuka S. Reverse-phase protein lysate microarrays for cell signaling analysis. Nat Protoc. 2008;3:1796–808.

46. Ciaccio MF, Wagner JP, Chuu C-P, Lauffenburger DA, Jones RB. Systems analysis of EGF receptor signaling dynamics with microwestern arrays. Nat Methods. 2010;7:148–55.

47. Maisel AS, Duran JM, Wettersten N. Natriuretic peptides in heart failure: atrial and B-type natriuretic peptides. Heart Fail Clin. 2018;14:13–25.

48. Rodríguez-Yáñez M, Sobrino T, Blanco M, de la Ossa NP, Brea D, Rodríguez-González R, et al. High serum levels of pro-brain natriuretic peptide (pro BNP) identify cardioembolic origin in undetermined stroke. Dis Markers. 2009;26:189–95.

49. Rost NS, Biffi A, Cloonan L, Chorba J, Kelly P, Greer D, et al. Brain natriuretic peptide predicts functional outcome in ischemic stroke. Stroke. 2012;43:441–5.

50. García-Berrocoso T, Giralt D, Bustamante A, Etgen T, Jensen JK, Sharma JC, et al. B-type natriuretic peptides and mortality after stroke: a systematic review and meta-analysis. Neurology. 2013;81:1976–85.

51. Nigro N, Wildi K, Mueller C, Schuetz P, Mueller B, Fluri F, et al. BNP but not s-cTnln is associated with cardioembolic aetiology and predicts short and long term prognosis after cerebrovascular events. PLoS One. 2014;9:e102704.

52. Bai J, Sun H, Xie L, Zhu Y, Feng Y. Detection of cardioembolic stroke with B-type natriuretic peptide or N-terminal pro-BNP: a comparative diagnostic meta-analysis. Int J Neurosci. 2018;128:1100–8.

53. Sudoh T, Kangawa K, Minamino N, Matsuo H. A new natriuretic peptide in porcine brain. Nature. 1988;332:78–81.

54. Jameson JL, Kopp P. Principles of human genetics. In: Jameson JL, Fauci AS, Kasper DL, Hauser SL, Longo DL, Loscalzo J, editors. Harrison's principles of internal medicine. 20th ed. New York: McGraw-Hill Education; 2018.

55. Peirson SN, Butler JN. RNA extraction from mammalian tissues. Methods Mol Biol. 2007;362:315–27.

56. Talebi R, Seighalani R, Qanbari S. A handmade DNA extraction kit using laundry powder; insights on simplicity, cost-efficiency, rapidity, safety and the quality of purified DNA. Anim Biotechnol. 2019:1–7. https://doi.org/10.1080/10495398.2019.1684933.

57. Weil PA. Molecular genetics, recombinant DNA, & genomic technology. In: Rodwell VW, Bender DA, Botham KM, Kennelly PJ, Weil PA, editors. Harper's Illustrated Biochemistry. 31st ed. New York: McGraw-Hill Education; 2018.

58. He SL, Green R. Northern blotting. Method Enzymol. 2013;530:75–87.

59. Tajadini M, Panjehpour M, Javanmard SH. Comparison of SYBR Green and TaqMan methods in quantitative real-time polymerase chain reaction analysis of four adenosine receptor subtypes. Adv Biomed Res. 2014;3:85.

60. Bumgarner R. Overview of DNA microarrays: types, applications, and their future. Curr Protoc Mol Biol. 2013;Chapter 22:Unit 22.1.

61. Eichler EE. Genetic variation, comparative genomics, and the diagnosis of disease. N Engl J Med. 2019;381:64–74.

62. Lander ES, Linton LM, Birren B, Nusbaum C, Zody MC, Baldwin J, et al. Initial sequencing and analysis of the human genome. Nature. 2001;409:860–921.

63. International HapMap Consortium. The International HapMap Project. Nature. 2003;426:789–96.

64. Ozaki K, Ohnishi Y, Iida A, Sekine A, Yamada R, Tsunoda T, et al. Functional SNPs in the lymphotoxin-alpha gene that are associated with susceptibility to myocardial infarction. Nat Genet. 2002;32:650–4.

65. Buniello A, MacArthur JAL, Cerezo M, Harris LW, Hayhurst J, Malangone C, et al. The NHGRI-EBI GWAS catalog of published genome-wide association studies, targeted arrays and summary statistics 2019. Nucleic Acids Res. 2019;47:D1005–12.

66. International Human Genome Sequencing Consortium. Finishing the euchromatic sequence of the human genome. Nature. 2004;431:931–45.

67. Schneider VA, Graves-Lindsay T, Howe K, Bouk N, Chen H-C, Kitts PA, et al. Evaluation of GRCh38 and de novo haploid genome assemblies demonstrates the enduring quality of the reference assembly. Genome Res. 2017;27:849–64.

68. Quail MA, Smith M, Coupland P, Otto TD, Harris SR, Connor TR, et al. A tale of three next generation sequencing platforms: comparison of Ion Torrent, Pacific Biosciences and Illumina MiSeq Sequencers. BMC Genomics. 2012;13:341.

69. Adams DR, Eng CM. Next-generation sequencing to diagnose suspected genetic disorders. N Engl J Med. 2018;379:1353–62.

70. Metzker ML. Sequencing technologies—the next generation. Nat Rev Genet. 2010;11:31–46.

71. Lu H, Giordano F, Ning Z. Oxford nanopore MinION sequencing and genome assembly. Genomics Proteomics Bioinformatics. 2016;14:265–79.

72. Lowe R, Shirley N, Bleackley M, Dolan S, Shafee T. Transcriptomics technologies. PLoS Comput Biol. 2017;13:e1005457.

73. Barros-Silva D, Marques CJ, Henrique R, Jerónimo C. Profiling DNA methylation based on next-generation sequencing approaches: new insights and clinical applications. Genes (Basel). 2018;9:429.

74. 1000 Genomes Project Consortium, Auton A, Brooks LD, Durbin RM, Garrison EP, Kang HM, et al. A global reference for human genetic variation. Nature. 2015;526:68–74.

75. Wetterstrand KA. DNA sequencing costs: data from the NHGRI Genome Sequencing Program (GSP). https://www.genome.gov/sequencingcostsdata. Accessed 15 Aug 2020.

76. Yates AD, Achuthan P, Akanni W, Allen J, Allen J, Alvarez-Jarreta J, et al. Ensembl 2020. Nucleic Acids Res. 2020;48:D682–8.

77. Phan L, Jin Y, Zhang H, Qiang W, Shekhtman E, Shao D, et al. ALFA: allele frequency aggregator. Bethesda, MD: National Center for Biotechnology Information, US National Library of Medicine; 2020. https://www.ncbi.nlm.nih.gov/snp/docs/gsr/alfa/. Accessed 15 Aug 2020.

78. Traylor M, Farrall M, Holliday EG, Sudlow C, Hopewell JC, Cheng Y-C, et al. Genetic risk factors for ischaemic stroke and its subtypes (the METASTROKE collaboration): a meta-analysis of genome-wide association studies. Lancet Neurol. 2012;11:951–62.

79. NINDS Stroke Genetics Network (SiGN), International Stroke Genetics Consortium (ISGC). Loci associated with ischaemic stroke and its subtypes (SiGN): a genome-wide association study. Lancet Neurol. 2016;15:174–84.

80. Malik R, Traylor M, Pulit SL, Bevan S, Hopewell JC, Holliday EG, et al. Low-frequency and common genetic variation in ischemic stroke: the METASTROKE collaboration. Neurology. 2016;86:1217–26.

81. Malik R, Chauhan G, Traylor M, Sargurupremraj M, Okada Y, Mishra A, et al. Multiancestry genome-wide association study of 520,000 subjects identifies 32 loci associated with stroke and stroke subtypes. Nat Genet. 2018;50:524–37.

82. Markus HS, Mäkelä K-M, Bevan S, Raitoharju E, Oksala N, Bis JC, et al. Evidence HDAC9 genetic variant associated with ischemic stroke increases risk via promoting carotid athero-sclerosis. Stroke. 2013;44:1220–5.

83. Shroff N, Ander BP, Zhan X, Stamova B, Liu D, Hull H, et al. HDAC9 polymorphism alters blood gene expression in patients with large vessel atherosclerotic stroke. Transl Stroke Res. 2019;10:19–25.

84. Prestel M, Prell-Schicker C, Webb T, Malik R, Lindner B, Ziesch N, et al. The atherosclerosis risk variant rs2107595 mediates allele-specific transcriptional regulation of HDAC9 via E2F3 and Rb1. Stroke. 2019;50:2651–60.

85. Wang W, Sun G, Zhang L, Shi L, Zeng Y. Circulating microRNAs as novel potential biomark-ers for early diagnosis of acute stroke in humans. J Stroke Cerebrovasc Dis. 2014;23:2607–13.

86. Li P, Teng F, Gao F, Zhang M, Wu J, Zhang C. Identification of circulating microR-NAs as potential biomarkers for detecting acute ischemic stroke. Cell Mol Neurobiol. 2015;35:433–47.

87. Xie Q, Zhang X, Peng S, Sun J, Chen X, Deng Y, et al. Identification of novel biomarkers in ischemic stroke: a genome-wide integrated analysis. BMC Med Genet. 2020;21:66.

88. Li P, Shen M, Gao F, Wu J, Zhang J, Teng F, et al. An antagomir to microRNA-106b-5p ameliorates cerebral ischemia and reperfusion injury in rats via inhibiting apoptosis and oxidative stress. Mol Neurobiol. 2017;54:2901–21.

89. Steiner T, Juvela S, Unterberg A, Jung C, Forsting M, Rinkel G, et al. European Stroke Organization guidelines for the management of intracranial aneurysms and subarachnoid haemorrhage. Cerebrovasc Dis. 2013;35:93–112.

90. Steiner T, Al-Shahi Salman R, Beer R, Christensen H, Cordonnier C, Csiba L, et al. European Stroke Organisation (ESO) guidelines for the management of spontaneous intracerebral hemorrhage. Int J Stroke. 2014;9:840–55.

91. Kobayashi A, Czlonkowska A, Ford GA, Fonseca AC, Luijckx GJ, Korv J, et al. European Academy of Neurology and European Stroke Organization consensus statement and practical guidance for pre-hospital management of stroke. Eur J Neurol. 2018;25:425–33.

92. Turc G, Bhogal P, Fischer U, Khatri P, Lobotesis K, Mazighi M, et al. European Stroke Organisation (ESO)–European Society for Minimally Invasive Neurological Therapy (ESMINT) guidelines on mechanical thrombectomy in acute ischemic stroke. J Neurointerv Surg. 2019;11:535–8.

93. Powers WJ, Rabinstein AA, Ackerson T, Adeoye OM, Bambakidis NC, Becker K, et al. Guidelines for the early management of patients with acute ischemic stroke: 2019 update to the 2018 guidelines for the early management of acute ischemic stroke: a guideline for healthcare professionals from the American Heart Association/American Stroke Association. Stroke. 2019;50:e344–418.

94. Casolla B, Caparros F, Cordonnier C, Bombois S, Hénon H, Bordet R, et al. Biological and imaging predictors of cognitive impairment after stroke: a systematic review. J Neurol. 2019;266:2593–604.

95. Martin AJ, Price CI. A systematic review and meta-analysis of molecular biomarkers associated with early neurological deterioration following acute stroke. Cerebrovasc Dis. 2018;46:230–41.

96. Donkel SJ, Benaddi B, Dippel DWJ, Ten Cate H, de Maat MPM. Prognostic hemostasis biomarkers in acute ischemic stroke. Arterioscler Thromb Vasc Biol. 2019;39:360–72.

97. Dolmans LS, Rutten FH, Koenen NCT, Bartelink M-LEL, Reitsma JB, Kappelle LJ, et al. Candidate biomarkers for the diagnosis of transient ischemic attack: a systematic review. Cerebrovasc Dis. 2019;47:207–16.

98. Jickling GC, Sharp FR. Biomarker panels in ischemic stroke. Stroke. 2015;46:915–20.

99. Misra S, Kumar A, Kumar P, Yadav AK, Mohania D, Pandit AK, et al. Blood-based protein biomarkers for stroke differentiation: a systematic review. Proteomics Clin Appl. 2017;11 https://doi.org/10.1002/prca.201700007.

100. Bustamante A, López-Cancio E, Pich S, Penalba A, Giralt D, García-Berrocoso T, et al. Blood biomarkers for the early diagnosis of stroke: the stroke-chip study. Stroke. 2017;48:2419–25.

Approach for Genetic Studies

Gie Ken-Dror and Pankaj Sharma

13.1 Introduction

A suspicion for a genetic aetiology of a disease starts with the recognition of patterns of variation in disease risk and changes in risk among migrants, race/ethnicity, socioeconomic class, time trends, age effects, and gender variation [1, 2]. The first steps are assessing family history, twin, and adoption studies (familial aggregation) at the phenotype level to demonstrate that the disease tends to run in families more than would be expected by chance and examining how that familial tendency is modified by the degree or type of relationship, age, or environmental factors [1, 3]. The results are expressed as a correlation matrix that is analysed by variance component analysis (used as nested analysis of variance to estimate a part of the total variability accounted for by a specified source of variability) or path analysis (used as multiple regression analysis to look at the relationship between variables graphically and explicitly at the causal factors by path coefficients) to estimate the proportion of variance due to shared environmental and genetic influences. The next step, still at a phenotype level in pedigree data, is study of the families of a population-based series of cases to determine whether the pattern of disease among relatives is compatible with one or more major genes, polygenes, or shared environmental factors (segregation analysis to estimate penetrance and allele frequency parameters).

G. Ken-Dror
Institute of Cardiovascular Research Royal Holloway, University of London (ICR2UL), London, UK
e-mail: Gie.KenDror@rhul.ac.uk

P. Sharma (✉)
Institute of Cardiovascular Research Royal Holloway, University of London (ICR2UL), London, UK

Department of Clinical Neuroscience, Imperial College Healthcare NHS Trust, London, UK
e-mail: pankaj.sharma@rhul.ac.uk

© Springer Nature Switzerland AG 2021
A. C. Fonseca, J. M. Ferro (eds.), *Precision Medicine in Stroke*,
https://doi.org/10.1007/978-3-030-70761-3_13

Table 13.1 The genetic research methods

Phenotype level		Genotype level	
Study	Statistical analysis	Study	Statistical analysis
Family history study Twin study Adoption study	Familial aggregation Variance component analysis Path analysis	Family study (members of multiple case families)	Linkage analysis LOD score Identical by descent (IBD)
Family study (pedigree)	Segregation analysis	Unrelated cases and controls	Linkage disequilibrium mapping (haplotype analysis)
		Genetic association studies and genetic wide association studies (GWAS)	Linear/logistic regression Mendelian randomisation Meta-analysis Polygenic risk score
		Next-generation sequences (NGS) and gene expiration (GE)	Likelihood ratio test (LRT) of the maximum likelihood estimates (MLE) or empirical Bayes procedure

If major genes seem to be involved, then the parameters of the corresponding genetic model are estimated [2, 3]. The genetic research methods are presented in Table 13.1.

We then move on to the genotype level, to collect blood samples from potentially informative members of multiple case families and types of genetic markers at known locations (linkage analysis to determine the approximate chromosomal location of a gene by looking for evidence of co-segregation with other genes whose locations are already known). Markers that are transmitted through families in a manner that parallels the transmission of the disease (co-segregation) provide evidence for the general chromosomal location of the gene [1, 3]. Extended families with many cases are particularly informative for this purpose and do not need to be population based, although large series of pairs of affected siblings can also be used. This search may begin before one has any idea of even which chromosome to examine, let alone where on that chromosome. Beginning with a widely spaced array of markers scattered over the entire genome, one narrows down the search as leads develop, a process known as a genome scan. Linkage is reported as a logarithm of the odds (LOD) score representing chromosomal position measured in centimorgan (cM). Large positive scores are evidence for linkage (co-segregation), and negative scores are evidence against. Different method to estimate the alleles shared by two relatives that were transmitted from the same ancestor is Identical By Descent (IBD) [2, 3].

As the search region narrows, other techniques are used to narrow it further (linkage disequilibrium mapping). Unrelated cases and controls can be compared on a dense panel of markers over the candidate region to look for associations that could reflect linkage disequilibrium with the causal gene (population associations between the alleles at two loci). Within linked families, haplotypes can be constructed from a series of closely spaced, highly polymorphic markers (genes that vary between individuals) in the hope of identifying flanking markers that represent "convincing" recombinants in single individuals [1, 2]. The linked region may include a number of genes with known functions that could be relevant to the aetiology of the disease (association with candidate genes). By comparing the genotypes at these candidate loci between cases and controls (population or family based), one can test hypotheses about whether they are actually associated with the disease. The association could also be noncausal, reflecting linkage disequilibrium with the truly causal gene, as in fine mapping, the process to discover a gene and identify mutations done in the polymorphic region in the DNA. With various molecular techniques, or more recently the established sequence databases from the Human Genome Project, coding sequences are identified, and each can then be screened for polymorphisms. Polymorphisms in cases that are rare in controls are considered to be possibly causal mutations. A causal mutation could also occur in a non-coding region (such as a regulatory region); in this case, sequencing of the candidate region, a very labour-intensive process, may be necessary. Once the gene has been identified, its structure, the function of each exon, regulatory elements, and other features are studied with molecular methods (characterising the gene). The genetic epidemiologist then estimates the frequency of various mutations and the effect of each on disease risk, including any interactions with age, host, or environmental factors [1, 3].

13.2 Family Studies

Historically, family-based studies have been the primary approach to detecting disease-causing genes [1, 4]. Diseases tend to run in families and this clustering of disease is often attributed to the genes shared within families. The number of relatives studied can range from two family members to enormous pedigrees. A main advantage of family-based association studies is the control for confounding bias due to population stratification, albeit at a potential loss of power [5, 6]. The results express familial correlation and compare the overall population prevalence with the risk of disease to other family members when there is an identified affected individual in the family [1, 3]. The degree of risk can be computed for different types of family members on the basis of their relatedness to the case as first- or second-degree relative. This risk can also be based on additional factors for the case age of onset. Moreover, family members may be easier to recruit for some disorders than unrelated individuals, since they can have higher motivation to participate given their affected family member. In addition, when genotyping is performed, it allows to check for Mendelian inheritance [4]. The traditional family study uses case and both parent (trios) analysed by the transmission disequilibrium test (TDT). The study starts with an affected individual as the case and recruits their parents as the controls. These are not conventional controls, however, as one compares the alleles transmitted from the parents to the case versus those not transmitted—the controls. These controls are often referred to as pseudo-sibs or pseudo-controls. The data are arranged as a matched case-control study, cross tabulating the alleles that each parent transmitted to the case versus those not transmitted. The transmission disequilibrium test (TDT, McNemar test) used to test whether a particular allele is transmitted more frequently than expected by chance [1, 4]. In the Case-Sibling Association Study Design each case is matched to one or more unaffected sibling. In general, eligible controls should be those unaffected siblings who have reached the age of diagnosis for the case. The study of twin pairs has played a major role in trying to distinguish between genetic and environmental factors for disease, taking advantage of the natural experiment created by the formation of two different types of twins, identical and fraternal. The classical twin method involves identifying twin pairs through affected members and comparing the concordance rates (the probability that twin pairs with shared genes will develop the same disease) of identical (monozygotic) and fraternal (dizygotic) twins. Assuming that identical and fraternal twins share environmental factors to a similar degree but differ in their genetic similarity, this comparison allows the estimation of heritability, the proportion of variance on an underlying liability to disease that is due to common genes, and environmentally the proportion due to shared environment. Various extensions of the twin design include comparisons of twins reared apart and twin family studies [1, 4].

13.3 Association Studies

Genetic association studies are used to detect association between one or more genetic markers with continuous or discrete phenotype [7]. They allow us to compare different alleles with the phenotype in a similar manner across the unrelated individuals or families, whereas linkage allows different alleles to be associated with the phenotype among different families. In addition, they have greater power than linkage studies to detect small effects but require more markers to be examined [7, 8]. The simplest study design used to test for association is the case-control study, in which a series of cases affected with the disease of interest are collected together with a series of control individuals. In this case the phenotype is a binary variable such as presence (prevalence) or occurrence (incidence) of a disease. Association studies find candidate genes or genome regions that contribute to a specific disease by testing for a correlation between disease status and genetic variation. They are the major tools for identifying genes conferring susceptibility to complex disorders where both genetic and environmental factors contribute to the susceptibility risk [1, 3].

Genetic markers (polymorphisms) are measurable variations at the DNA level, a chromosome region where differences in nucleotide sequences occur between individuals of the same species. Various types of markers have been used to detect DNA variability, the most common being restriction fragment length polymorphism (RFLP), random amplification of polymorphic DNA (RAPD), amplified fragment length polymorphism (AFLP), single-stranded conformation polymorphism

(SSCP), copy number variation (CNV), microsatellites, and single-nucleotide polymorphism (SNP). SNP is the most commonly used; a polymorphism occurs when different individuals have many genetic variants at the same location (loci) of their genomes [1, 9]. Every possible variant is called allele, and if only one nucleotide has changed, the variant is named single-nucleotide polymorphism (SNP). A higher frequency of a SNP allele or genotype in a series of individuals affected with a disease can be interpreted as meaning that the tested variant increases the risk of a specific disease. There are two possibilities for each locus (biallelic); every individual carries two alleles of every locus, one for each of the 22 autosomal chromosomes inherited independently from his/her parents. A genotype is an observed couple of individual alleles for some loci; there are three potential genotypes 1/1, 1/2, and 2/2. Two identical alleles (1/1 or 2/2) are homozygous; otherwise they will be heterozygous [2, 3].

The statistical analysis of a polymorphism is based on estimating the prevalence of each allele, by doing it for each genotype, and estimating the genotype and allele frequencies. To estimate the genotype frequencies, use the observed rate of genotypes. To calculate allele frequencies, double the sample chromosomes and count every allele rate. The Hardy-Weinberg equilibrium (HWE) test to assess independence between the alleles inherited from the parents needs to be done before the association analysis between genetic polymorphisms and diseases. The statistical tests compare the observed allele frequency with the expected one under the assumption of independence and have a chi-square distribution with one degree of freedom [1, 3].

The analysis of association between polymorphisms and disease describes polymorphism as a categorical variable with one level for each possible genotype, and the reference category is the homozygous form. The genotypes of a single, biallelic SNP on a set of cases and controls can be summarised in a 2×3 contingency table of the genotype counts for each group. Several different statistical analysis methods can be applied to this table. Pearson's chi-square test is used to assess departure from the null hypothesis that case and controls have the same distribution of genotype counts [7, 10]. This test statistic has a chi-square distribution with two degrees of freedom. This approach provides a valid statistical analysis; however column order is not used in the test statistic, and reordering the column table gives the same value of the test statistic and P-value. An alternative test is the Cochran–Armitage test for trend (CATT). It tests for a trend in differences in cases and controls across the ordered genotypes in the table. These tests are the primary analysis tool for genetic disorders. The estimation of the odds ratio (OR) for each genotype with respect to the reference genotype will give a measure of effect size. To include confounder variables in the model and adjust for clinical covariates logistic regression models can be used and provide adjusted odds ratios, and in addition allow to assess interaction between the polymorphism and the other factors. Logistic regression is an extension of linear regression where the outcome of a linear model is transformed using a logistic function that predicts the probability of having case status given a genotype class [1, 3, 10].

Continuous phenotypes such as protein S [11] or factor IIX [12] are characterised by quantitative measures. These measures can be tested for association in a linear regression framework, assessing whether the genotypes (as an explanatory variable) predict trait value. The genotypes 11, 12, and 22 are coded as a three-level factor, or as a count of alleles carrying 0, 1, and 2, respectively. The results describe as a beta coefficient, the additive effect of each copy of allele 2. Quantitative measures can be analysed in a case-control framework by dichotomising the sample. However, this method may result in a loss of power because all information on the distance of an individual's observed phenotype from the dichotomising threshold is lost. The power of a quantitative trait association study may be increased by ascertaining individuals only from the extremes of the distribution [2, 10].

Further tests can be used to test specific genetic hypotheses; there are five inheritance models: Co-dominant model is the most general model and it allows every genotype to give a different and nonadditive risk. This model compares heterozygous 1/2 and homozygous for the variant allele 2/2 genotypes to the homozygous for the most frequent allele 1/1. This model estimates two ORs, one for heterozygous 1/2 and the other for homozygous 2/2. Dominant model assumes that a single copy of allele 2 is enough to modify the risk. The model compares the combination of these two possible genotypes 1/2 + 2/2 to the homozygous 1/1. The recessive model assumes that two copies of 2 are necessary to change the risk. Hence, 1/2 and 1/1 genotypes have the same effect. A combination of both 1/1 + 1/2 is compared to the variant allele homozygous genotype 2/2. The overdominant model assumes heterozygous individuals have a higher fitness than homozygous individuals. The model compares the homozygous genotype 1/2 with pool of both homozygous genotypes 1/1 + 2/2. The additive model assumes that each copy of 2 modifies the risk in an additive form; homozygous 2/2 have double risk than heterozygous 1/2. Compare a combination of the two genotypes with weights 2 and 1, respectively, 2(2/2) + 1/2 to 1/1 [2, 13].

To decide the best inheritance model, every model may be compared to the general model (the co-dominant) by likelihood ratio test (LRT). The likelihood ratio test is a statistical test of the goodness of fit between two models, and compares the likelihood scores of the two models to assess if it fits a data set better. The statistic follows a chi-square distribution with degrees of freedom equal to the number of additional parameters in the models. The simplest model with the smallest number of predictors done by Akaike information (AIC) estimator or cross validation (CV) technique to estimate the accuracy of the model [2, 14]. The analysis of interactions with covariates includes the genotype and an environment variable or two genotype variables can be used by logistic regression model. The beta-coefficients describe the association between each polymorphism and the disease by ORs and the corresponding 95% confidence intervals (CI) [13, 14].

The statistical correlation between different polymorphisms located closer in the same chromosome is called linkage disequilibrium (LD) [1, 15]. The D statistic is used to test the tendency of two loci to be associated with each other in the population more than would be expected by chance. In addition, the D' statistic is equal to

D scaled in between -1 and 1 or the correlation coefficient between alleles r [2]. The set of polymorphisms transmitted together in every chromosome is called haplotype [1, 16]. Given the sample genotypes, every individual has two possible haplotypes, one per chromosome. The genotypes are given with non-chromosomal location, because of limitations of laboratory techniques. Due to this lack of information, when an individual has at least two heterozygous loci his/her couple of haplotypes is unknown and in practice, estimation methods like the expectation maximisation (EM) algorithm or Markov chain Monte Carlo (MCMC) methods are used [1, 16]. EM algorithm is the two-stage iterative method. First, initial values for the haplotype frequencies are given. Then, the E-pass consists of recalculating the expected genotype frequency for the genotypes with uncertainty haplotypes under Hardy-Weinberg equilibrium using the haplotype frequency. The M-pass calculates the genotype frequencies and counts the compatible haplotypes for every genotype. At the end, the algorithm converges the count to the haplotype frequencies. The method repeats with different start points to avoid local maximums. MCMC is an effective method; for each individual one samples a possible haplotype resolution with probability and then updates the haplotype frequencies using the current frequencies of haplotype assignments. The sampling for each subject can be done without having to enumerate all possible haplotype assignments by using the Metropolis-Hastings method, a flip of the alleles at a single locus or a single segment, and then accepting or rejecting the proposal with probability [1, 16, 17].

The analysis of association between haplotypes and disease is done by chromosome analysis instead of treating individuals because every individual has a couple of haplotypes. The sample is duplicated and then each individual is doubly represented with his/her two haplotypes. The risk for every haplotype will be compared with respect to the reference category (the most frequent haplotype) by logistic regression model. The analysis of haplotypes includes uncertainty due to the lack of chromosomal information and missing values in the data. To include the uncertainty of the haplotype in the analysis among individuals with more than two options every haplotype takes a different weight in the logistic regression mode [1, 15, 16].

Genetic association studies often involve testing a large number of hypotheses: multiple SNPs or haplotypes, multiple phenotypes, multiple analytical models, and testing of multiple strata such as sex, age, and ethnicity. Replicating the results with another set of independent data is highly desirable for all association studies, particularly for studies where extensive multiple testing means that study-wide significance is not clear. However, replication should only be claimed when it addresses the same variant, phenotype, and genetic model; otherwise other phenotypes or variants within a gene are offered as evidence of replication. The results of genetic association studies are interpreted as direct association; the genotyped SNP is the true causal variant conferring disease susceptibility. In direct association, the genotyped SNP in linkage disequilibrium (LD) with the true causal variant is genotyped. The results are considered as false positive by chance or by systematic confounding as population stratification or admixture [2, 7, 14].

13.4 Mandelman Randomising Functional Analysis

The major aims of genetic association studies are to identify risk factors or intermediate phenotypes, which are causal to the manifestation of a specific disease initiation, disease progression, or response to therapy. When identified, causal risk factors can enable preventive measures and represent attractive therapeutic targets. Randomised, controlled trials (RCTs) are the gold standard to establish causal relationships [18–20]. RCTs cannot always be conducted, because they can be excessively costly, impractical, or even unethical. When RCTs are not feasible, risk factors can be investigated in observational studies: cohort study, case-control study, or cross-sectional study [18]. These studies do differ not only in the risk factor of interest but also in several observed and unobserved characteristics. Differences between the groups may be attributed to any of these characteristics and do not directly establish causality that arises as the result of confounding [18, 20] or reverse causation [21]. Confounding can be addressed statistically by including known and measured confounders into regression models (multivariable regression). However, when confounders are unobserved, unmeasured, or unknown, or the number of confounders is too large, regression methods may fail to provide unbiased estimates of the true association [18]. The instrumental variable method is an alternative statistical method to examine causality while controlling for any confounder. An instrumental variable is chosen to replace the randomised allocation of individuals to the suspected risk factor and ensure comparability of groups with respect to any known and unknown confounder [18, 22]. Genetic variants, such as single-nucleotide polymorphisms (SNPs), can be used as instrumental variables, because alleles are assigned to individuals before any risk factor or disease. Genetic instruments are nonmodifiable, ensuring lifelong exposure and mitigating concerns about reverse causation. The alleles of a given SNP are randomly allocated inherited variants independent of potentially confounding environmental risk factors. Because of the relation to Mendel's laws, the term Mendelian randomisation was coined [18, 23].

The choice of the genetic instrumental variable is essential to a successful Mendelian randomisation study. To allow unbiased estimation of the causal effect of the risk factor on the disease, a valid genetic instrumental variable fulfils three assumptions: (1) It must be reproducibly and strongly associated with the risk factor. (2) It must not be associated with confounders (other risk factors). (3) It must be only associated with the disease through the risk factor [18, 19, 24]. Genetic instrumental variables can be identified by scanning published databases or reports evaluating genetic associations with the risk factor of interest as genome-wide association studies (GWAS) because they represent hypothesis-free scans, where the risk factor and/or the disease are tested for association with millions of SNPs. SNPs can represent instruments that replace the randomised allocation of a risk factor and can be used to assess causality. It is preferable to select those that are located in genes with biologic function that is best understood. A well-understood biologic mechanism simplifies the examination of the second and third assumptions of Mendelian randomisation. An alternative is the use of different genetic instrumental variables and the comparison of analysis results obtained for each of them or the generation of a genetic score composed of multiple genetic instrumental variables [18, 22].

Mendelian randomisation analysis comprises two steps: first, the examination of the three assumptions and second, the evaluation of the causal effect between risk factor and disease. Only the first assumption of genetic instrumental variable that the genetic variant is strongly associated with the risk factor of interest can be directly tested using the data available for the Mendelian randomisation study. The association is empirically tested using linear or logistic regression (F statistic, partial r^2, odds ratio, risk ratio, or risk difference) [20, 25, 26]. The second assumption of no association between genetic instrumental variable and confounders is often considered fulfilled because of the random allocation of alleles to gametes [20, 27, 28]. This assumption can be tested empirically by assessing associations between the genetic instrumental variable and observed confounders [20, 26]. However, the absence of such associations cannot be considered a proof that confounding is absent [18, 20]. Statistical tests for the third assumption, that is, genetic variant must not affect disease other than through the specific risk factor, have also been proposed (Sargan test, Q test) [18, 29].

Different methods have been proposed to carry out the actual Mendelian randomisation analysis and estimate the magnitude of causal effects, with the choice of method depending on the practical setting [19, 28, 30]. The standard approach for effect estimation is a linear model. The causal effect of the risk factor on the disease via the genetic instrumental variable can then be estimated by Wald ratio estimate (β_{MR}) that represents the causal effect estimate obtained from the regression coefficients obtained from the regression of the disease on the genetic instrumental variable ($\beta_{Y\sim G}$) divided by the regression of the risk factor on the genetic instrumental variable ($\beta_{X\sim G}$) [18, 31]. Another approach obtained the regression of the disease on the genetic instrumental variable ($\beta_{Y\sim G}$), and the expected effect estimate is calculated as the product of the effect estimates obtained from the regression of the risk factor on the genetic instrumental variable ($\beta_{X\sim G}$) and the disease on the risk factor ($\beta_{Y\sim X}$) [18, 31].

Mendelian randomisation can be done using summary statistics to facilitate the use of results from published GWAS studies and does not require a separate study in which to carry out the Mendelian randomisation analysis. In this approach, ratios on the basis of published summary statistics (regression coefficients that represent the $\beta_{Y\sim G}$ and $\beta_{X\sim G}$) are used to assess the causal effect of a risk factor represented by a single or multiple genetic instrumental variable [32]. Two-sample Mendelian randomisation can be done where the association estimates (summary statistics) between the genotype and the risk factor and between the genotype and the disease are generated or collected from two different data sets without or only with a limited number of overlapping individuals [18, 33]. Bidirectional Mendelian randomisation can be used to address the directionality of a causal association [34] because reverse causation is a common problem in observational studies. Network Mendelian randomisation can be used to investigate more complex causal relationships between variables, when some of the risk factors' effect on the disease occurs through a mediator variable (provides a link between risk factor and disease) [35]. The simplest network can be done by a two-step Mendelian randomisation, where a genetic instrumental variable for the risk factor is used to estimate the causal effect of a risk factor on the mediator variable in a first step, and another genetic instrumental variable for the mediator variable is used to estimate the effect of the mediator on the disease in a second step [20, 36]. Also Mendelian randomisation can be done by testing all pairwise relationships within large multidimensional data sets; associations can be identified that are then followed up to test specific hypotheses about causality in a Mendelian randomisation setting [18, 20, 37].

13.5   Genome-Wide Association Studies

Genome-wide association studies (GWAS) use chip technology to genotype hundreds of thousands of common single-nucleotide polymorphisms (SNPs), which are then analysed for association with a disease or trait [38]. GWAS are hypothesis-free methods for identifying associations between genetic regions (loci) and traits (including diseases). There are many different chips available for human applications [39]. Some chips are designed to test as many SNPs as practically possible up to about 5 million. Some chips are specifically designed to test SNPs in coding regions of genes, which make up about 2% of the genome. Other chips may test relatively small numbers of SNPs that have been carefully selected to efficiently represent worldwide haplotype diversity. Some chips are designed for specific ethnic groups or may be enriched with SNPs from genes implicated in particular diseases. In selecting a genotyping chip, it is important to consider the goals of the current project, compatibility with data from past or planned future studies, and the budget available [2, 38, 40].

The statistical analysis of genome-wide association can begin once samples have been collected and genotyped. The process begins with a thorough quality control (QC) analysis to confirm the accuracy of the genotype data [38, 41, 42]. Without extensive QC, GWAS will not generate reliable results because raw genotype data are inherently imperfect. Errors in the data can arise for numerous reasons, due to poor quality of DNA samples, poor DNA hybridisation to the array, poorly performing genotype probes, and sample mix-ups or contamination. The QC procedure includes seven steps consisting of filtering out of SNPs and individuals: (1) Individual and SNP missingness: excludes SNPs and individuals that are missing in a large proportion of the subjects and the genotype (>20%) SNP filtering done before individual filter. (2) Inconsistencies in assigned and genetic sex of subjects: Checks for discrepancies between sex of the individuals recorded in the data set and their sex based on X chromosome heterozygosity/homozygosity rates (>0.8 for males and <0.2 for females). (3) Minor allele frequency (MAF) includes only SNPs above the set MAF threshold (>0.05 or >0.01 depending on sample size). SNPs with a low MAF are rare; therefore power is lacking for detecting SNP-phenotype associations. These SNPs are also more prone to genotyping errors. (4) Deviations from Hardy-Weinberg equilibrium (HWE) exclude markers which deviate from

Hardy-Weinberg equilibrium (*P*-value <1e−10 in cases and <1e−6 in controls or quantitative traits): Common indicator of genotyping error and may also indicate evolutionary selection. (5) Heterozygosity excludes individuals with high or low heterozygosity rates (deviate ±3 SD from the sample's heterozygosity rate mean). Deviations can indicate sample contamination and inbreeding. (6) Relatedness, defined as family relatedness, calculates identity by descent (IBD) of all sample pairs (pi-hat >0.2). The analysis includes independent SNPs after pruning (select a subset of markers that are in approximate LD uncorrelated, based on a specified threshold of LD, and do not take the *P*-value of a SNP into account) and limits it to autosomal chromosomes only. (7) Ethnic outliers and population stratification produce a *k*-dimensional representation of any substructure in the data, based on IBS. Presence of multiple subpopulations and individuals with different ethnic backgrounds in a study can lead to false-positive associations and/or mask true associations because allele frequencies can differ between subpopulations [38, 41, 42].

Standard GWAS test statistics assume that all samples in the analysis are unrelated and selected from a uniform, random mating population. Any departure from this assumption can cause unexpected results, especially in large study cohorts [2, 38, 41]. A statistical hypothesis test is performed for each SNP, with the null hypothesis of no association with the phenotype. There are a number of association tests available depending on which type of trait is being tested. Continuous phenotype traits are generally analysed using linear regression approaches with the assumptions that the trait is normally distributed, variance within each group is the same, and the groups are independent. Popular analyses include analysis of variance (ANOVA) and general linear model (GLM). Binary traits are commonly analysed using logistic regression, or tests such as a chi-square or Fisher's exact test, and logistic regression that allows adjustment for other covariates. Specialised tests are available for study designs with family-based collection [38, 41, 43].

Statistical power and multiple test correction are important and inseparable issues for GWAS. False-positive associations are a great risk when testing large numbers of SNPs, so statistical evidence for association must be held to a high standard. The typical significance threshold used in human GWAS studies is *P*-value less than 5e−8, equivalent to a standard Bonferroni correction for 1 million independent tests. Populations with greater genetic diversity, such as African populations, require even greater stringency to determine that a test result is statistically significant [2, 41]. Very large sample sizes may be required to achieve such significance levels, especially for rare disease alleles and alleles with small effect sizes. Statistical power of GWAS is affected by the genetic architecture of the phenotype, frequency and effect size of the disease allele, accuracy of phenotypic measurements, homogeneity of the phenotype, and LD relationships between causal variants and genotyped SNPs. The results include location of each *P*-value graph in a Manhattan plot to see the data visually relative to genomic context [2, 38].

Principal component analysis (PCA) can be used to stratify subjects based on genomic similarity and is often used to assess population stratification in GWAS cohorts [38, 41]. It is a common practice to adjust GWAS tests for principal components in order to account for the structure of the population. An alternative to PCA-based correction is to account for pairwise allele sharing among all study subjects using mixed linear model (MLM) regression. MLM methods such as efficient mixed-model association expedited (EMMAX, each locus explains only a small fraction of the phenotype and avoids repetitive variance component estimation procedure) and genome-wide efficient mixed model association (GEMMA, fits a univariate linear mixed model (LMM) for marker association tests with a single phenotype to account for population stratification and sample structure) effectively account for population structure in both human and agricultural populations [2, 38, 40, 41].

Meta-analysis can be used to compare between different published results or compare results between different populations for an alternative to PCA correction or mixed-model analysis. It takes the results from existing studies and performs analysis on those results, not directly on the original data. The results visualised by forest plot to compare the effect sizes and confidence intervals for the individual studies overlap between them as well as the meta-analysis summary effect sizes and confidence interval [38, 44].

GWAS is the first step toward understanding the genetic architecture of traits; successful GWAS will result in one or many SNPs found to be associated with the trait of interest. Researchers may then evaluate the functional consequences of each associated SNP, examine other variants in LD with that SNP, study the function of the gene where the SNP is positioned, and study the biological pathways in which the gene participates. A great number of experiments are required to fully understand the results of a GWAS. As the biology of the trait is elucidated, it may be possible to develop assays to test for disease risk or to improve disease treatment and prevention programmes. GWAS method needs to improve by increasing statistical power, reducing false-negative rates, and incorporating biological context [38, 42, 43].

Single-variant association analysis has been the primary method in GWAS but it requires very large sample sizes to detect more than a handful of SNPs for every phenotype. Polygenic risk score (PRS) analysis does not aim to identify individual SNPs but instead aggregates genetic risk across the genome in a single individual polygenic score for a trait of interest [41]. A large discovery sample is required to reliably determine how much each SNP is expected to contribute to the polygenic score ("weights") of a specific phenotype [41, 45]. In an independent target sample, which can be more modest in size, polygenic scores can be calculated based on genetic DNA profiles and these weights. As a rule of thumb, a target sample of around 2000 subjects provides sufficient power to detect a significant proportion of variance explained. Furthermore, the discovery and target samples should have the same number of subjects until the target sample includes 2000 subjects [41, 45]. If more samples are available, additional subjects should be included in the discovery sample to maximise the accuracy of the estimation of the effect sizes. Although PRS is not powerful enough to predict disease risk on the individual level, it has been successfully used to show significant associations both within and across traits. To conduct PRS analysis, trait-specific weights (beta for continuous traits and log of the odds ratios for binary traits) are obtained from a discovery GWAS. In the target sample, a PRS is calculated for each individual based on the weighted sum of the number of risk alleles that he/she carries multiplied by the trait-specific weights. For many phenotypes, SNP effect sizes are publicly available in the NHGRI-EBI catalogue of human genome-wide association studies. Although in principle all common SNPs could be used in a PRS analysis, it is customary to first clump (only the most significant SNP with the lowest P-value in each LD block is identified and selected for further analyses; this reduces the correlation between the remaining SNPs, while retaining SNPs with the strongest statistical evidence) the GWAS results before computing risk scores. P-value thresholds are typically used to remove SNPs that show little or no statistical evidence for association only keeping SNPs with P-values <0.5 or <0.1. Usually, multiple PRS analyses will be performed, with varying thresholds for the P-values [41].

13.6 Next-Generation Sequences and Gene Expiration

Next-generation sequencing (NGS), also known as high-throughput sequencing, is the catch-all term used to describe a number of different modern sequencing technologies. These technologies allow for sequencing of DNA and RNA much more quickly and cheaply than the previously used Sanger sequencing, and as such revolutionised the study of genomics and molecular biology. Analysis of NGS data consists of a sequence of steps. Depending on the application, these include a combination of quality monitoring, base calling, alignment to a reference genome, de novo genome assembly, and estimating of transcript abundance. Each of these steps requires sophisticated mathematical and statistical techniques [9, 46].

The sequencing data analysis starts from files containing DNA sequences and quality values for each base. Check the overall success of the sequencing process by counting the raw reads, spots (clusters/beads) on the images, and fraction of reads accepted after base calling (filtered reads). These counts could be looked up in a results file generated by the base calling software. A low number of filtered reads could be caused by various problems during the library preparation or sequencing procedure. Only the filtered reads should be used for further processing. The sequenced DNA fragments are sometimes called "inserts" because they are wrapped by sequencing adapters. The adapters are partially sequenced if the inserts are shorter than the read length, for example, in small RNA sequencing. In these occasions, it is necessary to remove the sequenced parts of the adapter from the reads, which could be achieved by removing all read suffixes that are adapter prefixes [9, 46].

Many applications of next-generation sequencing require a reference sequence to which the sequenced reads could be aligned. Read mapping means to find the position in the reference where the read matches with a minimum number of differences. This position is hence most likely the origin of the sequenced DNA fragment. The detection of different variation types requires different sequencing formats and analysis strategies. There are systematic difficulties with the reads obtained from next-generation sequencing platforms and the reliability and reproducibility of the next-generation sequencing platforms. High correlation between gene counts provides strong evidence for the reliability of the replicates [9, 46].

Gene expression is the process where the DNA is converted into a functional product, such as a protein. There are two key steps involved in making a protein, transcription and translation. Transcription is when the DNA in a gene is copied to produce an RNA transcript called messenger RNA (mRNA). Translation occurs after the messenger RNA (mRNA) has carried the transcribed "message" from the DNA to protein-making factories in the cell, called ribosomes. There are two main platforms for expression profiling: microarrays and direct sequencing of transcripts (RNA-seq). The RNA-sequence is the dominant platform; RNA-seq uses next-generation high-throughput sequencing platforms to sequence RNA transcripts and generates millions of short raw sequence reads which then have to be assembled most commonly aligned against a reference [9, 47].

Pre-processing and quality control are paramount in expression studies. In terms of quality control, the key objective is to identify slides of bad quality and remove them from further analyses. Pre-processing is another interesting feature of array study which aims to remove technical noise from the data. With RNA-seq the objective is to remove reads or parts of reads of poor quality (reads that have sequencing errors) and sequences that do not belong to our samples (adapters and barcodes) [9, 46].

The primary focus of these studies is to identify genes (or at least gene expression signals) associated with differences between traits (or conditions). For example, compare gene expression levels between normal and CVT patients and try to identify which genes are differentially expressed between the two. And evaluate expression levels of different tissues of an organism to understand which genes are expressed in which tissues. Also study population variability, test how new drugs affect gene expression levels, contrast resistant and susceptible individuals to identify genes that confer resistance (or susceptibility), test how exposure to environmental stressors affects gene expression levels and how gene expression changes over time (time-course analysis), and the list goes on. In livestock, global gene expression analysis has been used to search for genes involved in disease resistance, marbling, meat yield, feed intake, and many other traits. In a nutshell, most expression studies will, at least initially, try to identify the subset of genes that are differentially expressed between two or more conditions; simplistically, it is a contrast analysis (differential gene expression (*DGE*) analysis) [46, 47].

RNA-seq is a next-generation sequencing (NGS) procedure of the entire transcriptome by which one can measure the expression of several features such as gene expression, allelic expression, and intragenic expression. The number of reads mapped to a given gene or transcript is considered to be the estimate of the expression level of that feature using this technology. Microarray technology has been the method of choice to measure gene expression since the 1990s. RNA-seq has a wider range of signal detection, evaluated at single-base resolution and more suitable for the discovery of novel transcripts. The end product of a RNA-seq experiment is a sequence of read counts, typically represented as a matrix with rows representing genes and columns representing samples from one or more populations. When RNA-seq data are generated from two or more populations, interest often is in the detection of differentially expressed genes among the populations, genes for which read count distributions differ among populations. Tests of differential expression are derived through a likelihood ratio test (LRT) or t-tests of the maximum likelihood estimates (MLE) of the expression parameters [9, 46, 47].

The challenge in the detection of differential expression for RNA-seq data results from the way in which reads are mapped to features such as genes, transcripts, or exons. One of the issues is that the expression quantification from short reads using RNA-seq data depends on the length of the features; longer features usually produce more reads. Normalisation by dividing the length of the transcript alleviates this problem somewhat but not completely. The expression value is referred to as reads per kilobase per million reads (RPKM). Differential RNA-seq analysis using an empirical Bayes procedure by the *limma* method uses log-counts per million (log-cpm), analogous to the log intensity values in microarray studies [9, 48–50].

Differential expression analysis is affected by the sequence depth of the NGS data generation. Sequence depth can be calculated as $N \times L/G$, where N is the number of reads, L is the average read length, and G is the length of the original genome. This is also equivalent to the percentage of genome covered by reads and the average number of times a base is read. Higher coverage can improve the power to identify differential expression using RNA-seq data. However, read counts are subject to technical variation in which the overall read count for a sample, referred to as the library size, can substantially vary among repeated NGS experiments on the same sample. In order to accommodate this source of variability, log-cpm values need to be adjusted by accounting for mean variance trends typically observed in RNA-seq data, particularly among genes with lower counts. Zero counts are augmented by a small positive value to avoid taking the logarithm of zero, ensuring non-missing log-cpm and reducing the variability at lower count values [9, 47, 48].

13.7 Pharmacogenetics in the Future

Pharmacogenetics is the study of how people respond differently to drug therapy based upon their genetic sequence or genes. Diet, overall health, and environment also have significant influence on medication response, but none are stronger indicators of how to process medication than genetics. Personal genotype information is increasingly being made available directly to the consumer. This is likely to increase the demand for personalised prescription and it means that prescribers need to take pharmacogenetic information into account. Projects such as 100,000 Genomes (UK Government project that is sequencing whole genomes from National Health Service patients; the project, initiated in 2013 and completed in 2018, is focusing on rare diseases, some common types of cancer, and infectious diseases) are providing complete genome sequences that can form part of a patient medical record. This information will be of great value in personalised prescribing [43, 51].

Current pharmacogenetics knowledge can be considered on an individual gene, therapeutic area, or individual drug basis. In addition to using already well-established pharmacogenetics knowledge more efficiently, developments in genomics including genome-wide association studies provide well-replicated data on genetic risk factors for complex diseases. Some of these novel risk factors may be useful therapeutic targets for either newly developed or existing drugs. Knowledge of patient genotype for these targets is likely to be important in prescribing these drugs in the future. There has been development of new drugs targeting particular genetic risk factors for disease. These could be prescribed to those with an at-risk genotype [43, 51].

## 13.8	Genetics of Cerebral Venous Thrombosis

Cerebral venous thrombosis (CVT) is a rare cerebrovascular condition accounting for <1% of all stroke cases and mainly affects young adults [52, 53]. Its genetic aetiology is not clearly elucidated. CVT is the result of undesirable interaction between multiple environmental, physical, social, and genetic risk factors. The phenotypic complexity of a clinical diagnosis of stroke makes a simple genetic risk assessment only partially informative on an individual basis. Family studies do not usually find clusters in families and there is no direct evidence to suggest a Mendelian inheritance [52].

The genetic component of CVT has so far been assessed mainly by candidate gene studies. Approximately 22% of cases are known to have inherited thrombophilia [53], explaining why most candidate gene studies have assessed mutations associated with this condition such as factor V Leiden and prothrombin G20120A mutation [54]. Other mutations investigated by candidate gene studies have included the MTHFR C677T polymorphism (risk factor for hyperhomocysteinaemia) [55], plasminogen activator inhibitor-1 (PAI-1) 4G/5G polymorphism (risk factor for thrombosis) [56], protein Z G79A polymorphism (involved in formation of blood clots) [57], and Janus kinase-2 V617F mutation (involved in making haematopoietic cells more sensitive to growth factors) [58]. However, the results from such individual candidate gene studies have been conflicting mainly because of lack of sufficient power due to the low number of cases.

One large meta-analysis on 1183 CVT cases and 5189 controls that pooled together results from 26 candidate gene studies highlighted significant associations of factor V Leiden G1691A mutation (OR = 2.40; 95% CI = 1.75–3.30; $P < 10^{-5}$) and prothrombin G20120A mutation (OR = 5.48; 95% CI = 3.88–7.74; $P < 10^{-5}$) in adult populations [59]. Interestingly, this study also found that genes involved in the clotting cascade provide a greater level of thrombosis risk in the cerebral venous circulation compared to its arterial circulation implying a larger genetic liability for CVT compared to sporadic ischaemic stroke [59]. Moreover, previous studies suggested a stronger genetic component in younger stroke patients compared to older stroke cases providing additional evidence to support a strong genetic susceptibility to CVT [52, 60].

The genetic susceptibility of CVT likely involves many genes and most of them have small effects. No single genome-wide association study (GWAS) has been conducted to find genetic markers of CVT susceptibility, although about a dozen have been undertaken for the more common forms of venous thromboembolism, deep-vein thrombosis, and pulmonary embolism. The establishment of large international consortia such as BEAST (Biorepository for Establishing the Aetiology of Sinovenous Thrombosis) is likely to yield positive results [52].

References

1. Thomas DC. ProQuest. In: Statistical methods in genetic epidemiology. Oxford: Oxford University Press; 2004.
2. Smith GD, Palmer LJ, Burton PR. An introduction to genetic epidemiology. Bristol: Policy Press; 2011.
3. Ziegler A, König IR. ProQuest. In: Pahlke F, editor. A statistical approach to genetic epidemiology: with access to e-learning platform. Weinheim an der Bergstrasse: Wiley-VCH Verlag GmbH & Co.; 2010.
4. Rebbeck TR, Ambrosone CB, Shields PG. Molecular epidemiology: applications in cancer and other human diseases. New York: Informa Healthcare; 2008.
5. Witte JS, Gauderman WJ, Thomas DC. Asymptotic bias and efficiency in case-control studies of candidate genes and gene-environment interactions: basic family designs. Am J Epidemiol. 1999;149(8):693–705.
6. Thomas DC, Witte JS. Point: population stratification: a problem for case-control studies of candidate-gene associations? Cancer Epidemiol Biomark Prev. 2002;11(6):505–12.
7. Lewis CM, Knight J. Introduction to genetic association studies. Cold Spring Harb Protoc. 2012;2012(3):297–306.
8. Foulkes AS. Applied statistical genetics with R: for population-based association studies. New York: Springer; 2009.
9. Datta S, Datta S, Nettleton D, Datta S. Statistical analysis of next generation sequencing data. Cham: Springer International Publishing; 2014.
10. Laird NM, Lange C. The fundamentals of modern statistical genetics. New York: Springer; 2011.
11. Ken-Dror G, Cooper JA, Humphries SE, Drenos F, Ireland HA. Free protein S level as a risk factor for coronary heart disease and stroke in a prospective cohort study of healthy United Kingdom men. Am J Epidemiol. 2011;174(8):958–68.
12. Ken-Dror G, Drenos F, Humphries SE, et al. Haplotype and genotype effects of the F7 gene on circulating factor VII, coagulation activation markers and incident coronary heart disease in UK men. J Thromb Haemost. 2010;8(11):2394–403.
13. Sole X, Guino E, Valls J, Iniesta R, Moreno V. SNPStats: a web tool for the analysis of association studies. Bioinformatics. 2006;22(15):1928–9.
14. Cordell HJ, Clayton DG. Genetic association studies. Lancet. 2005;366(9491):1121–31.
15. Neale BM. Statistical genetics : gene mapping through linkage and association. London: Taylor & Francis; 2008.
16. Schaid DJ. Genetic epidemiology and haplotypes. Hoboken, NJ: Wiley-Liss; 2004.
17. Ken-Dror G, Hastings IM. Markov chain Monte Carlo and expectation maximization approaches for estimation of haplotype frequencies for multiply infected human blood samples. Malar J. 2016;15(1):430.
18. Sekula P, Del Greco MF, Pattaro C, Kottgen A. Mendelian randomization as an approach to assess causality using observational data. J Am Soc Nephrol. 2016;27(11):3253–65.
19. Lawlor DA, Harbord RM, Sterne JA, Timpson N, Davey SG. Mendelian randomization: using genes as instruments for making causal inferences in epidemiology. Stat Med. 2008;27(8):1133–63.

20. Evans DM, Davey SG. Mendelian randomization: new applications in the coming age of hypothesis-free causality. Annu Rev Genomics Hum Genet. 2015;16:327–50.
21. Jansen H, Samani NJ, Schunkert H. Mendelian randomization studies in coronary artery disease. Eur Heart J. 2014;35(29):1917–24.
22. Burgess S, Thompson SG, Burgess S. Mendelian randomization: methods for using genetic variants in causal estimation. Boca Raton, FL: CRC Press; 2015.
23. Bennett DA. An introduction to instrumental variables—part 2: Mendelian randomisation. Neuroepidemiology. 2010;35(4):307–10.
24. Verduijn M, Siegerink B, Jager KJ, Zoccali C, Dekker FW. Mendelian randomization: use of genetics to enable causal inference in observational studies. Nephrol Dial Transplant. 2010;25(5):1394–8.
25. Davies NM, Smith GD, Windmeijer F, Martin RM. Issues in the reporting and conduct of instrumental variable studies: a systematic review. Epidemiology. 2013;24(3):363–9.
26. Swanson SA, Hernan MA. Commentary: how to report instrumental variable analyses (suggestions welcome). Epidemiology. 2013;24(3):370–4.
27. Davey Smith G, Hemani G. Mendelian randomization: genetic anchors for causal inference in epidemiological studies. Hum Mol Genet. 2014;23(R1):R89–98.
28. Hernan MA, Robins JM. Instruments for causal inference: an epidemiologist's dream? Epidemiology. 2006;17(4):360–72.
29. Greco MF, Minelli C, Sheehan NA, Thompson JR. Detecting pleiotropy in Mendelian randomisation studies with summary data and a continuous outcome. Stat Med. 2015;34(21):2926–40.
30. Burgess S, Small DS, Thompson SG. A review of instrumental variable estimators for Mendelian randomization. Stat Methods Med Res. 2017;26(5):2333–55.
31. Teare MD, Teare MD. Genetic epidemiology. Totowa, NJ: Humana Press; 2011.
32. Burgess S, Butterworth A, Thompson SG. Mendelian randomization analysis with multiple genetic variants using summarized data. Genet Epidemiol. 2013;37(7):658–65.
33. Pierce BL, Burgess S. Efficient design for Mendelian randomization studies: subsample and 2-sample instrumental variable estimators. Am J Epidemiol. 2013;178(7):1177–84.
34. Palmer TM, Nordestgaard BG, Benn M, et al. Association of plasma uric acid with ischaemic heart disease and blood pressure: mendelian randomisation analysis of two large cohorts. BMJ. 2013;347:f4262.
35. Burgess S, Daniel RM, Butterworth AS, Thompson SG, Consortium EP-I. Network Mendelian randomization: using genetic variants as instrumental variables to investigate mediation in causal pathways. Int J Epidemiol. 2015;44(2):484–95.
36. Relton CL, Davey SG. Two-step epigenetic Mendelian randomization: a strategy for establishing the causal role of epigenetic processes in pathways to disease. Int J Epidemiol. 2012;41(1):161–76.
37. Evans DM, Brion MJ, Paternoster L, et al. Mining the human phenome using allelic scores that index biological intermediates. PLoS Genet. 2013;9(10):e1003919.
38. Scherer A. GWAS. Bozeman, MT: Golden Helix, Inc.; 2016.
39. Cortes A, Brown MA. Promise and pitfalls of the immunochip. Arthritis Res Ther. 2011;13(1):101.
40. Bush WS, Moore JH. Chapter 11: Genome-wide association studies. PLoS Comput Biol. 2012;8(12):e1002822.
41. Marees AT, de Kluiver H, Stringer S, et al. A tutorial on conducting genome-wide association studies: quality control and statistical analysis. Int J Methods Psychiatr Res. 2018;27(2):e1608.
42. Teo YY. Common statistical issues in genome-wide association studies: a review on power, data quality control, genotype calling and population structure. Curr Opin Lipidol. 2008;19(2):133–43.
43. Motsinger-Reif AA, Jorgenson E, Relling MV, et al. Genome-wide association studies in pharmacogenomics: successes and lessons. Pharmacogenet Genomics. 2013;23(8):383–94.
44. Willer CJ, Li Y, Abecasis GR. METAL: fast and efficient meta-analysis of genome-wide association scans. Bioinformatics. 2010;26(17):2190–1.

45. Dudbridge F. Power and predictive accuracy of polygenic risk scores. PLoS Genet. 2013;9(3):e1003348.
46. Gondro C. Primer to analysis of genomic data using R. Cham: Springer International Publishing; 2015.
47. Kukurba KR, Montgomery SB. RNA sequencing and analysis. Cold Spring Harb Protoc. 2015;2015(11):951–69.
48. Anders S, McCarthy DJ, Chen Y, et al. Count-based differential expression analysis of RNA sequencing data using R and bioconductor. Nat Protoc. 2013;8(9):1765–86.
49. Liu JX, Gao YL, Xu Y, Zheng CH, You J. Differential expression analysis on RNA-Seq count data based on penalized matrix decomposition. IEEE Trans Nanobioscience. 2014;13(1):12–8.
50. Rapaport F, Khanin R, Liang Y, et al. Comprehensive evaluation of differential gene expression analysis methods for RNA-seq data. Genome Biol. 2013;14(9):R95.
51. Daly AK. Pharmacogenetics: a general review on progress to date. Br Med Bull. 2017;124(1):65–79.
52. Cotlarciuc I, Marjot T, Khan MS, et al. Towards the genetic basis of cerebral venous thrombosis—the BEAST Consortium: a study protocol. BMJ Open. 2016;6(11):e012351.
53. Ferro JM, Canhao P, Stam J, Bousser MG, Barinagarrementeria F, Investigators I. Prognosis of cerebral vein and dural sinus thrombosis: results of the International Study on Cerebral Vein and Dural Sinus Thrombosis (ISCVT). Stroke. 2004;35(3):664–70.
54. Martinelli I, Sacchi E, Landi G, Taioli E, Duca F, Mannucci PM. High risk of cerebral-vein thrombosis in carriers of a prothrombin-gene mutation and in users of oral contraceptives. N Engl J Med. 1998;338(25):1793–7.
55. Martinelli I, Battaglioli T, Pedotti P, Cattaneo M, Mannucci PM. Hyperhomocysteinemia in cerebral vein thrombosis. Blood. 2003;102(4):1363–6.
56. Junker R, Nabavi DG, Wolff E, et al. Plasminogen activator inhibitor-1 4G/4G-genotype is associated with cerebral sinus thrombosis in factor V Leiden carriers. Thromb Haemost. 1998;80(4):706–7.
57. Le Cam-Duchez V, Bagan-Triquenot A, Barbay V, Mihout B, Borg JY. The G79A polymorphism of protein Z gene is an independent risk factor for cerebral venous thrombosis. J Neurol. 2008;255(10):1521–5.
58. Passamonti SM, Biguzzi E, Cazzola M, et al. The JAK2 V617F mutation in patients with cerebral venous thrombosis. J Thromb Haemost. 2012;10(6):998–1003.
59. Marjot T, Yadav S, Hasan N, Bentley P, Sharma P. Genes associated with adult cerebral venous thrombosis. Stroke. 2011;42(4):913–8.
60. Cheng YC, Cole JW, Kittner SJ, Mitchell BD. Genetics of ischemic stroke in young adults. Circ Cardiovasc Genet. 2014;7(3):383–92.

Part VI

Conclusion

Precision Medicine Versus Personalized Medicine

14

Louis R. Caplan

Every illness is not a set of pathologies but a personal story
Anne Fadiman [1]

Precision refers to a mode of action, being exact and accurate, while *personalized* refers to attention to an individual person. These words are quite different—one refers to a *process* of care and the other to the *target* of care. Unfortunately, the terms *precision medicine* and *personalized medicine* are often confused and used differently and sometimes even interchangeably by physicians and commenters. Dr. Francis Collins, the director of the National Institutes of Health in the USA, and Dr. Harold Varmus, a Nobel laureate, characterize precision medicine as emphasizing the application of genetics and other biological data to medical care especially to cancer.

> The prospect of applying this concept (i.e. precision medicine) broadly has been dramatically improved by the recent development of large-scale biologic databases (such as the human genome sequence), powerful methods for characterizing patients (such as proteomics, metabolomics, genomics, diverse cellular assays, and even mobile health technology), and computational tools for analyzing large sets of data [2].

The definition used in Wikipedia is "Precision medicine is a medical model that proposes the customization of healthcare, with medical decisions, treatments, practices, or products being tailored to the individual patient." This definition seems to confuse precision and personalized.

L. R. Caplan (✉)
Beth Israel Deaconess Medical Center, Boston, MA, USA

Neurology, Harvard University, Boston, MA, USA
e-mail: lcaplan@bidmc.harvard.edu

© Springer Nature Switzerland AG 2021
A. C. Fonseca, J. M. Ferro (eds.), *Precision Medicine in Stroke*,
https://doi.org/10.1007/978-3-030-70761-3_14

Herein I will discuss personalized care, that is, care directed to individual persons whether or not it is precise. I will use cerebrovascular disease as an example of choosing treatment. Optimally treatment should be both precise and personalized.

14.1   What Information Is Used to Consider Treatment and Care for an Individual Patient?

I follow, and urge others to use, a concept, the comprehensive medical diagnosis, disease, and personality—the double diagnosis [3, 4]. This construct, originally proposed and described by Lisansky and Shochet, and illustrated in Fig. 14.1, involves drawing lines to organize the collection of clinical information. The physical symptoms, signs, and manifestations of disease are noted above the line. Below the line are the personal relationships and feelings of the patient, and along the line in a

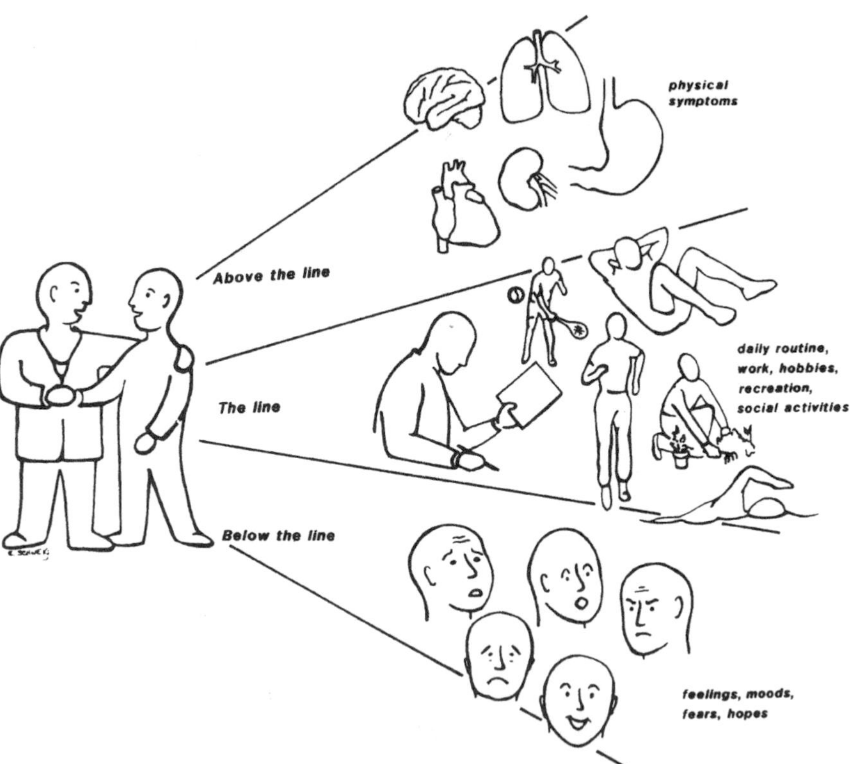

Fig. 14.1 A conceptualization of the medical interview rather than components of the medical interview. (Adapted from Lisansky ET, Schochet BR. Comprehensive Medical Diagnosis for the internist. Med Clin N Amer 1967;51) and illustrated by Evie Schweig and reproduced in Caplan LR, Hollander J. The effective Clinical Neurologist, 3rd edition People's Medical Publishing House USA. Shelton CT 2011

"neutral" zone are the important social and environmental factors. Physicians should arrive at a double diagnosis: (1) What medical disease does the patient have? (2) What kind of a person is this and how do personality and life experiences and the environment relate to the illness, its etiology, recurrence, chronicity, and management?

Patients live in a very complex social, civic, cultural, economic, religious, and philosophic environment. Treating physician must try to understand and diagnose the cause of the patient's symptoms and illness—the disease material above the line, in as much detail as possible. The physician must also understand the person and the milieu. Cultural differences and education and training also influence patients' compliance and response to discussions of potential treatments. Many illnesses including stroke cannot be understood using only biomedical concepts. Physicians can divide clinical data into four categories: (1) strictly medical information relating to the pathology and mechanisms of the disease and its symptoms and signs; (2) social, in the broadest sense of the word information about the patient's environment (Where does the patient live, work, and play? Who are the significant others in the patient's life? What are the patient's cultural, religious, and economic attributes and resources?); (3) personal, interpersonal, and psychological information about the patient's feelings, stresses, and choice of lifestyle; and (4) when ordering investigations and prescribing various treatments—the patient (and sometimes their important others) preferences and biases regarding alternative choices after these have been explained.

The physician's training, expertise, and the environment in which he or she operates also impacts the care of the individual patient. Not all consultants, investigations, and treatments are always available.

14.2   What Is the Patient's Medical Problem?

Defining precisely a patient's cerebrovascular disease is complex. Hinman and colleagues have detailed many of the genetic and biomedical information that contribute to precision in stroke management [5]. The patient has symptoms and examination may or may not show signs. The clinical deficits may be slight, moderate, or severe. The clinical findings may be stable, improving, or worsening. The patient may have comorbidities that affect their ability to communicate, walk, work at their job, drive a car, and perform activities of daily living. Brain imaging can show the extent of recent brain infarction and/or hemorrhage. There may be other older lesions or coexistent disease (atrophy, meningioma, enlarged ventricles, etc.). Vascular imaging can identify lesions that explain the symptoms and signs and brain imaging lesions or may be incidental but important. The patient likely has a number of potential vascular risk factors that need to be considered for optimal management (hypertension, hyperlipidemia, diabetes, obesity, inactivity, smoking, use of drugs, etc.). To provide the best care, the treating physician should define as many of these variables as possible—precision and detail are important.

14.3 The Patient and Their Environment

Many details about the patient and his or her milieu are important in choosing treatment. Age, actual and relative, is always relevant. How much will the patient's medical problem, if untreated or unresponsive to treatment, cause morbidity and mortality and alter his or her lifestyle and life goals? Medical and surgical procedures and many treatments are less well tolerated as patients age. Where does the patient live? A large house, apartment, or a room? What floor do they live on? If on a high floor are there elevators available? Is there a spouse or significant other to care for the patient and if so are they well and capable? Are there resources—money, a car, insurance, friends, and relatives—that can help with care delivery and treatment?

What does the patient do on a daily basis? Work, shop, read, watch TV, exercise? How will the medical condition and/or treatments affect these activities? What are the patient's and significant others' goals of care?

14.4 Treatment and the Role of Therapeutic Trials in Choosing Treatment for an Individual Patient

Recently there has been increasing pressure on clinicians to choose treatment that is "evidence based." Much pressure comes from insurers and managed-care organizations who pay for treatments. Often the only evidence recognized in determining the evidence base is that garnered from randomized controlled trials (RCTs) especially those that are double blinded [6, 7]. This emphasis on the results of RCTs has been overstated especially in relation to neurology [8–10]. Many, if not most, treatment dilemmas have not been studied in RCTs. Many medical and neurological conditions are unsuitable for trials. Statisticians love numbers. To provide statistically valid results, randomized trials must contain large numbers of patients with enough end points for analysis, and those end points must be reached in a short period of time. The condition studied must be acute and cause adverse end points or rapid improvement within a short time. Chronic conditions must be severe enough to cause clear end points within 1–5 years of follow-up. Patients who are too ill, too old, too young, female and "of childbearing age," incapable of giving informed consent, too complex, or too full of coexisting illnesses are not included in trials.

Randomized trials have important limitations that reduce their applicability to individual patient therapeutic decisions. By definition, randomized trials consider only large groups of patients with relatively common conditions. For trials to yield results that are statistically valid, they must include many patients—*numbers*. These are needed to power the trial to avoid errors in interpretation [11–13]. For the results to be useful to practicing physicians, the data must *specifically* apply to individual patients with the conditions studied. To achieve enough patients, a *lumping* strategy must predominate over *splitting*. For example, to study the effectiveness of a treatment to prevent brain embolism in patients with mitral valve prolapse, a study would not be able to obtain enough individuals with mitral valve prolapse, mitral regurgitation, and mitral valve fibrinoid degeneration who had prior brain or systemic emboli and congestive heart failure although this group is at highest risk and would be most likely to respond to prophylaxis. The study would have to include all patients with mitral valve prolapse to accrue enough patients.

The greater the numbers of patients needed, the more the pressure there is to adopt a lumping strategy. The more a study lumps diverse subgroups, the more *general* are the results and their applicability to specific patient's declines. For practicing neurologists, treatment must be very specific. Physicians are faced with individual patients for whom they must make therapeutic decisions. To be useful, trial results must help physicians treat individual patients in given situations. Can I recognize my patient within the trial? The "evidence" derived from RCTs does not consider the personal—the complexities of the individuality of each patient.

The results of RCTs provide a guide for public health officers faced with an ultimatum to give all patients who have a given risk factor or condition the same treatment ("group medicine"). But for clinicians faced with making treatment decisions for individuals ("personalized medicine"), many factors apply, only one of which is the results of RCTs. George Thibault said it well in a discussion about choosing treatment in the New England Journal of Medicine [14]:

> We then need to decide which approach in our large therapeutic armamentarium will be most appropriate in a particular patient, with a particular stage of disease and particular coexisting conditions, and at a particular age. Even when randomized clinical trials have been performed (which is true for only a small number of clinical problems), they will often not answer this question specifically for the patient sitting in front of us in the office or lying in the hospital bed [14].

Decisions about treatment should always be a shared experience between the doctor and the patient. The final decision must rest with patients, their families, and their caregivers.

References

1. Fadiman A. The spirit catches you and you fall down: a Hmong child, her American doctors, and the collision of two cultures. New York: Farrar, Straus and Giroux; 1997.
2. Collins FS, Varmus H. A new initiative on precision medicine. N Engl J Med. 2015;372:793–5.
3. Lisansky ET, Shochet BR. Comprehensive medical diagnosis for the internist. Med Clin North Am. 1967;51:1381–97.
4. Caplan LR, Hollander J. The effective clinical neurologist. 3rd ed. Shelton, CT: People's Medical Publishing House; 2011.
5. Hinman JD, Rost NS, Leung TW, et al. Principles of precision medicine in stroke. J Neurol Neurosurg Psychiatry. 2017;88:54–61.
6. Sackett DL, Richardson WS, Rosenberg W, Haynes RB. Evidence-based medicine. How to practice and teach EBM. London: Churchill Livingstone; 1996.
7. Sackett DL. Evidence-based medicine: what it is and what it isn't. BMJ. 1996;312:71–2.
8. Caplan LR. Evidence-based medicine. Concerns of a clinical neurologist. J Neurol Neurosurg Psychiatry. 2001;71:569–76.

9. Caplan LR. Is the promise of randomized control trials ("evidence-based medicine") overstated? Curr Neurol Neurosci Rep. 2002;2:1–8.
10. Caplan LR. How well does "evidence-based" medicine help neurologists care for individual patients? Rev Neurol Dis. 2007;4:75–84.
11. Meinert CL. Clinical trials: design, conduct, and analysis. New York: Oxford University Press; 1986.
12. Straus SE, Glasziou P, Richardson WS, Haynes RB. Evidence-based medicine: how to practice and teach EBM. 5th ed. Edinburgh: Elsevier; 2018.
13. Mayer D. Essential evidence-based medicine with CD-Rom. 2nd ed. Cambridge: Cambridge University Press; 2010.
14. Thibault G. Clinical problem solving. Too old for what? N Engl J Med. 1993;328:946–50.

Index

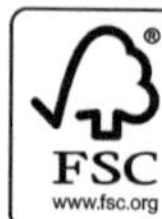